Hormones and Vitamins in Cancer Treatment

Author

Aurel Lupulescu, M.D., Ph.D.
Senior Research Scientist
Formerly Associate Professor
Wayne State University
School of Medicine
Detroit, Michigan

CRC Press
Boca Raton   Ann Arbor   Boston

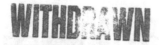
Library of Congress Cataloging-in-Publication Data

Lupulescu, Aurel.
    Hormones and vitamins in cancer treatment / author, Aurel
Lupulescu.
      p. cm.
    Includes bibliographical references.
    ISBN 0-8493-5973-2
    1. Cancer—Hormone therapy. 2. Cancer—Diet therapy. 3. Vitamin
therapy. I. Title.
    [DNLM: 1. Hormones—therapeutic use. 2. Neoplasms—drug therapy.
3. Vitamins—therapeutic use. QZ 267 L966h]
RC271.H55L87 1990
616.99'4061—dc20
DNLM/DLC
for Library of Congress
90-1490
CIP

Direct all inquiries to CRC Press, Inc., 2000 Corporate Blvd., N.W., Boca Raton, Florida 33431.

© 1990 by CRC Press, Inc.

International Standard Book Number 0-8493-5973-2
Library of Congress Card Number 90-1490
Printed in the United States

PREFACE

Hormones and vitamins have been used in cancer treatment for a long time, mainly on an empirical basis. However, recent advances in cancer biology and endocrine pharmacology have dramatically changed their role as therapeutic agents over conventional therapies in cancer management. Discovery of new hormones and hormone antagonists (antiestrogens, steroid synthesis inhibitors, and LHRH agonists), hundreds of times more active than natural hormones, with less toxic effects than cytotoxic agents and radiation therapy, will make hormonotherapy a more acceptable treatment for cancer patients, providing similar beneficial effects.

Recently, isolation of a myriad of hormone-like substances (growth factors, interferons, interleukins, and prostaglandins), generally termed cytokines, which control cancer development by paracrine and autocrine mechanisms, also exert potential therapeutic effects. Using recombinant DNA technology and genetic engineering, it would be possible to synthesize great amounts of hormonomimetic substances and thus use them on a large scale in clinical trials. It is likely that these new substances will have a major role, not only in clinical oncology, but in general medicine as well.

Isolation and discovery of new vitamins, their synthetic analogs, some of them acting as hormone-like substances, increases our knowledge regarding hormones and vitamins as chemotherapeutic and chemopreventive agents. These important advances in hormone, cytokine and vitamin physiologies, as well as a better understanding of their *modus operandi* at cellular and molecular levels, will significantly increase our knowledge regarding the therapeutic role of hormones, cytokines, and vitamins in cancer treatment in the next decade. Thus, an exciting field in cancer research will just begin in the coming years and will offer physicians better methods for cancer treatment.

The newest information regarding hormones, hormone antagonists, cytokines, vitamins and monoclonal antibodies, are included in this book, and it is hoped it will be useful for cancer researchers, physicians, and their patients.

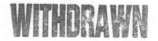

THE AUTHOR

Aurel Lupulescu, M.D. (Internal Medicine), Ph.D. (Molecular Biology), is a cancer researcher and author of almost 300 scientific articles, 5 books, and 4 chapters in books, regarding the role of hormones and vitamins in cancer development and regression.

His name and biography are published in *Who's Who in Frontiers Science and Technology,* first and second editions; *Who's Who in the World,* seventh and eighth editions, and *Personalities of America.* Dr. Lupulescu is also an active member in 12 scientific and medical societies. Formerly, he was an Associate Professor at Wayne State University, School of Medicine, Detroit, Michigan.

Dr. Lupulescu has worked for over 30 years in endocrinology and cancer biology, studying the effects of various hormones and vitamins on cancer growth and regression. He has studied the mechanism of action of hormones and vitamins at cellular and molecular levels (DNA, RNA, and protein synthesis), as well as the cell surface structure, extending our knowledge of hormones and vitamins on cancer biology and treatment.

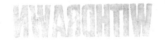

TABLE OF CONTENTS

Chapter 1

PRINCIPLES AND RATIONALE FOR HORMONE AND VITAMIN THERAPY IN CANCER

I. GENERAL CONSIDERATIONS

Hormonal and vitamin treatment in cancer patients has rapidly increased over the last two decades. Recent advances in cancer biology have revealed that hormones and vitamins are important modulators in controlling tumor growth and regression; by controlling neoplastic cell differentiation and proliferation, dramatic changes can be made in cancer evolution and the overall survival rate in cancer patients. Although both hormones and vitamins have been used for several years in cancer treatment, they are still used, in many cases, on an empirical basis only. The data presented in this chapter will provide a more specific and rational basis for their use in cancer treatment.

Hormones, vitamins, and growth factors are important modulators of cancer cell growth and proliferation because they change the "milieu intérieur". They are also potential "cell environmental factors" in cancer cell growth and proliferation and lead ultimately to tumor regression or extinction (see Figure 1). We believe that cancer: (1) is not always an autonomous and self-perpetuating process, and (2) can be stimulated or inhibited in its propagation by hormones, vitamins, and growth factors. Thus, cancer is a controllable process, and endocrine-induced regression of it is possible.[1] Therefore, in the last two decades there has been a resurgence and reassessment of the role of hormones and vitamins in cancer therapy and prophylaxis, due to the revolutionary changes that have taken place in endocrine pharmacology, such as the discovery of new hormone and vitamin products, a better understanding of their mechanism of action, and their advantages as compared to chemotherapy and radiation therapy.

A. PRINCIPLES AND RATIONALE FOR HORMONE THERAPY IN CANCER
1. Historical Review and Classification

Interestingly, long ago it was assumed that cancer is a systemic disease due mainly to a hormonal disequilibrium and can be hormonally controlled. Cummings[2] assumed that cancer is a systemic disease due mainly to a hormonal imbalance. Local treatment by surgery or radiation is not satisfactory; the only satisfactory treatment is endocrine therapy. He stated that "no progressive physician or surgeon can afford to ignore its role in cancer treatment."[2] Later, Lacassagne (1932) demonstrated the induction of mammary cancer in mice after hormone administration; in his experiment, weekly injections of estrone benzoate induced cancer of the breast (mammary adenocarcinomas) in male mice in 5 to 6 months.[3] However, the scientific concepts and rational basis for hormonotherapy in cancer started with Huggins (1941).[4] He found that hormones are crucial factors not only in cancer development but also in tumor regression and extinction. Thus, the cancer of man can be controlled by endocrinologic methods, and the era of hormonotherapy in cancer treatment began.[4] Spontaneous prostate cancer in aged dogs is hormonally dependent (androgen-dependent); it is stimulated by testosterone administration and is regressed after castration (orchiectomy) or estrogen therapy. Since then, hormonotherapy has undergone considerable changes.

During the 1960s and 1970s, the selection of cases for hormonotherapy was still largely clinical. The clinical decision to use hormonal therapy vs. chemotherapy was based on two major criteria: (1) the site and the number of metastases and (2) the disease-free interval site. At present, the choice of therapy and success of hormone responsiveness depends upon the objective criteria, which can predict the outcome of hormonal treatment and the prognosis

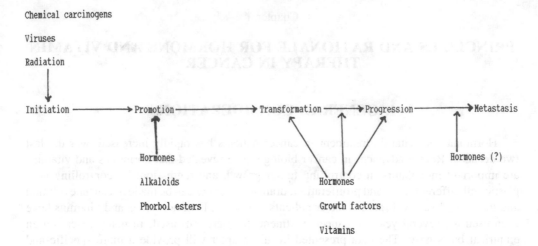

FIGURE 1.   Role of hormones, vitamins, and growth factors in carcinogenesis.

TABLE 1
Most Important Factors in Patient Selection and Their Response to Hormonotherapy

a.   Hormone receptor status
b.   Growth factor receptors
c.   Lymph node involvement
d.   Tumor size and metastases
e.   Heterogeneity of cell tumor population
f.   Menopausal status
g.   DNA content
h.   Histologic differentiation: improved diagnostic methods
i.   Tumor markers and ectopic hormones
j.   Oncogene amplification
k.   Monoclonal antibodies (mAbs): using radiolabeled mAb for tumor detection and its response to hormon-
       otherapy
l.   Screening procedures

and also can identify the subgroup of high risk patients not responding to endocrine therapy. Based on these objective and accurate criteria, new strategies can be developed in cancer treatment by using hormones alone, hormone combinations, or hormone antagonists.

2. Objective and Scientific Criteria for Hormone Therapy

The major criteria for patient selection for hormonotherapy and prediction of their hormone response and disease prognosis are listed in Table 1.

a. Hormone Receptor Status

Over the past several years, it has become evident that the assessment of hormone receptor status in cancer is an important prognostic indicator as well as an indicator of response to hormonal therapy.[5] Hormone receptors are cytosol or cell membrane proteins, and their presence is critical for the hormone function at target tissues. Thus, the hormones bind to their receptor sites before entering the cells and then translocate to nuclear chromatin (DNA) as hormone-receptor(s) complexes $H + R \rightarrow HR \rightarrow E$. After they combine with DNA, a new RNA messenger (m-RNA) is released that will govern the synthesis of new proteins in the ribosomes or microsomes. These new proteins initiate a specific cellular response. It is postulated that hormones have hydrophobic regions that propel them out of the circulation at their specific receptor sites. The receptors are randomly distributed at the cell membrane, but the target cells accept only the appropriate hormone, while rejecting all others. After the hormones are translocated as hormone-receptor complexes to the nuclear DNA, they have to remain a certain length of time before the messenger RNA production is activated. This can explain the different time intervals before their physiologic action takes place: estriol remains 3 to 6 h; estradiol, almost 24 h; and estrone, for a period between the other two.

It is also suggested that there is a regulatory system that maintains this homeostasis between hormones and their receptors at the cellular level by: (1) downregulation, which modulates the effect of excessive hormones by applying a "brake" with the loss of a number of receptors; and (2) negative cooperativity, which occurs when the receptors do not decrease, but become inactive. Receptor studies in biopsies removed from cancer patients showed that not all receptor-positive tumor cells are hormone-responsive, and also that 10% or less from receptor-negative cases still respond to hormone therapy. By using recombinant DNA techniques, it is possible to induce and increase the receptors in receptor-negative tumors, and thus enhance the hormone responsiveness.

Thus, for a protein to become a receptor, it has to fulfill at least four criteria: it must (1) be specific, (2) have high affinity, (3) be saturable, and (4) be able to elicit a physiologic response. After the hormone is propelled toward a target cell and enters it, the following intracellular events take place:

1. Hormone uptake — a small vesicle, or receptosome, on the cell membrane engulfs the hormone in a phenomenon called micropinocytosis.
2. Transformation and activation — the hormone meets and attaches to its cytosol receptor to form a hormone-receptor complex ($H + R \rightleftharpoons HR$).
3. Translocation — the hormone-receptor steroid complex (HR) is translocated to the nucleus.
4. Retention — HR is retained in the nuclear chromatin for a certain length of time.
5. Transcription — a new messenger RNA (m-RNA) is synthesized from DNA.
6. Translation — this is the action of m-RNA on ribosomes to form new proteins.
7. Physiologic action — this is brought about by the newly synthesized proteins (biological effectors) called effectors (E).

There are two major groups of hormone receptors: (1) steroid hormone receptors, located intracellularly (cytosol receptors) and (2) polypeptide hormone receptors, located mainly on the cell surface or membrane (membrane receptors). Generally, the receptors belong to a common class of acrylic proteins of 80,000 to 100,000 mol wt. Receptor proteins are found in concentrations ranging from 50 to 50,000 sites in target cells, but they are absent in nontarget tissues. Major steroid hormone receptors are the estrogen receptor (ER), progesterone receptor (PR), androgen receptor (AR), and glucocorticoid receptor (GR). Polypeptide hormone receptors include the prolactin receptor (PLR), insulin receptor (INR), thyrotropin receptor (TSH-R), and gonadotropin-releasing hormone receptor (GnRH-R).

At present, the most assessed hormone receptors used for selection of cancer patients for endocrine therapy are estrogen receptors, progesterone receptors, and androgen receptors. The determination of ERs, PRs, and ARs is usually routinely performed on all breast cancer and prostate cancer biopsy tissues for evaluation of hormonal responsiveness. It is generally accepted that monoclonal antibodies (mAbs) are immunogenic for the ER and PR proteins. By using these techniques, we can detect both "free" or cytosol ER and "filled" (nuclear) ER receptors; while using the previous biochemical techniques, only free ER were determined. It was also found that tumors containing ER only in the cytosol (or free ER) have lower response rates to hormonal treatment, as compared to tumors containing both cytosol ER and nuclear (filled) ER.[6,7]

Recently, using monoclonal or polyclonal anti-ER antibodies, it was found that defective estrogen receptors (which are unable to bind to the nucleus in a hormone filled state) in human as well as in mouse hormone-resistant breast cancers and defective PRs in human mammary cancers, are unable to bind to the nuclei. Approximately 65 to 70% of breast carcinomas contain estrogen receptors and approximately 50% of tumors contain progesterone receptors. Since synthesis of PR is estrogen-dependent, it mediates a more favorable prognosis and a better response. Thus, PR may actually be more important than ER as a prognostic factor. There is a good relationship between receptor status and menopausal status, age, progression of disease, and responses to various types of endocrine therapy. For instance, both ER and PR are higher in postmenopausal women than in premenopausal. There also is a relationship between estrogen receptor status and response to additive and ablative endocrine therapy.

	ER +	ER −
Additive hormone therapy	56%	11%
Ablative hormone therapy	55%	8%
Total	56%	10%

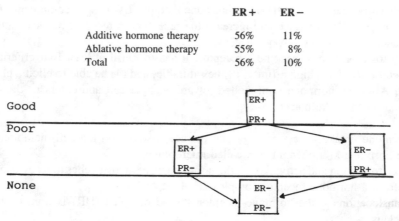

Thus, hormone responsiveness can be more accurately predicted according to the presence or absence of ER and PR in a given tumor tissue. During neoplastic transformation some tumor cells lose their hormone receptors (ER, PR) and change from good hormone-responsive, to poor-responsive, or even to autonomous (hormone-nonresponsive). Also, progression of the disease and relapses can be predicted by ER and PR content in tumor tissues. Thus, the role of estrogen and progesterone receptor estimation in the hormonal management of breast cancer is well established.[8,9] The postmenopausal patients have a greater content of ER and PR in their tumor tissue then the premenopausal women; well-differentiated tumors are more often receptor positive than undifferentiated, and lobular carcinomas are more often positive than ductal or medullary types. It has also been observed that up to 50% of patients with negative estrogen receptors, but positive progesterone receptors, respond to hormone therapy. These findings indicate that the progesterone receptor may be more important than the estrogen receptor as a prognostic factor. Therefore, women with small tumors (≤ 2 cm diameter), negative lymph node status, and positive ER and PR receptors have the best chance and response to hormonal therapy.

Prolactin receptors (PLRs), androgen receptors (ARs), glucocorticoid receptors (GRs), insulin receptors (INRs), and epidermal growth factor receptors (EGF-Rs) were found in variable amounts in tumor tissues. Thus, PLRs have been detected in approximately 50% of human breast cancers. ARs are usually positive in about 30% of the tumors, and GRs have been found to be positive in 50% of mammary carcinomas in some studies. Prolactin receptors are specific membrane receptors, and their prognostic significance in human breast cancer is still under investigation.[10] However, recently androgen receptors have been found to be predictive of hormone-responsive breast cancer.[11] For accurate determination of all hormone receptors, specimens should be frozen immediately in liquid nitrogen. Surgical ischemia decreased the hormone-receptor level.

Recently, it has been shown that in stage I of breast cancer, the lack of estrogen receptor

(ER −) seems to be the most important factor for predicting the earlier recurrence and poorer survival; whereas in stage II of the disease, the PR appears to be better than ER in predicting disease-free and overall survival. A correlative study regarding the predictive value of ER and PR concentrations and the clinical behavior of breast cancer on 547 patients revealed that the correct prediction percentages of the response of patients to hormonal treatment were 77% if ER +, 69% if PR +, and 80% if both ER + and PR +.[12-14] Glucocorticoid-receptor levels in leukemic blasts from peripheral blood of patients with acute lymphoblastic leukemia (ALL) are predictive in response to combination chemotherapy. Epidermal growth factor receptors (EGF-Rs) were detected in 36% of human breast cancers in the ductal and medullary carcinomas, but not in lobular and colloid tumors. Levels of epidermal growth factor receptor and insulin-like growth factor receptor (IGF-R) were evaluated and correlated with steroid receptors (ER, PR) in human breast cancer. Thus, EGF-R correlated negatively to the ER and PR, whereas the IGF-R correlated positively to ER and PR. Growth factors also act on restriction points in the cell cycle of transformed cells, allowing the cells to progress. Thus, platelet-derived growth factor (PDGF) allows cells to pass a restriction point in G_1, epidermal growth factor, and the related transforming growth factor-α (TGF-α) act later; while insulin-like growth factor (IGF-1) acts even later on, and these last ones are termed "progression" factors.

Recent studies also revealed an important correlation between the progesterone receptor and antiestrogen (tamoxifen) therapy. Thus, antiestrogen therapy with tamoxifen in 200 stage II postmenopausal breast cancer patients reveals that significant therapeutic benefits were seen in the PR + group and no tamoxifen benefits were observed in the PR − group. Androgen receptors were detected and measured as nuclear androgen receptors and dihydrotestosterone (DHT) in the prostate cancer cells. Thus, prostate gland is androgen-dependent and 80% of prostate cancers are hormone-dependent.

Usually the classical 8 S receptor complex is an oligomer made up of dissimilar subunits. It seems that the 8 S cytosol receptor (250 to 300 kDa) is made up of one ligand-binding unit plus two 90 kDa nonhormone-binding units. Each steroid hormone has its own high-affinity receptor. GR_1 has a molecular weight of 94 to 98 kDa, and estrogen, 65 to 70 kDa. Thus, the hormone-receptor status provides: (1) the ability to "target" therapy for hormones as well as for antiestrogen drugs (tamoxifen); (2) their lack of toxicity as compared to other therapeutic agents, cytotoxic agents, or radiation therapy; and (3) the decreased risk and sequelae as compared with the surgical techniques of ovariectomy, adrenalectomy, and hypophysectomy.

Hormone-receptor profiles are now recommended for all breast cancer patients and these should be obtained before mastectomy. At present, improved techniques in hormone-receptor measurements reveal that approximately 50 to 65% of breast tumors are ER positive. Premenopausal women have a lower incidence of ER-positive tumors than postmenopausal women (30% vs. 60%). The synthesis of PR is originated and governed by ER (see Figure 2). The best prognosis is for patients with small primary tumors (≤2 cm), negative lymph nodes, positive ER and PR, well-differentiated (low) aneuploidy, and low DNA content (S-phase fraction). One of the most used antiestrogens is tamoxifen.[14] This drug has mild side effects and is associated with a response rate of up to 75% in ER-positive tumors (see Figure 3). Tamoxifen (Nolvadex) became the drug of choice for postmenopausal women with lymph node involvement and ER + receptors.

It is interesting that hormone receptors, e.g., ER, PR, AR, and GR, were found in other nondependent cancers, such as lung, colon, melanoma, meningioma, neuroblastoma, and pancreatic tumors. Their presence may indicate some beneficial therapeutic effects of hormonotherapy in these patients. The dynamics of hormone receptors can indicate more accurately the change and "shift" of certain hormone-dependent tumors to hormone independence. Only free-serum testosterone (free T) is capable of passing through the prostatic cell membrane passively and is converted enzymatically to dehydrotestosterone (DHT),

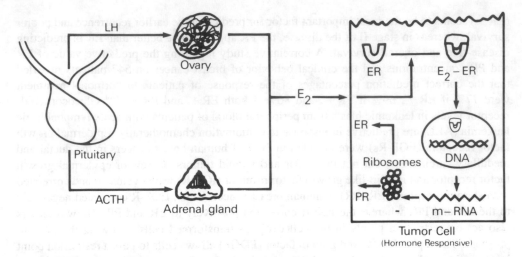

FIGURE 2.   Effect of estrogens on hormone sensitive cells.

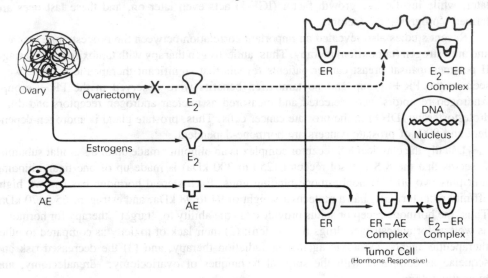

FIGURE 3.   Effects of ovariectomy, estrogens, and antiestrogens on tumor cells. (Modified from Netter, F. H., *Clin. Symp. Ciba-Geigy,* 39, 25, 1987. With permission.)

which combines with a cytoplasmic androgen receptor. This complex enters the nucleus, causes and increase in messenger RNA (mRNA) synthesis followed by protein synthesis, and thus elicits the biologic effect. Antiandrogens (flutamide and cyproterone acetate) compete with DHT for the cytoplasmic androgen receptor, and consequently they inhibit the interaction between DHT and AR (see Figure 4).[15] However, it seems unlikely that the gonadotropin-releasing hormone-receptor sites in human breast tumors modify the evolution of disease.

b. Growth Factor Receptors: Their Significance for Hormonotherapy

Many tumor cells show an abnormal expression of receptor for growth factors and also an abnormal production of growth factors.[16] In recent years several growth factors have been discovered. All are believed to exert their initial effect on a target cell by specific receptors at the cell surface and are extremely active biologically in a very low concentration, e.g., within the range of picograms (pg) per ml. Thus, the receptors of growth factors play an important role in neoplastic cell physiology and the response pattern of cancer cells to

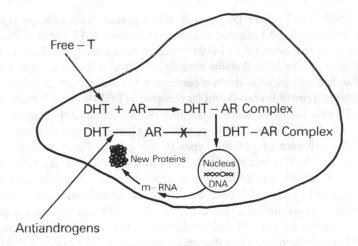

FIGURE 4.   Mechanism of action of androgens and antiandrogens on the receptors in the prostate cell.

TABLE 2
Growth Factors and Their Receptors in Cancer and Normal Cells

Epidermal growth factor (EGF) or transforming growth factor-alpha (TGF-α)
Transforming growth factor β (TGF-β)
Platelet-derived growth factor (PDGF)
Fibroblast growth factors (FGF-α, β)
Insulin-like growth factors (IGF-1, IGF-2)
Tumor necrosis factor (TNF)/cachectin
Colony-stimulating factors (CSF)
Nerve growth factor (NGF)
Angiogenic factor (AGF)
Cytokines: interferons (α, β, γ)
   Interleukin-1 (IL-1)
   Interleukin-2 (IL-2)

different drugs, hormones, or other environmental cell factors. The most common peptide growth factors found in cancers and normal cells are listed in Table 2.

Epidermal growth factor receptors (EGF-R) — EGF is a 64-kDa polypeptide consisting of 53 amino acids and probably identical to urogastrone. EGF and TGF-α bind to the same receptor, a 170-kDa plasma membrane protein. These transmembrane receptors exhibit cytoplasmic tyrosine kinase activity. EGF receptors are expressed by many human cancer cell lines, particularly by squamous epithelial cell carcinomas, breast cancer cells, and glioblastomas.[16] Thus, the EGF receptor is a transmembrane glycoprotein and is encoded by the oncogene C-erb-B$_1$, which corresponds to the rat oncogenic "neu". Estradiol induced a four- to sixfold increase in EGF receptors in MCF-7 cells. Assays for determination of EGF receptors in human mammary carcinomas and their metastases revealed that 25% of the primary tumor and 48% of the metastases exhibit EGF-receptors at measurable levels. A correlation between EGF-R with steroid hormone receptors (ER, PR) in primary human breast cancer and axillary lymph node metastases was found from 89 primary breast cancers and 23 axillary lymph node metastases; about 87% of primary and 72.2% of metastatic tumors were EGF-R positive and EGF-R levels were higher in metastatic tissue than in primary breast tumor, whereas the steroid hormone receptors (ER and PR) were lower. Thus, EGF-R positive are only 39% progesterone receptor positive (PR+), whereas EGF-R negative tumors are 60% PR+.

Recently, an association between epidermal growth factor receptor (EGF-R) and a new oncogene C-erb-β-2 and cancer progression was reported. This new oncogene has been isolated from human cells and mapped to human chromosome 17 and is distinct from EGF-R gene located on chromosome 7. Furthermore, it was found that EGF-R (170 kDa) is composed of an extra cellular domain binding to mitogen EGF, a short transmembrane domain, and an intracytoplasmic domain containing tyrosine kinase activity.[17]

Transforming growth factor-β and its receptors (TGF-β-R) — Transforming growth factor-β is a 25-kDa secreted protein consisting of two identical 112 amino acid subunits held together by disulfide bonds.[18] Recently, more accurate purification of TGF-β has demonstrated the presence of multiple types of the growth factor TGF-β_1, TGF-β_2, and TGF-$\beta_{1,2}$. Thus, a 280-kDa receptor binds both TGF-β_1 and TGF-β_2 with equal and high affinity. However, the 65- and 85-kDa forms of the binding site prefer TGF-β_1. TGF-β is unique among growth factors because it exerts bifunctional (stimulating and inhibitory) effects on cell growth and differentiation. It is interesting that in hormone-dependent breast cancers, the estrogens decrease TGF-β production, whereas the antiestrogens (tamoxifen) increase TGF-β production, an effect that may contribute to their ability to inhibit the tumor growth. The hormonal resistance to antiestrogens may be due to the loss of the ability to make or respond to TGF-β.

Platelet-derived growth factor receptors (PDGF-R) — PDGF is a growth factor for fibroblasts, glial cells, and smooth muscle cells. PDGF is a dimer consisting of a 14- to 18-kDa chain and disulfide bonded to a 16 DB chain. The receptor for PDGF is a tyrosine protein kinase (180 kDa) with the capacity to phosphorylate itself and other proteins. Its receptor is also different from that of EGF-R and insulin. However, PDGF receptors are rarely detected on tumor cells that produce PDGF-like growth factors.

Fibroblast growth factor-receptors (FGF-R) — FGF exists under two closely related forms: basic (β-FGF) and acidic (α-FGF), which interact with common cell surface receptors. The ability to share receptors enable α-FGF and β-FGF to exert similar biologic effects on a wide range of mesoderm and neuroectoderm cells. The presence of β-FGF in ovarian tissue (granulosa cells) could be a contributing factor to tumor formation. Recently, three oncogenes have been shown to be structurally related to FGF and its receptors. These oncogenes were identified in Kaposi's sarcoma, a cancer that now frequently occurs in patients with Acquired Immunodeficiency Syndrome (AIDS), and also in human stomach and bladder cancers. Strong evidence also indicates a similar lineage between oncogenes and growth factors or their receptors.

Insulin-like growth factor-receptors (IGF-R) — The insulin family is the largest group of polypeptide growth factors, which in addition to insulin includes the insulin-like growth factors (IGF-1 and IGF-2), nerve growth factor (NGF), and relaxin. Human somatomedin C has been shown to be identical with IGF-1. Of these five peptides, only insulin and IGFs have been implicated in carcinogenesis. Insulin itself can increase the affinity of cell membrane receptors for IGF-2 (7.5 kDa) and is conducive for the action of several other polypeptide growth factor on cells. IGF-1, a 70 amino acid peptide (7.6 kDa) is synthesized by many tissues (e.g., kidney) and a variety of normal and tumor-derived cell lines (e.g., breast cell cancers and human lung tumors). The specificity of the receptors for IGF-I was documented by the findings that IGF-1 was 20-fold more potent than IGF-II and 2000-fold more potent than insulin. Recently, the presence of IGF-I receptors in normal and nodular goitrous tissue was reported. The IGF-I receptor content was higher in thyroid cancer extracts than that of normal thyroid tissue. These data suggest that the stimulatory effects of TSH on thyroid cell proliferation could be mediated by IGF-1 action as well as the goitrogenic process.[19]

Tumor necrosis factor (TNF)/cachectin receptors — TNF/cachectin is a cytokine or lymphokine (hormone-like) with pleiotropic cellular effect, such as a cachexia and tumor necrosis by inducing cytostatic or cytocidal effects on certain tumors, as well as tumor necrosis *in vivo*. It is assumed that macrophages are the principal source of this factor. Recently, it was shown that cachectin and TNF are identical chemically. TNF/cachectin has a subunit molecular mass of 17 kDa. In all three mammalian species (human, mouse, and rabbit), TNF/cachectin is synthesized as a prohormone, which is subsequently cleaved to yield the mature 17-kDa hormone.[20] Different cell types may carry between 1,000 and 10,000 copies of the receptor. Since the TNF receptors have been detected on TNF-sensitive cells as well as TNF-resistant cells, the presence of TNF receptors per se cannot be the basis of selective toxicity. Thus, the content of TNF-receptors cannot be correlated with TNF sensitivity and TNF receptors cannot be a predictive test for tumor necrotic response.

Colony-stimulating factors (CSF) and their receptors (CSF-R) — Colony-stimulating factors are a class of glycoproteins having molecular weights approximately 23,000 to 70,000 and are essential for proliferation and differentiation of normal and malignant hematopoietic progenitor cells. These hormone-like substances are known collectively as the colony-stimulating factors because of *in vitro* stimulation of progenitor cells to form discrete colonies of mature cells. The best characterized factors are granulocyte macrophage colony-stimulating factors (GM-CSF), granulocyte colony-stimulating factor (G-CSF), macrophage colony-stimulating factor (M-CSF), and erythropoietin (EPO). Some hematopoietic growth factor receptors appear to be related to oncogenes;[21] genes for CSF or their receptors have been mapped to altered chromosomal locations associated with malignancies, suggesting a possible role in pathogenesis. G-CSF has been reported on small cell carcinoma cells, and it is likely that other types of nonhematopoietic tumors will express receptors for these factors.

Nerve growth factor (NGF) — NGF was originally isolated from mouse salivary glands and has a potent effect on sympathetic neurons. Certain tumor cell lines, such as pheochromocytomas and melanomas, respond to NGF. β-NGF is a stable dimer that has some sequence similarity to IGF-1, but it does not bind to its receptors.

Other cytokines (interferons, interleukins) and their receptors — Interferons are glycoproteins that are synthesized by a variety of cells and act in a paracrine capacity on cancer cells, exerting pleiotropic effects that mimic the diversity of endocrine system. Although 20 interferons have now been identified in humans, they can be classified in three broad groups: (1) α-interferons (secreted by the leukocytes), (2) β-interferons (secreted by the fibroblasts), and (3) γ-interferon (secreted solely by T-cells). There are marked homologies between human α- and β-interferons; their genes cluster on chromosome 9. The receptor for γ-interferon is found on chromosome 6 and appears to be different from that of α- and β-interferons. There are specific receptors: one class of α- and β-interferons, another class for γ-interferons.

Interleukins — Of the several interleukins (ILs 1 to 8), which all are cytokines or lymphokines, Interleukin-2 (IL-2), previously called T-cell growth factor (TCGF), is well known as a central molecular regulator in the expression of cellular immune response. Biochemically IL-2 is a glycoprotein with a single molecular size of 15.5 kDa. IL-2 is known to act on the cell surface by IL-2 specific receptors. The molecular nature of the high affinity IL-2 receptor has been completely defined. IL-2 is bound to two different binding proteins (p75 and p55), which are independent but cooperative.[22] After they cross the cell membrane and become intracellular, since the p75-α chain contains the structures responsible for signaling internalization and cell growth, its cytoplasmic domain is larger than the small cytoplasmic domain of p55-β chain that contains only 13 residues. Interleukins, interferons, TNF, and colony-stimulating factor all are an important part of the "lymphokine cascade". The practical application of this information is that the role of the p55 molecule, which is induced with activation, is to interact with the p75 to produce a receptor very sensitive to even low concentrations of IL-2.[23] NK cells bear only the low affinity p75 molecule and require high IL-2 concentrations for activation, whereas activated T-cells express the high affinity receptor p55 and require only low concentrations of IL-2. Thus, it is possible that tumors responding through T-cell mechanisms would require lower IL-2 doses than those in which NK-cell cytotoxicity is the central mechanism. It is equally important that growth factor receptors be determined on tumor tissue. Most of the growth factor receptors contain three domains: (1) an extracellular domain, which binds to specific receptors on the cell surface, (2) a short transmembrane domain, and (3) an intracytoplasmic domain, which usually contains tyrosine kinase activity. Recently, abnormal or defective steroid hormone receptors were found in human cultured cells and consequently can explain the therapeutic failure of glucocorticoids in leukemias or lymphomas. These steroid-receptor mutations may include (1) glucocorticoid nuclear deficient receptors (lower affinity), and (2) nuclear transfer increased (high-affinity or wild-type) receptors, where they bind to DNA 10- to 100-fold higher than their counterparts. These receptor mutations can account for a defective receptor function and probably the hormone resistance. It is possible that steroid receptors from cancer cells may differ from their normal counterpart cells.[24,25]

c. *Lymph Node Involvement*

Lymph node status, the presence (node positive) or absence (node negative) and the number of lymph nodes are important factors in staging the disease, predicting survival rate, and selecting patients for hormonal therapy or chemotherapy. Axillary node status and TNM (tumor, nodes, metastasis) classification (stages I to IV) give accurate information, the same as hormone receptor status, on the proportion of patients likely to respond to hormonal therapy. In fact, the hormone receptor status, lymph node involvement, and tumor size are reported by many experts to be the most important factors for hormonal therapy. The lymph node status correlated with hormone-receptor status, growth factors, and tumor size can predict more accurately the hormonoresponsiveness of patients and, in general, the cancer aggressiveness. Breast cancers without lymph node metastases or with one to three lymph nodes are considered to have a better prognosis than those tumors that have four or more lymph nodes (the worst being those with eight to nine lymph node metastases). There is a negative correlation between hormone receptor status and lymph node positivity; the hormone receptors (ER and PR) decrease with increased number of lymph nodes. The content of peptide growth factors (EGF, insulin-like factor, INF, and PGDF) is always positively correlated with the number of lymph nodes. Correlative studies showed that patients with small tumors (<2 cm), negative lymph nodes, and positive hormone-receptor status, have the most favorable prognosis, low risk, and longer survival. Studies using computerization of different factors have shown that the most reliable prognostic factors for cancer patients are the tumor size, lymph node status, hormone receptors, differentiation of the tumor, and the DNA content in tumor cells.[24]

Thus, the evaluation of lymph node status should include (1) number of lymph nodes, (2) loco-regional distribution, and (3) histological examination. The number of positive regional nodes found at surgery is an important factor in predicting systemic spread and incidence of recurrent disease. Thus, in patients with 0 nodes (node negative) at surgery, the incidence of recurrent disease will be 0 at 18 and 36 months and only becomes 20% at 60 months (5 years). A significant increase in recurrent disease occurs in patients with one to three nodes (node positive), from 15 to 17% at 18 months, 40% at 36 months, and 50% at 5 years. Thus, the inspection of regional lymph nodes helps to determine: (1) the stage of disease (local or systemic) and (2) the prognosis or prediction for the incidence of relapses and survival rate. Loco-regional distribution includes (1) axillary lymph nodes; (2) internal mammary and supraclavicular nodes; and (3) infraclavicular and distant metastatic lymph nodes. Axillary lymph nodes, which occur along the axillary vein and its tributaries, are a critical prognostic factor. Patients with negative axillary lymph nodes do considerably better than patients with any degree of axillary nodal involvement. Patients with involved infraclavicular, internal mammary, and supraclavicular lymph nodes usually have edema of the arm, skin ulcerations, and fixation to the chest wall called "peau d'orange", and they have a very poor prognosis. Absence of palpable lymph nodes (node negative) does not completely rule out the spread of cancer cells and micrometastases in the loco-regional lymph nodes.

In conclusion, the recommendations for patients taking into account node status and menopausal status are

Node Status	Premenopausal	Postmenopausal
Positive		
HR+	Chemotherapy (tamoxifen)	Tamoxifen ± chemotherapy
HR−	Chemotherapy	Chemotherapy ± tamoxifen
Negative		
High risk	Chemotherapy (tamoxifen)	Chemotherapy ± tamoxifen
Low risk		Tamoxifen

It seems likely that lymph node status is an important and independent prognostic factor, and lymph node involvement is an important factor in staging and prognosis of other types of hormone-dependent cancers, such as prostate cancer, endometrial (uterine), ovarian, and kidney carcinomas. Prostate cancer most commonly metastasizes to the lymph nodes, spreads to pelvic lymph nodes, and has critical prognostic and therapeutic implications. Within 3 years of diagnosis, approximately 50% of patients with positive pelvic nodes have a progression of disease, usually with bone metastases, and 85% have a progression within 5 years. The spread of ovarian cancer occurs mainly to the para-aortal nodes, but occasionally also to the pelvic or inguinal nodes. As anticipated, in many patients with breast cancer the number of positive lymph nodes was the most important factor for predicting early recurrence ($p < .0001$), followed by progesterone receptor (PR). The third factor of borderline statistical significance was the size of the primary tumor ($p = .07$)[5,9]

d. Tumor Size and Metastases

It is assumed that tumor size, tumor growth, and metastatic lesions are important factors for determining the therapeutic response to hormonal treatment. Smaller tumors are more responsive than larger ones to various types of therapies, such as chemotherapy, hormonotherapy, and radiation. Recently, it has been shown that tumor mass negatively influences the outcome of surgery, radiotherapy, and cancer chemotherapy. Also, because mutation toward resistance is mass-related, patients with large tumor masses have a high possibility of developing one and probably more resistant cell lines, and would be more resistant to therapy than microscopic tumors growing exponentially.[25] The concept that "small is sensitive" has been recently challenged. In order to prevent drug or hormone resistance, the hormones or drugs are better administered at full doses. There is a dose-effect relationship. Well-differentiated tumors respond three times more frequently than those with poorly differentiated disease.

These differences in tumor response suggest that hormonal therapy and chemotherapy have independent targets of action at the cellular level. The primary tumor size and lymph node involvement have the same prognostic significance in men as in women. The pattern of metastasis is similar to that in women with bone (48%), soft tissue (60%), and various visceral sites. Soft tissue (or visceral) metastases are less hormonoresponsive and have a more unfavorable prognosis as compared to bone and skin metastasis in both men and women. Metastases in liver and brain rarely respond.

TABLE 3
Factors Predicting Frequency of Response to Hormonotherapy and Chemotherapy

	Hormonotherapy	Chemotherapy
Disease-free interval	+ +	±
Tumor grade (differentiation)	+ +	±
Tumor hormone receptors	+ +	±
Tumor size	− −	+ +
Site of tumor	− −	− −

e. Heterogeneity of Cancer Cell Population

Important advances in tumor cell biology were recently made by using modern methods (electronmicroscopy, autoradiography — light and high resolution, immunohistochemistry, hormone receptor assays, and monoclonal labeled antibodies). These methods revealed that tumor cellular pattern is not homogenous, but a heterogenous pattern composed of different phenotypically clonal subpopulations; most tumors are a "mosaic" of cell populations. The exact number of phenotypically distinct clonal cell subpopulations in different malignant tumors is not known, but is probably very high. This can explain why a malignant tumor, originally a hormonally responsive or hormone-dependent cancer, loses its responsiveness and finally becomes a hormonally unresponsive or autonomous tumor. It can also explain the hormonal escape from treatment or drug resistance. Tumor cell heterogeneity is not a random and uncontrolled process. Of considerable importance to clinical oncologists is the fact that much of this cell heterogeneity may be generated prior to clinical detection of the tumor.[26] It is likely that drug or hormone resistance during treatment occurs partially by adaptation and largely by random somatic mutation.

There are two possible explanations for hormonoresistance: adaptation and selection. According to the theory of adaptation, the tumor has a homogeneous receptor cell population, but after ablation or suppression of hormonal source, a majority of the cells die and only a small fraction will adapt to the new environment and proliferate independently of hormones. According to the theory of selection, the tumor has a heterogenous cell population with hormone-sensitive and hormone-resistant clones; and the hormone resistance reflects the selection of hormone-resistant clones. This knowledge has a profound therapeutic implication, suggesting a combination of drugs or hormones and cytotoxic agents, or chemo-hormonotherapy in order to overcome the hormono- or drug resistance only by combination therapeutic modalities. This suggests an inherited (genetic) capacity of bacteria to mutate toward resistance to organisms they have never seen. Thus, tumor cell heterogeneity, which is commonly observed in most human and experimental cancers, can explain the hormone and drug resistance by the occurrence of mutant-resistant cell lines.

Hormone-like growth factors can play an important role in "cellular therapy" of cancers because they act on a particular kind of cell. These are recently isolated, growth inhibitor substances that might inhibit growth factors by altering the genes involved in their synthesis. One in particular is PDGF, which stimulates certain cells to divide and inhibits others. Thus, it can be a stimulator and inhibitor, depending on the cell system.

f. Menopausal Status

It has been suggested that menopausal status and menstrual patterns are important factors in making therapeutic decisions and patient selection for hormonotherapy vs. chemotherapy, their response to hormonal treatment, and the prediction of relapses. Thus: (1) for premenopausal women with positive nodes, regardless of hormone receptor status, the recommended treatment is chemotherapy; (2) for premenopausal women with negative nodes, adjuvant therapy is not recommended; (3) for postmenopausal women with positive nodes and positive hormone receptor status, tamoxifen is the treatment of choice; (4) for postmenopausal women with positive nodes and negative hormone receptor status, chemotherapy may be considered, and (5) for postmenopausal women with negative nodes, regardless of hormone receptor status, there is no indication for adjuvant therapy. The histology of human breast is very sensitive to endogenous hormone production. Thus, there are dramatic changes in histology of the breast in the follicular, luteal, and late luteal phases of the menstrual cycle. Examination of mammograms may often show concentric decrease of dense tissue as the menopause progresses.

In late menopause, the alveolar tissue disappears to the point of a vestigial ductal system similar to the prepubescent breast. Aberrations of cyclic changes in ovarian function may produce cystic conditions or fibroadenomas. In most cases, premenopausal women have a lower incidence of ER+ tumors (30%) compared to 60% in postmenopausal patients. The perimenopausal tumors have the lowest rate (<20%). In an extensive study by the Danish Breast Cancer Cooperative Group (DBCCG), 3735 patients were registered in relation to age, menopausal status, tumor size, lymph node involvement, and grade of anaplasia. The data revealed that both ER and PR status were found to be significant prognostic variables for premenopausal women under 50 years of age. In contrast, in the postmenopausal women neither ER nor PR status was a significant prognostic factor in the low risk group (tumor <5 cm and negative lymph nodes). However, in high risk postmenopausal women, ER status is a significant prognostic factor for disease-free survival (DFS), and appears to be independent of lymph node status.[27] It seems that the production of estrogen receptor protein (ERP) is suppressed at the time of ovulation in the normal breast epithelial cells of premenopausal women. In contrast, breast carcinoma cells either synthesize this ERP continuously throughout the menstrual cycle or fail to express it despite fluctuations of serum hormone concentrations.[28]

g. Evaluation of DNA Content and Its Significance for Hormonotherapy

Recent observations suggest that other factors, such as DNA content (S-phase) measured by [³H]-thymidine labeling index (TLI) or by flow cytometry, tumor markers, and oncogene amplification, work in concert on tumor responsiveness to hormone or cytotoxic agents and might identify subsets or groups of patients at high risk for recurrence in whom endocrine therapy and chemotherapy are strongly recommended. A review and update of published studies on hormone receptors as prognostic factors in breast cancer revealed that in stage I the estrogen negative receptor (ER −) seems to be the most important predicting factor for recurrence and poor survival; whereas in stage II breast cancer, the progesterone positive receptor (PR +) is more important in predicting the outcome of hormone therapy. Thus, the benefits of hormonotherapy are better predicted by the presence or absence of PR rather than by ER.[29]

It was found that the median percentage of S-phase is markedly higher in almost all breast tumor specimens lacking both receptors (ER − and PR −) and is the lowest in tumors containing both receptors (ER + and PR +). Thus, the thymidine labeling index studies with percentage of S-phase and ploidy estimation can identify a high risk patient subset for recurrence in stage I. TLI can be determined on fresh tumor material, which is minced into small fragments of about 1 mm, immediately following surgery. These fragments are placed in a medium with fetal calf serum, antibiotics, and [³H]-thymidine. It has been reported that TLI of tumors can identify high and low risk groups of patients with negative nodes; there was a 37% difference in disease-free survival at the 4-year followup among those with high and low risk.[30] High TLI was the most significant and only independent predictor of relapse when TLI, estrogen receptor status, and tumor size were compared in a multivariate analysis of 215 node-negative patients. The 5-year relapse-free survival again was 85% for low TLI patients and 62% for those with a high TLI. In this study, high TLI was defined as a value above the median of 4.6% for premenopausal women and only 1.4% for postmenopausal patients.

A multivariate analysis study indicated that epidermal growth factor receptor (EGF-R) is also a powerful discriminant factor in primary breast cancer, particularly in those with negative nodes.[39] Thus, TLI is more associated with EGF-R than ER in predicting the prognosis of patients with node negative and poor differentiated tumors. In operable node-negative women treated surgically, predicted survival at 5 years was 89% for 81 patients with low TLI (≤3%), 64% for 101 with mid-TLI (3.1 to 8%), and 66% for 86 with high TLI (>8%).[32]

Breast cancer is a heterogenous tumor in which the TLI defines high and low risk prognostic subgroups. Patients with aneuploid tumors or with high S-phase diploid tumors are at increased risk for relapse. Also, a strong correlation between TLI and K_1-67 growth fraction (KGF) was found in breast cancer, mainly in malignant tumors. In double-labeled sections of breast carcinoma the mean TLI was 6.1 and KGF was 16.4. Tumors with high TLI or KGF are frequently estrogen receptor negative. Therefore, both TLI and K_1-67 growth factor (KGF) are valuable indicators of proliferative activity in breast cancer.[33] Flow cytometry (FCM) is the simultaneous measurement of several cellular parameters while a cell suspension flows past a light source and can analyze 5,000 to 10,000 cells per second and can estimate DNA content, aneuploidy, surface marker phenotype, enzyme content and immunoglobulins, cellular RNA, protein content, calcium flux, and membrane permeability. Thus, FCM will become an important tool for tumor pathologists in establishing a diagnosis, determination of cancer prognosis, and selection and followup of patients for endocrine therapy and chemotherapy.

Several studies have been performed to elucidate the correlation between DNA content and steroid receptors. Lack of steroid receptor expression (ER − and PR −) in breast cancer cells, is correlated with a more aggressive clinical course and also requires more aggressive therapeutic approaches. Tumors with a normal diploid DNA content have the highest level of estrogen receptors, whereas hyperdiploid tumors show reduced ER levels. DNA analysis of cervical carcinomas revealed that the majority (78%) of specimens with severe dysplasia or carcinoma *in situ* are reported to have aneuploid DNA levels and progression to invasive carcinoma. In colorectal carcinoma, the DNA content has been described as having prognostic significance and defining distinctive histologic grade of the tumor. In all Dukes' stage A, B, or C colorectal carcinoma, the disease-free and overall survival lines of the patients with diploid or near-diploid tumors was nine times better than that of patients with aneuploid tumors, over a 5-year period.[34] It has also been shown that the induction of DNA synthesis by different estrogens occurs only when a sufficient amount of steroid-receptor is retained on the chromatin for at least 12 h. Thus, there is a direct relationship between increased protein synthesis at 12 h. and increased DNA synthesis at 24 h.

In previous studies we investigated the effect of various hormones and vitamins on neoplastic epithelial cells of squamous and basal cell carcinomas chemically induced in rodents, following 3-methylcholanthrene (3-MCA) administration. The DNA synthesis was quantitatively estimated by light and electron microscopic autoradiography following [³H]-thymidine administration. Quantitative estimation with light and electron microscopic autoradiography revealed that estradiol, thyroxine, calcitonin, and prostaglandin $F_{2\alpha}$ ($PGF_{2\alpha}$) markedly stimulated the DNA synthesis within the nuclei of neoplastic cells, whereas a notable inhibition occurred after hydrocortisone administration or hormone deprivation (castration and hypophysectomy). Electron microscopic autoradiography revealed that most of the developed grains are located in the dense chromatin (heterochromatin) or genetic chromatin (chromosomes) and not in the euchromatin (or metabolic chromatin). Estradiol induced a peripheral distribution of developed grains.[35] Vitamin A (retinol) administration produced a marked inhibition of DNA synthesis in the nuclei of neoplastic cells, whereas Vitamin E (α-tocopherol) and Vitamin C (ascorbic acid) produced only a moderate one.

These findings indicate that certain hormones and vitamins markedly influence the DNA synthesis in epithelial cancer cells, acting on the S-phase of the cell cycle. Thus, determination of the thymidine labeling index (TLI) by autoradiography, flow cytometry, and aneuploidy by FCM should be recommended to be performed routinely in tumor specimens.

h. Histologic Differentiation: Improved Diagnostic Methods

It is generally accepted that the most accurate way to predict hormone responsiveness of tumors is to combine biochemical and morphological methods. Thus, the importance of histologic grade (HG) and its nuclear grade (NG) are significant prognostic indicators. Patients with well-differentiated tumors have a better disease-free survival than those tumors with poor differentiation. In a recent study including 1157 histologically node-negative breast cancer patients, treated only surgically, without adjuvant systemic therapy, histologic grade and nuclear grade indicated that NG is a more important single marker of prognosis than is tumor ER and PR.[36] Recent studies revealed that breast carcinomas are heterogenous neoplasms.

All the transitional stages between carcinoma *in situ* and invasive carcinomas cannot be accurately detected by light microscopy only. Ultrastructural studies are more precise and can reveal early invasive changes in what appears by light microscopy to be carcinoma *in situ*. In my opinion, the combination of ultrastructural and cell surface studies by using scanning electron microscopy can better detect the early cell atypia with the occurrence of more aggressive, less differentiated cells having a high propensity to metastases and a high degree of aneuploidy or heteroploidy. Therefore, ultrastructural cellular characteristics and cell surface pattern are important criteria in differentiated distinct subgroups with hormone-dependent or hormone-independent cells, and they are important diagnostic and prognostic indicators. Aneuploid tumors exhibited a higher SPF (S-phase fraction) than ER/PR negative tumors.

Most grading systems in prostate cancer are based on the degree of anaplasia of the cancer cells or the arrangement and appearance of malignant glands. Thus, one widely accepted classification is the Gleason system, which considers the degree of glandular differentiation of the tumor and its relationship to the prostate stroma under low power magnification. On the basis of histologic differentiation, tumors are classified as grades 1 to 5, and the range is from well differentiated to poorly differentiated. Thus, there is a strong correlation between histologic differentiation of tumor and its hormone dependency and responsiveness to hormone therapy.

i. Tumor Markers and Ectopic Hormones

It has long been known that malignant tumors are associated with abnormal production of proteins, enzymes, and circulating hormones, but only recently has it been found that some of these substances can act as tumor markers. Classically, a tumor marker is a substance synthesized by the tumor and released into the circulation of patients with cancer. Several characteristics define the ideal tumor marker:

1. It should be produced by the tumor cells and be readily detectable in body fluids.
2. It should be tumor specific so that the marker will not be present in healthy bodies or benign disease.
3. It should be useful in the screening of different cancers; thus, it should be present frequently and early enough in the development of a malignancy.
4. It should be detectable when a tumor is present, but not clinically appreciable.

5.   The quantity of the tumor marker should directly reflect and be indicative of the bulk of malignancy.
6.   The level of the ideal marker should correlate with the results of anticancer therapy.

Tumor markers should have both "specificity" and "sensitivity" and thus play a potential role in screening, diagnosing, staging, and following patients during the course of their illness, or monitoring the anticancer therapy. A variety of substances or cellular products are described as tumor markers. They may be oncofetal antigens, such as alpha-fetoprotein (AFP), and carcinoembryonic antigen (CEA); hormones, such as human chorionic gonadotropin (HCG) and ectopic hormones; enzymes, such as prostatic acid phosphatase (PAP); or tissue-associated antigens, such as prostatic-specific antigen (PSA). At present, due to technological advances, such as radioimmunoassays (RIA) and monoclonal antibodies, a great number of tumor markers are detected in tumor tissue, in serum, or in body fluids of cancer patients, but some of them have only a limited value. Oncofetal proteins are expressed during embryonic development, and usually they occur in malignant tissue. The most widely used are carcinoembryonic antigen (CEA) and α-fetoprotein (AFP) (see Table 4).

Carcinoembryonic antigen (CEA) — CEA was found to be a glycoprotein (45% protein and 55% carbohydrate) with a molecular weight of 180 to 200 kDa, and it is located on the luminal surface (glycocalyx) of the tumor cell membrane.[37] CEA is frequently found in the serum of patients with adenocarcinomas of the colon, e.g., in 4% of the patients with Dukes' Grade A. Particularly high volumes of CEA were found in the blood serum of patients with colon carcinomas with liver metastases. Usually CEA is evaluated by both radioimmunoassays and the enzyme-linked immunoabsorbent assays (ELISA), which is more sensitive. Normal values commonly used are between 2.5 and 5.0 ng/ml depending upon the assay used. Also, raised plasma levels of CEA or CEA-like materials have been described in various other carcinomas. Despite some controversy regarding the specificity and sensitivity of CEA, the measurements of circulating CEA are recognized as a valuable tool for the postoperative surveillance.[38] Potentially, the CEA test could be used for: (1) screening populations for cancer, (2) monitoring the success of surgery and other forms of therapy such as chemotherapy and endocrine therapy, (3) detecting localized cancer earlier, (4) determining the onset of neoplastic change in premalignant conditions (ulcerative colitis, familial polyposis), (5) noninvasive identification of tumors, (6) staging of tumors, (7) determining clinical status, and extent of disease, (8) deciding preoperative prognosis and, (9) predicting tumor recurrence or regression following surgery or other forms of therapy. Patients with breast cancer surviving less than 6 months showed a higher rate of elevated CEA assays than those who survived 6 to 18 months. In recent years, more than 30 different monoclonal anti-CEA antibodies have been described, and they are directed against various epitopes of the CEA. Serum tests can be improved significantly.

α-Fetoprotein (AFP) — Human AFP is a single polypeptide chain glycoprotein, with a molecular weight of approximately 70 kDa, consisting of 590 amino acids with about 40% sequence homology to human albumin. The production of AFP is maximal during the 12th to 15th weeks of gestation and falls dramatically after birth; AFP reaches levels of 8.5 μg/l in adult serum and has an approximate half-life of 3.5 to 6.0 d. AFP binds to a large variety of substances (e.g., copper, zinc, estrogens, and long-chain fatty acids) although the physiological significance of this is unknown. An elevation of serum AFP levels occurs in patients with liver cell carcinomas and germ-cell neoplasms and occasionally other endodermally derived tumors.[39] Values of AFP can be used to monitor response to therapy in gynecologic malignancies. However, the diagnostic value of the currently used AFP tests are of limited value due to the fact that increased AFP levels are also found in 20 to 40% of patients with acute or chronic hepatitis and in 5 to 30% of the patients with liver cirrhosis. Recently a new AFP test was reported to be more specific using two monoclonal antibodies;

TABLE 4
Tumor Markers and Their Clinical Use in Cancer Patients

Marker	Type(s) of tumor identified
Carcinoembryonic antigen (CEA)	Colorectal cancer; various other carcinomas (choriocarcinoma, breast cancer, medullary thyroid carcinoma, prostate cancer, etc.)
α-Fetoprotein (AFP)	Hepatomas, germ-cell neoplasms, endodermal sinus tumor, ovarian cancer
CA-125	Nonmucinous ovarian carcinomas, various carcinomas
CA-50	Squamous cell carcinoma of the esophagus
CA19-9	Tumors from gastrointestinal tract, colorectal carcinoma
CA15-3	Metastatic breast cancer, ovarian cancer
Prostatic acid phosphatase (PAP)	Prostate carcinomas
Prostatic-specific antigen (PSA)	Prostate carcinomas
Ovarian cancer antigen (OCA)	Ovarian carcinoma
Human chorionic gonadotropin (HCG)	Trophoblastic tumors, ovarian carcinoma
Neuron-specific enolase (NSE)	Neuroblastomas
Plasminogen activator (PA)	Prostate cancer
Ectopic adrenocorticotropic hormone (ACTH)	Carcinoma of the lung, oat cell carcinoma
Ectopic melanin-stimulating hormone (MSH)	Mediastinal carcinoma, oat cell carcinomas
Ectopic parathyroid hormone (PTH)	Lung tumors (squamous cell CA), hepatomas
Ectopic calcitonin (CT)	APUD cell tumors, medullary thyroid carcinoma
Ectopic gonadotropins (HCG)	Lung, breast, liver and ovarian tumors; testicular germ cell tumor
Ectopic antidiuretic hormone (ADH)	Oat cell carcinoma of the lung, pancreas, and thymus
Ectopic insulin-like activity (ILA)	Tumors of mesenchymal origin
Ectopic erythropoietin (ESH)	Kidney tumors, hepatomas, cerebellar hemangioblastoma
Ectopic thyrotropin (TSH)	Trophoblastic tumors, epidermoid carcinoma of the lung, mesotheliomas
Ectopic prolactin (PRL)	Renal cell carcinoma, bronchogenic carcinoma
Ectopic human placental lactogen (HPL)	Trophoblastic tumors, other tumors
Ectopic growth hormone (GH)	Bronchogenic carcinoma, gastric cancer
Ectopic glucagon	Bronchogenic carcinoma, ovarian carcinoma, kidney tumors
Ectopic and VIP (vasoactive intestinal polypeptides)	Pancreas tumors, bronchus carcinoids, VIPomas
Ectopic growth hormone-releasing factor (GRF)	Pancreas and lung tumors
Ectopic serotonin	Pancreas and bronchus endometrial carcinoids
Tachykinins (substance P, SP neurokinin A)	Ileal and lung carcinoid tumors, carcinoid tumors, ovarian tumors
Tetranectin	Metastatic tumors
Fibronectin	Embryonal cell tumors, melanoma
Laminin	Squamous and basal cell carcinoma, metastatic tumors, tumors of mesenchymal origin
Somatostatin (SRIF) and chromogranin	Medullary thyroid carcinoma, breast cancer, argyrophilic carcinoma, small cell carcinoma
Melatonin	Breast cancer
Inhibin	Hydatidiform mole
Alkaline phosphatase	Bone tumors and bone metastases
Bombesin; neurophysin	Small cell carcinoma of lung
Ferritin	Liver tumors (primary hepatocellular carcinoma)
Proteoglycans	Melanomas, astrocytomas, gliomas, neuroblastomas
52K-cathepsin D	Breast tumors (after tamoxifen treatment); endometrial carcinoma
Catecholamines and their metabolites	Neuroblastomas, pheochromocytomas
Bence-Jones proteins	Myelomas and some lymphomas, nonlymphoid tumors
5-Hydroxyindolacetic acid (5-HIAA)	Carcinoid tumors, APUDomas, bronchial carcinoma

TABLE 4 (CONTINUED)
Tumor Markers and Their Clinical Use in Cancer Patients

Marker	Type(s) of tumor identified
Serotonin	Carcinoid tumors
Neurotensin (NT)	Pancreatic endocrine tumors, prostatic adenocarcinoma, fibrola-mellar hepatoma

at least one of these antibodies appears to recognize only AFP, but not albumin which occurs in the course of hepatitis. Elevated AFP values (over 200 ng AFP/ml) were found only in patients with liver carcinomas.

CA-125 — Recently a new glycoprotein CA-125 has been found in colonic epithelium in embryogenesis, has a high molecular weight (>500 kDa), and is recognized by the monoclonal antibody OC-125. The CA-125 antigen is found in 82% of nonmucinous epithelial ovarian carcinomas, and its titers can be correlated with disease in 93% of patients and 5% of patients with benign disease (e.g., endometriosis and pelvic inflammatory diseases). CA-125 is not affected by smoking, but is affected by pregnancy, menstruation, and other benign diseases. CA-125 can be used as a screening test of benign and malignant gynecologic tumors, and in most cases with elevated CA-125 (>50 to 65 µg/ml) and pelvic masses is a strong indication for malignancy in 80 to 90% of cases. A comparative study between CA-125 and CEA in ovarian cancer revealed that CA-125 levels were increased in 91.5% of the cases with recurrent or progressive disease, whereas only 34% of these patients had increased CEA levels.[40] Thus, the CA-125 serum test is of diagnostic and prognostic value, mainly in ovarian cancer. However, increased preoperative CA-125 levels in patients with pelvic masses are highly suggestive of a malignant tumor.

CA-50, CA19-9, and CA15-3 — These are other tumor markers (all glycoproteins) that circulate as heterogenous species with a molecular weight ranging from 300 to 450 kDa. Elevated levels of CA-50 (above 17 u/ml) were frequently found in patients with squamous cell carcinoma of the esophagus and can be used as a predictor of response to therapy of esophageal cancer. Normal values of CA19-9 are approximately ≤37 µm/ml. Increased CA19-9 levels (≥37 µm/ml) were found in patients with esophageal cancer (13%); in patients with localized colon carcinomas (4 to 8%), in patients with advanced carcinomas of the pancreas (76%), the bile ducts (73%), and less frequently of the stomach (42%) or the liver (22%).[41] CA15-3 is a glycoprotein with a molecular weight of 300 to 450 kDa found on the cell membrane and sometimes in the cytosol. It has been found at elevated levels (which are considered to be above 220.0 u/ml) in 72% of women with metastatic breast cancer. In a correlative study between CA15-3 and CEA in patients with metastatic breast cancer, it was found that significantly more patients had elevated circulating levels of CA15-3 than CEA. Also, CA15-3 increased more often than CEA in patients with progressive disease and decreased more often than CEA in patients with regressive disease.

Prostatic acid phosphatase (PAP) — Acid phosphatase is a monoester phosphohydralase present in large amounts in the prostate tissue. Although the PAP serum values can be elevated in a variety of conditions, such as nonmalignant diseases, it has been known since 1936 that a strong association exists between elevated serum acid phosphatase and advanced prostatic cancer and that serum PAP measurements are useful both in diagnosing prostate cancer and in determining response to therapy. PAP is more elevated in advanced prostate carcinoma with bone metastases.

Prostatic-specific antigen (PSA) — PSA is a specific antigen, a glycoprotein of 34 kDa identified with antisera or monoclonal antibodies in the cytoplasm of prostatic epithelial cells. PSA is produced by the normal, hypertrophic prostate and by most prostate carcinomas. In the serum of healthy individuals, usually only trace amounts of PSA can be found.

Increased PSA serum levels were found in patients with prostate carcinomas in 58% of patients in stage A and B, in 68% of patients in stage C, and in 92% of patients in stage D. Comparative studies of prostatic specific antigen and prostatic acid phosphatase demonstrated that PSA is more sensitive and more specific than PAP in detecting the prostate cancer. It was established that the upper normal limit is 10 ng/ml for PSA and 2.5 ng/ml for PAP. The sensibility of PSA was 87% in prostate carcinoma and only 64% for PAP.[42] Others reported even higher values, e.g., 96% for PSA and only 45% for PAP. PSA levels higher than 40 ng/ml are associated with at least 63% nodal metastases. A massive increase in PSA values following a treatment can indicate a recurrence.

Human chorionic gonadotropin (HCG) — HCG contains two chains: the α-chain, which is shared by luteinizing hormone (LH) and thyroid-stimulating hormone (TSH), and the β-chain, which contains unique C-terminal residues that confer its antigenic identity. The use of HCG as a tumor marker is mainly restricted to trophoblastic tumors, nongestational ovarian carcinoma, and embryonal cell carcinoma. Elevated HCG levels have also been reported in up to 35% of patients with ovarian or cervical malignancies. Since the α-chain is identical to other hormones (LH, FSH), the β-chain is specific only to HCG; therefore, when it is tested, it is the only β-HCG that is assayed. High levels are found in patients with choriocarcinoma (up to 80 to 100%) and with teratoma of testis (up to 40 to 60%). β-HCG is occasionally found in liver, breast, stomach, ovary, and bronchus carcinoma.

Neuron-specific enolase (NSE) — The neuron-specific enolase (NSE) is frequently found in patients with neuroblastomas. Children with stage-III and stage-IV neuroblastomas and with more than 100 ng/ml/NSE in their serum have a very bad prognosis; whereas serum NSE levels of <100 ng/ml in infants are associated with excellent long-term survival.[43]

Plasminogen activator (PA) — Plasminogen activators (PAs) are serum proteases catalyzing the conversion of plasminogen into plasmin. Increased secretion of PA has been observed in many malignant cells, indicating a role of PA in tumor progression and metastasis.

Ectopic hormones as tumor markers — Among the topics of great interest in the study of cancer is the inappropriate production of hormones (polypeptide hormones) by neoplasms of nonendocrine origin. To be considered an "ectopic" hormone, the polypeptide must be secreted by a tumor arising from an organ that does not normally secrete this hormone. That is in opposition to hormones secreted by the tumors developing in organs that are normally sites of hormone synthesis. The ectopic hormones are the same as natural hormones and cause metabolic and clinical effects that resemble oversecretion of the hormone from a specific endocrine gland. The detection of a hormone in the circulation or its presence in tumor extracts is not sufficient to establish an ectopic hormone or a paraendocrine syndrome. A number of criteria have been proposed; among them is *in vitro* demonstration of synthesis of the hormone by cultured human tumor cells, or the disappearance of the hormone excess after surgical removal of the tumors. The production of ectopic hormones and the occurrence of paraendocrine syndromes may be the first manifestation of the presence of cancer, which may be of more importance than the management of the underlying malignant disease itself. Failure to know that cancer may produce ectopic hormones and a clinical syndrome similar to those produced by endocrine glands may lead to incorrect diagnosis and treatment (see Table 3).

Ectopic adrenocorticotropic hormone (ACTH) — It is found as "big" and "little" ACTH in both plasma and tumor tissue of patients with ectopic ACTH-producing tumors, such as oat cell carcinoma, bronchogenic carcinoma, pancreas carcinoma, medullary carcinoma of the thyroid, and chronic obstructive lung disease. The big ACTH is considered the precursor of the little ACTH. Ectopic MSH appears as α-MSH, but generally biologic activity in most of the tumor extracts could be attributed to β-MSH, which is probably a lipoprotein. It was found in mediastinal carcinoma, oat cell carcinoma, and pancreatic tumors.

Ectopic parathyroid hormone (PTH) — Ectopic PTH is found in tumors other than parathyroid tumors, e.g., in lung carcinoma (squamous cell CA), hepatomas, hypernephroma, and carcinoma of the breast and pancreas. Using radioimmunoassay (RIA) it was found in lower levels of ectopic PTH in cancer patients, than those found in hyperparathyroidism for an equivalent increase in serum calcium. It was suggested that the ectopic PTH circulates more as an inactive form (inactive fragments) than the real (eutopic) PTH. Some immunological studies suggest that ectopic PTH is produced mainly as pro-PTH or even as a higher molecular component, prepro-PTH, which cannot be converted in the active PTH due to the absence of an enzyme that splits the molecule.

Ectopic gonadotropins — Because gonadotropins are normally produced by both pituitary and trophoblastic tissue, this implies that ectopic gonadotropins are secreted by nonpituitary or nontrophoblastic tumors. The most common tumors associated with excessive gonadotropin secretion are carcinomas of the lung, breast, and ovary, testicular germ cell tumors, and less commonly, hepatoblastomas and melanomas. Immunologic and biochemical studies revealed that human chorionic gonadotropin (HCG) has two chains: α-chain and β-chain. Since the α-chain is found also in pituitary gonadotropins, they share biochemical properties with each other and with HCG secreted by trophoblastic disease. By using a specific radioimmunoassay for the β-subunit, it is possible to determine more accurately only the β-HCG and thus it can be differentiated from pituitary FSH and LH.

Ectopic antidiuretic hormone (ADH) — Ectopic ADH appears to be biologically, chemically, and immunologically indistinguishable from original or eutopic ADH. Ectopic ADH is most commonly produced by oat cell carcinoma of the lung (almost one third of all cases), followed by cancer of the pancreas, duodenum, breast, and esophagus.

Ectopic insulin (or insulin-like) hormone — Ectopic insulin-like hormone, now called somatomedin, is mainly produced by extra-pancreatic tumors, especially of mesenchymal origin (fibrosarcomas, neurofibromas, mesotheliomas, and lymphosarcomas) followed by hepatomas (21%) and adrenal carcinoma (5%). The major symptoms are hyperglycemia with neurologic findings (mental confusion and coma).

Ectopic erythropoietin (ESH) — The most common tumors associated with ectopic ESH are solid and cystic tumors of the kidney (more than half of these). Other tumors associated with ectopic ESH are cerebellar hemangioblastoma (20%), fibromyomas of the uterus, hepatomas, pheochromocytomas, Wilms' tumors, and thymus carcinomas. Patients with ectopic ESH have an abnormal increase of red blood cells, hematocrit and hemoglobin (Hb).

Ectopic thyrotropin (TSH) — Ectopic TSH is mainly found in trophoblastic tumors; several patients with hyperthyroidism with trophoblastic tumors have been reported. There are four isolated substances with thyrotropic activity: pituitary TSH, LATS (long-acting thyroid stimulator), hCT (human chorionic thyrotropin), and mTSH (molar thyroid-stimulating hormone). The ectopic TSH syndrome has also been described in patients with epidermoid carcinoma of the lung and mesotheliomas; these patients also have clinical hyperthyroidism.

Ectopic prolactin (PRL) — High levels of ectopic prolactin have been found in patients with renal cell carcinoma, bronchogenic carcinoma, ovarian and testicular tumors, and medullary carcinoma of the thyroid.

Ectopic glucagon — Ectopic glucagon production was demonstrated in renal tumors that contain some APUD cells, in pancreatic islet α-cell tumors, glucagonomas, and also in bronchogenic and ovarian carcinoids. Clinically, it is characterized by severe constipation, malabsorption, and hyperglycemia.

Ectopic growth hormone (GH) — High levels of ectopic GH were found in some patients with bronchogenic carcinoma and gastric cancer associated with hypertrophic pulmonary osteoarthropathy.

Ectopic gastrin and vasoactive intestinal polypeptides (VIP) — Ectopic gastrin is produced by the pancreatic tumors (adenomas of Langerhans' cells) in most of the patients having Zollinger-Ellison syndrome with peptic ulcerations and diarrhea. Ectopic gastrin occurs in circulation in several forms, such as "big, big" gastrin, "big" gastrin, and "little" or "mini" gastrin. Patients with Zollinger-Ellison syndrome have in their sera, up to 50% "little" gastrin and the remainder, often the major position as "big" gastrin and only 20% as "big, big" gastrin.[44] Ectopic gastrin also is found in midgut carcinoma (VIPomas).

Ectopic serotonin — Ectopic serotonin production occurs in patients with pancreas and bronchus carcinoids and endometrial adenocarcinomas; it is clinically characterized by symptoms similar to that of carcinoid syndrome. Normally serotonin is secreted by the "argyrophill-cells" and ectopic serotonin by the "argyrophill-cell carcinomas". Thus, the production of these ectopic hormones may be used in early detection of tumors and also in monitoring the response to cancer therapy. They are valuable and accurate tumor markers.

Tachykinins (substance P and neurokinin A) — Both tachykinins, substance P and neurokinin A, are cleaved from the same precursor, called β-prepro-tachykinin. They are produced by midgut (ileal) and lung carcinoid tumors. Using RIA procedures, it was found that midgut carcinoid tumors and lung carcinoid contain both tachykinins or neurokinin A alone. Detection of tachykinins may prove to be a useful diagnostic for these tumors.[45]

Tetranectin, a novel protein, is a tetramer composed of four identical noncovalently bound 181 amino acid polypeptide chains, has a molecular weight of 20 kDa, and is related to the fibrinolytic system. It had a high predictive specificity and sensitivity and can be used as an important marker for metastatic and nonmetastatic cancer.

Fibronectin and Laminin — Cell surface-associated fibronectin consists of two or more disulfide-linked glycoproteins of 200 to 250 kDa. Often, the transformation of cells is associated with a reduction of fibronectin synthesis. Laminin is found in the basement membrane and is a valuable indicator for basement membrane integrity and cancer invasion. Both fibronectin and laminin can indicate an early cancer invasiveness and metastatic process. Recent studies in using ^{125}I-laminin found laminin receptor expression on murine tumor cells. Laminin may promote the metastases by interaction of cancer cells with basement membranes and also through NK (natural killer) cells decreasing the host antimetastatic activity.[46]

Somatostatin (SRIF) and other neuroendocrine markers — Somatostatin is a tetradecapeptide originally isolated from hypothalamus. Elevated levels of SRIF were found in the plasma and in the tumor tissue of patients with medullary thyroid cancer. Recently somatostatin receptors (SSR) were detected in human breast cancers, and a high correlation was established between the somatostatin receptors and neuroendocrine markers (chromogranin A and B and synaptophysin). There is also a relationship between ER and SSR, which indicates the existence of a defined group of breast cancer similar to neuroendocrine tumors.[47]

Alkaline phosphatase — Elevated alkaline phosphatase was found in 66% of patients with bone metastases. It is also raised in osteomalacia, liver metastases, Paget's disease, and cirrhosis.

Bombesin and neurophysin — These are synthesized in small cell lung carcinomas *in vivo* as well as *in vitro*. Bombesin is a tetradecapeptide and was originally found in frog skin.

Ferritin — Ferritin is the major cellular storage protein for iron; elevated serum ferritin is associated with inflammation, liver disease, and certain neoplasms, including neuroblastoma, Hodgkin's disease, and primary hepatocellular carcinoma (PHC).

Proteoglycans — These are glycosaminoglycans made up of a heterogenous group of long polysaccharide chains; they are found in almost all melanomas, and many astrocytomas, neuroblastoma, and human gliomas produce proteoglycans.

52K-cathepsin D — 52K-cathepsin and its precursor, the pro-cathepsin D of 52 kDa are regulated by estrogens via the estrogen receptor (ER) and is secreted by breast cancer cells *in vitro* and human endometrium.

Catecholamines and their metabolites (VMA and HVA) — Catecholamines and homovanillic acid (HVA) and vanillylmandelic acid (VMA) are often raised in neuroblastoma. Neuroblastomas release catecholamines into the blood; VMA and HVA, which are metabolites, are released in urine (in 75% of patients).

Bence-Jones proteins and immunoglobulins — These proteins are increased in myelomas and some lymphomas and can be detected in urine. In myeloma, 95% of cases have monoclonal immunoglobulins and 50% have Bence-Jones proteinuria. Elevated immunoglobulins can also be found in nonlymphoid tumors, autoimmune benign disease, and macroglobulinemia. Neurotensin (NT) is a 13-amino acid gut-brain peptide found in ileum and endocrine pancreatic tumors.

5-Hydroxyindolacetic acid (5-HIAA) — This metabolite is secreted by carcinoid tumors (which are apudomas arising in the midgut) and excreted in the urine of patients and may confirm the diagnosis of a carcinoid tumor. Tumor markers may be used in: (1) establishing the diagnosis, (2) monitoring response to treatment, (3) monitoring patients for relapse, (4) screening programs, (5) localizing of tumors, and (6) deciding a prognostic factor.[48,49]

j. Oncogene Amplification

There are at least three types of cellular genes: (1) oncogenes (c-oncogenes), which may induce cancer development when activated by regulatory or structural changes, (2) emerogenes (tumor suppression genes), which can counteract tumor development by acting as "brakes" and preventing the occurrence of cancers, and (3) modulatory genes, which can modulate secondary properties of the tumor, such as metastatic ability and immunogenicity.[50]

Oncogene amplification recently has been used in diagnostic and mainly as prognostic factors for various types of cancers (breast, lung, thyroid, and bladder) and most of solid tumors.[51] There are many oncogene types, such as ras oncogenes (H-ras, K-ras, and N-ras); myc oncogenes (c-myc, N-myc, and L-myc); erb-B family (C-erb-B, V-erb-B, and HER-2/neu); C-fos and sis oncogenes. The most clinically used in human cancers are ras oncogenes and erb-B, especially HER-2/neu and C-myc oncogenes. Members of the ras family of cellular oncogenes are the most frequently detected in human solid tumors, including carcinomas of the breast, colon, bladder, ovary, prostate, lung, and proliferative thyroid tissue. Thus, 25 of 28 breast tumors contained more ras p21 than the average of the values obtained for fibroadenomas, in 17 of the 19 cases studied, over 20% more ras p21 was observed in breast carcinomas compared with their normal counterparts.

In several types of cancer, amplification of a specific oncogene has been shown to correlate with advanced stages of tumor progression, suggesting that oncogene amplification and expression may be valid prognostic markers.[52] Examples of consistent tumor-specific oncogene amplification and expression include the HER-2/neu oncogene in breast carcinoma; N-myc in neuroblastoma; and C-myc, N-myc, and L-myc in small cell lung cancer. There is a belief that oncogenes are associated with cellular differentiation, through the growth factors and their receptors. More direct evidence comes from the fact that three of the twenty known protooncogenes are related to a growth factor or a growth factor receptor.

Recently, it has been shown that the HER-2/neu oncogene is significantly amplified in human breast cancer. Thus, alterations of this gene were investigated in 189 primary human breast cancers, and HER-2/neu was found to be amplified from 2- to > 20-fold in 30% of the tumors. Amplification of the HER-2/neu gene was a significant predictor of both overall survival and time of relapse in 86 patients with stage II breast cancer.[52] Amplification of HER-2/neu was significantly correlated with the stage of the disease. Thus, HER-2/neu amplification was observed in 18.5 and 38% of node-negative and node-positive patients,

TABLE 5
Potential Uses of Monoclonal Antibodies in Clinical Oncology

Diagnosis

Nuclear scanning with radiolabeled mAb (immunoscintigraphy)
  Detection of primary or metastatic tumors
Tumor markers
  Screening of body fluids for circulating or excreted tumor-associated antigens (TAAs)
Immunopathology
  Differential diagnosis of tumor type
Cytology: malignant vs. benign

Therapy

Direct cytotoxicity of mAb
Radionuclide conjugation to mAb
Systemic therapy
Bone marrow clearance

Prognosis

Predicted response to specific therapeutic regimens
Subclassification of tumors based on tumor-associated antigen expression
Differentiation antigens
Antigens associated with low or high metastatic potential
Antigens associated with different sites of metastasis

respectively.[53] Therefore, the oncogene amplification or overexpression is an important diagnostic factor and mainly a prognostic factor for the overall survival and recurrences of cancer patients within and following adjuvant systemic therapy such as hormonotherapy and chemotherapy. This oncogene is an independent prognostic factor, sometimes even more valuable than hormone receptor status, tumor size, or age at diagnosis. Furthermore, acting with other factors, such as DNA content, lymph node involvement, histological differentiation, and hormone receptors (ER, PR), HER-2/neu strongly increases the diagnostic and prognostic value in selecting patients for hormonotherapy and/or chemotherapy.

Interestingly, expression of protooncogenic C-fos in human breast cancer cells is significantly influenced by steroid hormones, peptide growth factors, and Vitamin D_3. Thus, 17β-estradiol increased C-fos mRNA level, whereas progesterone, Vitamin D_3, dihydrotestosterone, and dexamethasone had little effect on C-fos mRNA. The peptide growth factors, TGF-α and EGF increased C-fos expression sixfold above controls after 30 min of treatment.

k. Monoclonal Antibodies (mAbs)

The development of technology to produce monoclonal antibodies (hybridoma technology) generated substantial enthusiasm for using this approach in the diagnosis and treatment of cancer. Monoclonal antibodies are specific for single antigens, are target-specific or so-called "magic bullets", and can be efficiently coupled to isotopes, drugs, hormones, and toxins. Human monoclonal antibodies have two potential applications in the study of human cancer: (1) to define the humoral immune response of patients with cancer, (2) to provide diagnostic and therapeutic agents for administration to patients with cancer.[54] There are numerous potential applications for mAbs in the study and treatment of human cancer. The use of radiolocalization studies may be of considerable value especially in early cancer detection and in identification of metastases for those patients.[55] The following table shows the potential uses of monoclonal antibodies in clinical oncology (see Table 5).

However, the greatest excitement with monoclonal antibodies is their therapeutic potential, delivering high doses of drug, toxin or radioactivity to the site of the tumor. ^{131}I-radiolabeled mAbB72.3 administered intravenously is a positive tumor targeting colorectal, ovarian, gastric, breast and pancreatic carcinoma. Treatment of B-cell malignancies with a labeled [131]I Lym-1 monoclonal antibody has recently been reported. Clinical trials of murine monoclonal antibody therapy have been reported for acute T-cell leukemia, B-cell lymphoma, melanoma and colon carcinoma, but results are minimal, although some patients with B-cell lymphomas, melanoma, or colon carcinoma, have had significant improvement.

l. Screening Procedures for Cancer Detection

It is generally agreed that screening for detection of cancer in the early stage is a crucial factor for cancer treatment and prognosis of the disease. Unfortunately, almost 50% of cases are detected by a physician, when cancer has already spread to lymph nodes or distant organs, that is, when cancer is a systemic disease.

Breast Cancer — There are three main screening maneuvers for breast cancer: clinical breast examination (CBE), mammography, and breast self-examination (BSE). Breast self-examination is a simple, noninvasive, and inexpensive screening procedure for breast cancer. Despite the literature published, the quality of BSE is particularly difficult to assess because BSE is not a laboratory test, with a rigid protocol and quality control. As currently practiced, the BSE accuracy (sensitivity and specificity) is considerably low (20 to 30%) and is even lower among older women, compared with the combination of CBE and mammography. However, the guidelines developed by the American Cancer Society for early detection of breast cancer recommend that all women over 20 years should perform breast self-examination monthly; women between 20 and 40 should have a clinical breast examination every 3 years, and women over 40 should have a CBE every year. Also, women between the ages of 35 and 40 should have a baseline mammogram. Women over 50 should have a mammogram every year. Women at high risk (personal or family history of breast cancer) should have more frequent examinations or consult their physician about the need of mammography before the age of 50.[56] Thus, the U.S. Preventive Task Force suggests that physicians perform CBE annually. The mammography for women younger than 50 years is not recommended except in the context of studies designed to evaluate effectiveness. A recent randomized trial was performed in Sweden regarding the advantages of mammography in women of different age groups divided in women without breast cancer, women with breast cancer, those who died from breast cancer, and those who died from other reasons. It was concluded that screening mammography reduced by 20% the mortality of breast carcinoma only in women over 55 years. Furthermore, the results of this study do not strongly recommend mammography as a routine and obligatory procedure for all old women.[57] However, a recent study in the U.S. recommended an annual screening mammogram and CBE in symptomatic women over 50 years and also a mammogram at 1- to 2-year intervals in asymptomatic women aged from 40 to 49 years.[58]

Cervical, uterine, and endometrial invasive cancer — Cancers of the female reproductive tract are the fourth leading cause (after breast, lung, and colorectal cancers) among women in this country.[59] It can be stated unequivocally that the cervical smear is an effective procedure for cancer detection, perhaps the only effective cancer screening test known today. Generally, it is known as the Papanicolaou test (or Pap smear). The Pap smear can detect 90% of early cervical neoplasia, and its use has significantly reduced death from cervical cancer by >50% due to recognition and treatment of preinvasive neoplasia (carcinoma *in situ*).[60] According to the American Cancer Society, the test should be done at least every 3 years in normal asymptomatic women between the ages of 20 and 65 years. In women under 20, it should be done only in the sexually active. However, a recent study suggests that cervical cancer screening and Pap test should also be recommended in women beyond 65 years of age. Pap test results are grouped into four classes: Class I, no abnormal cells are seen; Class II, atypical (usually inflammatory) cells are seen; Class III, cells suspicious of carcinoma are found; Classes IV and V, atypical cancer cells and carcinoma cells are present. Colposcopy and biopsy are mandatory if a suspicious lesion is seen. Pelvic examination should be recommended every 3 years in women aged 20 to 40 years and every year in women over 40 years. However, the conventional Pap smear, considered 90% accurate for cervical cancer, is only 50% accurate for endometrial cancer. Of particular concern are women with "atypical" Papanicolaou smears, showing a significant cytologic abnormality but not at a diagnostic level. Technical and interpretation errors may occurs in 10-15% of cases.

Cancer of the prostate — This is the second most common cancer in males in the U.S. At present, there is no reliable screening test for prostate cancer. However, measurements of serum acid phosphatase, prostatic acid phosphatase (PAP), and prostatic-specific antigen (PSA) are useful in early detection of cancer and in response to therapy. Bone scans have been found to be more useful than X-rays, serum acid phosphatase, and tumor size in reflecting the early success or failure of treatment. Although the PSA is a sensitive test and especially valuable after total prostatectomy, PSA cannot be used for screening of early prostate cancer because it is elevated in 55 to 83% of patients with benign prostatic hyperplasia (BPH).[61] Because localized prostate cancer is mostly asymptomatic, routine rectal palpation is the most effective method now available for detecting early disease and should be done every year in men over 40 to 50 years old. A palpable prostate nodule or area of induration is always an indication for rectal ultrasonography and fine needle biopsy from the suspected area.

Ovarian cancer — Since the ovaries are relatively inaccessible to examination, ultrasonography is used for screening of early ovarian cancer. Ultrasonography is a sensitive, safe, and versatile imaging technique widely employed for detection of intra-abdominal masses. It can display normal ovaries in approximately 90% of patients as well as the presence of fluid or cyst-like material. Sigmoidoscopy is also recommended by the American Cancer Society as a procedure for early colorectal cancer detection.

3. Comments and Conclusions: Hormonoresistance

The evaluation of the 12 factors already described is crucial for a rational hormonotherapy. They are important parameters in determining the diagnosis, prognosis, and responsiveness to a certain type of hormonotherapy or endocrine manipulation. A main obstacle of hormonotherapy is still the occurrence of hormonoresistance. The mechanism of resistance to hormone therapy is complex and not yet well understood. Hormone resistance can occur spontaneously due to genetic instability or spontaneous mutations. The presence of hormone receptors is important. Not only receptor numbers, but function is important in eliciting the hormone response at the cellular level. There are tumors containing defective hormone receptors. This can explain why 10% of breast cancer that do not have hormone receptors respond to hormonal therapy; whereas, 50% of those that have the estrogen receptor (ER) and 25% that have both ER and PR sometimes fail to respond to hormonal therapy. Some of the neoplasms can secrete several growth factors and inhibitor substances by autocrine mechanisms.

B. PRINCIPLES AND BIOLOGICAL BASIS FOR VITAMIN THERAPY IN CANCER

1. General Considerations

Vitamins, due to their particular mechanism of action, offer a new approach to cancer therapy, which is different from those of chemotherapy, radiation therapy, surgery, and immunotherapy. Several experimental, epidemiological, and clinical studies revealed that vitamins are a new class of compounds with remarkable prophylactic and therapeutic activities

TABLE 6
Possible Mechanisms of Action of Vitamins in Carcinogenesis

Mechanism of action	Vitamin
Cellular receptors	Vitamin A (retinol), retinoids, Vitamin D (calciferol), $1\alpha,25(OH)_2D_3$
DNA synthesis	A, retinoids, E(α-tocopherol)
DNA replication	Vitamin B_{12}, D, niacin
Antioxidation	E, C (ascorbic acid), β-carotene
Cell differentiation	A, retinoids, D
Immune system	C, D, A, B_6 (pyridoxine), E
Cell membrane alterations and cytotoxicity	E, A, K, C
Free-radical scavengers	A, E
Reduction of mutagenicity	C, E, K_3 (menadione)
"Rescue" effect (citrovorum factor)	Folic acid
Collagen synthesis	C
N-Nitrosocompounds	C, E

for cancer patients. At present little is known regarding the therapeutic effects of vitamins in human cancers except how vitamins and provitamins exert their antitumor activity.

2. Possible Mechanisms of Action of Vitamins in Carcinogenesis

Studies using tissue culture models should be useful in order to elucidate the mechanism by which tumor cells resistant to vitamins develop and vitamin resistance occurs. Vitamins influence many cellular functions that are important in the induction and promotion of cancer, such as cell growth and cell differentiation, antioxidation, DNA synthesis, and cell membrane alterations.[62,63] Some vitamins and their possible mechanisms of action in carcinogenesis are given in Table 6.

3. Commonly Used Vitamins in Cancer Treatment and Prevention
a. Vitamin A (Retinol) and Its Analog Derivatives (Retinoids)

Vitamin A, a fat-soluble compound that cannot be synthesized within the body, is known for its importance on the growth and differentiation of epithelial tissues, visual function, reproduction, epithelial differentiation, and mucous secretion. (A detailed description of the therapeutic effects of vitamins is given in Chapter 5 of this book.) It is possible that retinoids act in a manner analogous to that of the steroid hormones and that specific intracellular-binding proteins (cellular retinol-binding and retinoic acid-binding protein) play a critical role in facilitating the interaction of retinoids with binding sites in the cell nucleus.[62] Recently, a human nuclear retinoic acid-receptor and its DNA sequence were described. The ability of retinoic acid (RA) to induce differentiation in several types of human tumor cells is associated with its ability to suppress the expression of the C-myc oncogenes or its related N-myc gene in carcinogenesis. It was shown that retinoids influence the immune response. Isotretinoin, for instance, enhances the secondary antibody response of IgG and IgE, but has no effect on IgM.[64]

b. Vitamins B (B_1, B_2, B_6, B_{12}, and Niacin)

The effects of Vitamin B in carcinogenesis are not clearly determined. Vitamin B_6 (pyridoxine) is a water-soluble vitamin that plays a crucial coenzymatic role in nucleic acid synthesis, protein metabolism, and cell proliferation. A deficiency of this vitamin in animals and humans has been correlated with impairment of both humoral and cell-mediated immunity. Breast cancer patients who excreted subnormal amounts of 4-pyridoxine acid had a significantly high probability of breast cancer recurrence after mastectomy. Vitamin B_{12}

(cyanocobalamin) occupies a key position as the coenzyme of the only reaction known to be involved in the metabolism of 1-carbon fragments. Clinical studies in humans revealed that Vitamin B_{12} deficiency decreased the evolution of hematopoietic malignancy associated with pernicious anemia. This supports the notion that patients with Vitamin B_{12} deficiency are at increased risk of developing hematopoietic malignancy. Thus, Vitamin B_{12} may act as a cocarcinogen, anti- and procarcinogen, depending on the dose and time when it is administered in the experiment.[65] Clinical studies revealed an improvement in bronchial squamous metaplasia in smokers treated with folate and Vitamin B_{12}.[66]

Studies concerning the effects of the essential vitamin niacin and its active form, nicotinamide, were evaluated. Conflicting results were produced when nicotinamide was administered at pharmacological doses concurrently with or following carcinogen administration to mice or rats. It has been suggested that diets relatively deficient in niacin, zinc, and possibly riboflavin, may play a role in the etiology of esophageal cancer.

c. Vitamin C (Ascorbic Acid)

In vitro studies have shown that Vitamin C can exert multiple mechanisms of action depending upon the cell type and experimental conditions. First, one of the mechanisms by which Vitamin C kills tumor cells and exerts its cytotoxicity is the formation of hydrogen peroxide (H_2O_2) at the cell surface, or within the cell:[67] ascorbate $+ 0_2 \rightarrow$ dehydroascorbate $+ H_2O_2$. Second, normal cells have both catalase and peroxidase activities. Sodium ascorbate inhibits only the catalase activity *in vitro,* and thus will kill only the tumor cells having predominantly catalase activity. Therefore, the efficacy of Vitamin C treatment also varies with the number of tumor cells having predominantly catalase activity in a tumor mass at the time of Vitamin C treatment. *In vitro* data also suggested that the presence of cupric ions forms hydroxyl-free radicals which are primarily responsible for DNA cleavage.

$$\text{Ascorbate} + 2Cu^{2+} \rightarrow \text{dehydroascorbate} + CU^{+}$$

Dehydroascorbate, a metabolite of Vitamin C, produced cytotoxic effects primarily in hypoxic cells. Third, Vitamin C can inhibit formation of nitrosamines from its precursors and this can inhibit tumors produced by nitrosamines. Vitamin C blocks the formation of nitrosamines both *in vitro* and *in vivo.* Humans are exposed to nitrosamines and also to a variety of nitrosating agents in food and water, and in polluted air. Fourth, Vitamin C reduces mutagenic activity by blocking the mutagenesis by nitroso-compounds. Finally, Vitamin C enhances the cellular and humoral defense reactions in the host as a biologic redox agent.

These inconclusive or conflicting results in animals may be because most studies of the effect of Vitamin C on carcinogenesis have used mice, rats, or hamsters, species that are able to synthesize ascorbic acid and have no dietary requirements. It should be used in animals incapable of synthesizing Vitamin C, such as guinea pigs, or Vitamin C-requiring rats. Epidemiological studies suggest that Vitamin C may lower the risk of cancer, particularly in the esophagus and stomach. In addition, Vitamin C is also involved in collagen synthesis protecting against infection, detoxification process, wound healing, chemotaxis, and phagocytosis.

d. Vitamin D and Its Endocrine Role

It has become apparent during the last few years that $1\alpha,25$-dihydroxy-Vitamin D, the steroid hormone that is formed from the biotransformation of Vitamin D in the body, plays a role in normal biology of the body as well as in cancer biology. Research effort during the last decade has disclosed that $1\alpha,25(OH)_2D$ mediates its actions via specific intracellular receptors in a similar manner to the estrogens and thyroid hormones. It is newly established that the $1\alpha,25(OH)_2D$ receptor is a protein well conserved with a molecular weight of 50 to 60 kDa. In addition to the classical targets of the hormone, intestine, bone, and kidney, hormone receptors were found in a variety of unsuspected tissues such as pancreas, pituitary, ovary, testes, mammary tissue, thymus, bone marrow, thyroid, skeletal muscle, T-lymphocytes, and cancer cell lines. Many cancer cells have now been found to possess receptors for $1\alpha,25(OH)_2D$ that are indistinguishable from the receptors found in the normal target tissues of the hormone. Indeed $1\alpha,25(OH)_2D$ receptors have been identified in cell lines derived from tumors of the breast, lung, and cervix; melanomas; osteogenic sarcomas; colon cancer; and leukemia. Interestingly, a relationship between oncogenes and $1\alpha,25(OH)_2D$ has emerged recently.[68] Thus, an association has been found between the myc gene and the $1\alpha,25(OH)_2D$ receptor protein expression, which can explain the ubiquity of this hormone and its role in cell growth and differentiation of malignant cells. A relationship exists between Vitamin D and the immune system, especially the potential role of $1\alpha,25(OH)_2D_3$ on cells of this system. The vitamin can inhibit T-lymphocyte proliferation and B-cell immunoglobulin production and also decrease interleukin-2 (IL-2) and interferon-gamma (IFN-γ) synthesis.[69]

e. Vitamin E, D-α-Tocopherol

This vitamin may exert inhibitory effects on chemical carcinogenesis. It has been shown in experimental animals and *in vitro* studies that Vitamin E can effectively inhibit the formation of carcinogenic nitrosamines. No definite links between dietary Vitamin E and human cancer have been demonstrated. Early results indicated a decrease of mixed tumor incidence by 50% in rats receiving i.p. injections of MCA and Vitamin E compared to those on a control diet. Later, a decreased incidence of fibrosarcomas, lymphomas, and hepatomas was also reported in mice after combined administration of methylcholanthrene and α-tocopherol. *In vitro* studies on tumor cells in culture showed that various tocopherol esters inhibited growth and caused morphological changes in mouse melanoma cells, B-16, mouse neuroblastomas, and rat glioma cells in culture. Clinical trials and studies regarding the role of Vitamin C in the etiology and therapy of human cancers suggest a role of Vitamin E in carcinogenesis.

In summary, Vitamin E may influence cancer development and management by: (1) inhibiting neoplastic cell growth, (2) inhibiting mutagenic activity, (3) serving as a strong antioxidant and free-radical scavenger, (4) being involved in cell integrity and cell membrane maintenance, (5) taking part in DNA synthesis and chromosomal breakage induced by carcinogenesis, (6) stimulating immune system activity, (7) preventing platelet aggregation release, and (8) modulating prostaglandin (PG) biosynthesis.

f. Vitamin K

Vitamin K is a fat-soluble antihemorrhagic agent comprising three similar compounds: Vitamin K_1 (phylloquinone) found naturally in higher plants; Vitamin K_2 (menaquinone) produced by bacteria; and Vitamin K_3 (menadione), a synthetic derivative. Despite some chemical differences, all Vitamins K share common properties, such as agents serving as electron acceptors for mammalian redox enzymes. A significant inhibition by Vitamin K_3 was also observed in several human cancer cell lines from the breast, ovary, colon, stomach, and kidney, and from primary and squamous cell carcinoma of the lung. This inhibition of cancer cells is a dose-dependent phenomenon. Clinical trials using Vitamin K_3 and 5-FU for patients with metastatic adenocarcinoma of the breast and colon showed some objective responses that have lasted more than 12 months in four responding patients.[70] It also has been suggested that Vitamin K_3 is an important radio sensitizing agent. The addition of Vitamin K_3 as synkavite to radiation therapy in patients with buccal carcinoma increased the survival rate at 5 years to 39% as compared to 20% in patients treated with radiation alone. The mechanism of cytotoxicity of Vitamin K is electron transfer mediated. Also, changes in the cytosol ionized calcium pool may be an important pathway of toxicity.

4. Comments and Conclusions

In conclusion, the preventive effect of certain vitamins has been well established by clinical, epidemiological, and experimental studies. Whether physiological, pharmacological or high doses (megadoses) of some vitamins (C, A, E) can have curative effects on cancers is still undetermined. Although most vitamins strongly influence cell growth and cell differentiation, DNA synthesis, mutagenicity, redox-oxidative and phosphorylation processes, all cornerstones in cancer development, their therapeutic effect in cancer patients is not similar to that demonstrated in laboratory animals. This controversy can be due to the animal species, type of tumors, and the dose used.

Some vitamins exert their mechanism of action through cellular receptors; after binding and forming vitamin-receptor complexes they are transformed to the nucleus where they couple with DNA. This steroid hormone-like function is mainly observed in Vitamin A and D. Recently, using the immunocytochemical method, the Vitamin D receptor status of tumors from patients with primary carcinoma of the breast was determined. Patients with receptor-positive tumors had significantly longer disease-free survival than those with receptor-negative tumors. It was found that more than 80% of breast tumors contain receptors for $1\alpha,25$-dihydroxy Vitamin D, the active hormonal form of Vitamin D.[71] Since certain vitamins (A, C, D, E, and B_6) have immune stimulatory effects, they may be used as immunoaugmentators in chemotherapy and radiation therapy, by enhancing the therapeutic effects of cytotoxic agents and radiation. Therefore, vitamins should be used as adjuvant therapeutic agents in combination with hormones, cytotoxic agents, and radiation. Patients with cancer will benefit from this combined hormone-vitamin therapy.

Furthermore, recent findings indicate that β-carotene, retinol, retinoic acid, and vitamin E succinate can inhibit expression of some molecular cancer risk factors and include certain oncogenes (C-myc and H-ras) in several cell lines *in vitro*. This suggests that expression of transformed cell phenotypes is inhibited by vitamins.[72] It was also found that new tumor markers, such as Cathepsin D, an estrogen-induced lysosomal protease, may be a very sensitive independent predictor of early recurrence and death in node-negative breast cancer patients.[73] The discovery of oncogenes opened a new era for cancer detection and prevention. Mutations of the C-RAS-Ki genes are sensitive molecular markers for early diagnosis of colon, pancreatic, and lung cancers, with a high sensitivity to one cancer cell in 10^5 or 10^6. Therefore, this ability to detect minimal residual malignant disease is likely to revolutionize the diagnosis and treatment of cancer.[74]

REFERENCES

1. **Huggins, C.,** Endocrine-induced regression of cancers, *Science,* 156, 1050, 1967.
2. **Cummings, C.,** The endocrine evolution and therapy of cancer, *Am. J. Cancer,* 2, 143, 1925.
3. **Lacassagne, A.,** Apparition de cancers de la mammelle chez la souris mâle soumise à des injections de folliculine, *C. R. Acad. Sci. (Paris),* 195, 630, 1932.
4. **Huggins, C. and Hodges, C. V.,** Studies on prostatic cancer: the effect of castration, of estrogen and of androgen injection on serum phosphatases in metastatic carcinoma of the prostate, *Cancer Res.,* 1, 293, 1941.
5. **Clark, G. M. and McGuire, W. L.,** Steroid receptors and other prognostic factors in primary breast cancer, *Semin. Oncol.,* 15 (Supp. 1), 20, 1988.
6. **King, R. J.,** Structure and function of steroid receptors, *J. Endocrinol.,* 114, 341, 1987.
7. **Thorpe, S. M.,** Estrogen and progesterone receptor determinations in breast cancer, *Acta Oncol.,* 27, 1, 1988.
8. **Muldoon, T. G. and Craig, E. A.,** Hormones and their receptors, *Arch. Intern. Med.,* 148, 961, 1988.
9. **Manni, A.,** Hormone receptors, in *Breast Cancer: Diagnosis and Treatment,* Ariel, I. and Clearly, J., Eds., McGraw-Hill, New York, 1987, 119.

10. **Bonneterre, J., Peyrat, J. P., Beuscart, R., Lefebvre, J., and Demaille, A.,** Prognostic significance of prolactin receptors in human breast cancer, *Cancer Res.,* 47, 4724, 1987.
11. **Dietel, M., Kostrouch, Z., Courtoy, P. J., Boonstra, J., and Toth, J.,** What's new in the importance of receptors in pathology, *Pathol. Res. Pract.,* 184, 116, 1989.
12. **Vollenweider-Zerargui, L., Barrelet, L., Wong, Y., Lemarchand-Béraud, T., and Gómez, F.,** The predictive value of estrogen and progesterone receptors' concentrations on the clinical behavior of breast cancer in women, *Cancer,* 57, 1171, 1986.
13. **Allegra, J. C., Lippman, M. E., Thompson, E. B., Simon, R., Barlock, A., Green, L., Huff, K., Do, H., and Aitken, S.,** Distribution; frequency and quantitative analysis of estrogen, progesterone, androgen, and glucocorticoid receptors in human breast cancer, *Cancer Res.,* 39, 1447, 1979.
14. **Townsend, C. M.,** Management of breast cancer: surgery and adjuvant therapy, *Clin. Symp. Ciba,* 39, 3, 1987.
15. **Huben, R. P. and Murphy, G. P.,** Prostate cancer: an update, *CA-Cancer J. Clinicians,* 36, 274, 1986.
16. **Libermann, T. A., Nusbaum, H. R., Razon, N., Kris, R., Lax, I., Soreg, H., Whittle, N., Waterfield, M. D., Ullrich, A., and Schlesinger, J.,** Amplification, enhanced expression and possible rearrangement of EGF receptor gene in primary human brain tumours of glial origin, *Nature (London),* 313, 144, 1985.
17. **Carpenter, G.,** Receptors for epidermal growth factor and other polypeptide mitogens, *Annu. Rev. Biochem.,* 56, 881, 1987.
18. **Knecht, M., Feng, P., and Catt, K. J.,** Transforming growth factor-beta: autocrine, paracrine and endocrine effects in ovarian cells, *Semin. Reprod. Endocrinol.,* 7, 12, 1989.
19. **Minuto, F., Barreca, A., Del Monte, P., Cariola, G., Torre, G., and Giordano, G.,** Immunoreactive insulin-like growth factor I (IGF-1) and IGF-1 binding protein content in human thyroid tissue, *J. Clin. Endocrinol. Metab.,* 68, 621, 1989.
20. **Sherry, B. and Cerami, A.,** Cachectin/tumor necrosis factor exerts endocrine, paracrine, and autocrine control of inflammatory responses, *J. Cell Biol.,* 107, 1269, 1988.
21. **Platzer, E. and Kalden, J. R.,** Human granulocyte colony stimulating factor, *Blut,* 54, 129, 1987.
22. **Smith, K. A.,** Interleukin-2: inception, impact and implications, *Science,* 240, 1169, 1988.
23. **Parkinson, D. R.,** Interleukin-2 in cancer therapy, *Semin. Oncol.,* 15 (Supp. 6), 10, 1988.
24. **Stoscheck, C. M. and King, L. E.,** Role of epidermal growth factor in carcinogenesis, *Cancer Res.,* 46, 1030, 1986.
25. **Goldie, J. H. and Goldman, A. J.,** Clinical implications of the phenomenon of drug resistance, in *Drug and Hormone Resistance in Neoplasia: Clinical Concepts,* Vol. 2, Bruchowsky, N. and Goldie, J. H., Eds., CRC Press, Boca Raton, FL, 1983, 111.
26. **Heppner, G. H. and Miller, B. E.,** Therapeutic implications of tumor heterogeneity, *Semin. Oncol.,* 16, 91, 1989.
27. **Thorpe, S. M. and Rose, C.,** Oestrogen and progesterone receptor determinations in breast cancer: technology and biology, *Cancer Surv.,* 5, 505, 1986.
28. **Markopoulos, C., Berger, U., Wilson, P., Gazet, J. C., and Coombes, R. C.,** Oestrogen receptor content of normal breast cells and breast carcinomas throughout the menstrual cycle, *Br. Med. J.,* 296, 1349, 1988.
29. **McGuire, W. L.,** Prognostic factors in primary breast cancer, *Cancer Surv.,* 5, 527, 1986.
30. **Meyer, J. S.,** Cell kinetics of histologic variants of *in situ* breast carcinoma, *Breast Cancer Res. Treat.,* 7, 171, 1986.
31. **Sainsbury, J. R., Farndon, J. R., Sherbet, G. V., and Harris, A. L.,** Epidermal growth factor receptors and oestrogen receptor in human breast cancer, *Lancet,* 1, 364, 1985.
32. **Meyer, J. S. and Province, M.,** Proliferative index of breast carcinoma by thymidine labeling prognostic power independent of stage, estrogen and progesterone receptors, *Breast Cancer Res. Treat.,* 12, 191, 1988.
33. **Gerdes, J., Pickartz, H., Brotherton, J., Hammerstein, J., Weitzel, H., and Stein, H.,** Growth factors and estrogen receptors in human breast cancers as determined *in situ* with monoclonal antibodies, *Am. J. Pathol.,* 129, 486, 1987.
34. **Kokal, W., Sheibani, K., Terz, J., and Harada, J. R.,** Tumor DNA content in the prognosis of colorectal carcinoma, *J. Am. Med. Assoc.,* 255, 3123, 1986.
35. **Lupulescu, A.,** Hormonal regulation of epidermal tumor development, *J. Invest. Dermatol.,* 77, 186, 1981.
36. **Fisher, B., Redmond, C., Fisher, E. R., and Caplan, R.,** Relative worth of estrogen or progesterone receptor and pathologic characteristics of differentiation as indicators of prognosis in node negative breast cancer patients: findings from national surgical adjuvant breast and bowel project protocol B-06, *J. Clin. Oncol.,* 6, 1076, 1988.
37. **Gold, P. and Freedman, S. O.,** Demonstration of tumor-specific antigens in human colonic carcinomata by immunological tolerance and absorption techniques, *J. Exp. Med.,* 121, 439, 1965.

38. **Sikorska, H., Shuster, J., and Gold, P.,** Clinical applications of carcinoembryonic antigen, *Cancer Detect. Prev.,* 12, 321, 1988.
39. **Tatarinov, Y. S.,** Detection of embryo specific alpha-globulin in the blood serum of patients with primary liver tumors, *Vopr. Med. Khim.,* 10, 90, 1964.
40. **Brioschi, P. A., Bischof, P., Rapin, C., DeRoten, M., Irion, O., and Krauer, F.,** Longitudinal study of CEA and CA 125 in ovarian cancer, *Gynecol. Oncol.,* 21, 1, 1985.
41. **Munck-Wikland, E., Kuylenstierna, R., Wahren, B., Lindholm, J., and Haglund, S.,** Tumor markers carcinoembryonic antigen, CA 50 and CA 19-9 and squamous cell carcinoma of the esophagus, *Cancer,* 62, 2281, 1988.
42. **Robles, J. M., Morell, A. R., Redorta, J. P., Mateos, J. A., and Rosello, A. S.,** Clinical behavior of prostatic specific antigen and prostatic acid phosphatase: a comparative study, *Eur. Urol.,* 14, 360, 1988.
43. **Zelzer, P. M., Marangos, P. J., Sather, H., Evans, A., Siegel, S., Wong, K. Y., and Hammond, D.,** Prognostic importance of serum neuron specific enolase in local and widespread neuroblastoma, in *Advances in Neuroblastoma,* Evans, A. E., D'Angio, J. D., and Seeger, R., Eds., Alan R. Lyss, New York, 1985, 319.
44. **Yalow, R. and Berson, S.,** Characteristic of "big ACTH" in human plasma and pituitary extracts, *J. Clin. Endocrinol. Metab.,* 36, 415, 1973,
45. **Bishop, A. E., Hamid, Q. A., Adams, C., Bretherton-Watt, D., Jones, P. M., Denny, P., Stamp, G. W., Hurt, R. L., Grimelius, L., Harmar, A. G., Valentino, K., Cedermark, B., Legon, S., Ghatei, M. A., Bloom, S. R., and Polak, J. M.,** Expression of tachykinins by ileal and lung carcinoid tumors assessed by combined *in situ* hybridization, immunocytochemistry, and radioimmunoassay, *Cancer,* 63, 1129, 1989.
46. **Laybourn, K. A., Hiserodt, J. C., and Varani, J.,** Laminin receptor expression on murine tumor cells: correlation with sensitivity to natural cell-mediated cytotoxicity, *Int. J. Cancer,* 43, 737, 1989.
47. **Papotti, M., Macri, L., Bussolati, G., and Reubi, J. C.,** Correlative study on neuro-endocrine differentiation and presence of somatostatin receptors in breast carcinoma, *Int. J. Cancer,* 43, 365, 1989.
48. **Kelly, W. M.,** Tumor markers, *Radiography,* 54, 14, 1988.
49. **Lamerz, R.,** Klinische relevanz von Tumormarkern, *Wien. Klin. Wochenschr.,* 101, 464, 1989.
50. **Klein, G.,** Oncogenes and tumor suppressor genes, *Acta Oncol.,* 27, 427, 1988.
51. **Alitalo, K. and Schwab, M.,** Oncogene amplification in tumor cells, *Adv. Cancer Res.,* 47, 235, 1986.
52. **Slamon, D., Clark, G. M., Wong, S. G., Levin, W. J., Ullrich, A. U., and McGuire, W. L.,** Human breast cancer: correlation of relapse and survival with amplification of the HER-2/neu oncogene, *Science,* 235, 177, 1987.
53. **Seshadri, R., Matthews, C., Dobrovic, A., and Horsfall, D. J.,** The significance of oncogene amplification in primary breast cancer, *Int. J. Cancer,* 43, 270, 1989.
54. **Houghton, A. N. and Cote, R. J.,** Human monoclonal antibodies, in *Monoclonal Antibodies in Cancer,* Sell, S. and Reisfeld, R., Eds., Humana, Clifton, NJ, 1985, 399.
55. **Schlom, J.,** Basic principles and applications of monoclonal antibodies in the management of carcinomas, *Cancer Res.,* 46, 3225, 1986.
56. **American Cancer Society,** Guidelines for the Use of Mammography, American Cancer Society, New York, 1989.
57. **Andersson, I., Aspergren, K., Janzon, L., Landberg, T., Ranstam, J., Lyungberg, O., Sigfusson, B., Lindholm, K., and Linell, F.,** Mammographic screening and mortality from breast cancer: the Malmö mammographic screening trial, *Br. Med. J.,* 297, 943, 1988.
58. **Council report:** mammographic screening in asymptomatic women aged 40 years and older, *J. Am. Med. Assoc.,* 261, 2535, 1989.
59. **Silverberg, E., and Lubera, J. A.,** Cancer statistics, 1989, *CA-Cancer J. Clinicians,* 39, 3, 1989.
60. **Koss, L. G.,** The Papanicolaou test for cervical cancer detection: a triumph and a tragedy, *J. Am. Med. Assoc.,* 261, 737, 1989.
61. **Gittes, R. F.,** Prostate-specific antigen, *N. Engl. J. Med.,* 317, 954, 1987.
62. **Stähelin, H. B.,** Vitamins and cancer, *Rec. Res. Cancer Res.,* 108, 227, 1988.
63. **Lupulescu, A.,** Inhibition of DNA synthesis and neoplastic cell growth by vitamin A (retinol), *J. Natl. Cancer. Inst.,* 77, 149, 1986.
64. **Barnett, J. B.,** Immunomodulating effects of 13-cis-retinoic acid on the IgG and IgM response of BALB/ c mice, *Int. Arch. Allerg. Appl. Immunol.,* 72, 227, 1983.
65. **Eto, I. and Krumdieck, C. L.,** Role of Vitamin B_{12} and folate deficiencies in carcinogenesis, *Adv. Exp. Med. Biol.,* 206, 313, 1986.
66. **Heimburger, D. C., Alexander, C. B., Birch, R., Butterworth, C. E., Bailey, W. C., and Krumdieck, C. L.,** Improvement in bronchial squamous metaplasia in smokers treated with folate and vitamin B_{12}, *J. Am. Med. Assoc.,* 259, 1525, 1988.

67. **Peterkofsky, B. and Prather, W.,** Cytotoxicity of ascorbate and other reducing agents towards cultured fibroblasts as a result of hydrogen peroxide formation, *J. Cell Physiol.,* 90, 61, 1977.
68. **Manolagas, S. C.,** Vitamin D and its relevance to cancer, *Anticancer Res.,* 7, 625, 1987.
69. **Amento, E. P.,** Vitamin D and the immune system, *Steroids,* 49, 55, 1987.
70. **Chlebowski, R. T., Akman, S. A., and Block, J. B.,** Vitamin K in the treatment of cancer, *Cancer Treat. Rev.,* 12, 49, 1985.
71. **Colston, K. W., Berger, U., and Coombes, R. C.,** Possible role for vitamin D in controlling breast cancer cell proliferation, *Lancet,* 1, 188, 1989.
72. **Prasad, K. N. and Prasad, J.-E.,** Expression of some molecular cancer risk factors and their modification by vitamins, *J. Am. Coll. Nutr.,* 9, 28, 1990.
73. **Tandon, A. K., Clark, G. M., Chamness, G. C., Chirgwin, J. M., and McGuire, W. L.,** Cathepsin D and prognosis in breast cancer, *N. Engl. J. Med.,* 322, 297, 1990.
74. **Cline, M. J.,** Biology of disease: molecular diagnosis of human cancer, *Lab. Invest.,* 61, 368, 1989.

Chapter 2

HORMONES AND HORMONOTHERAPY

I. GENERAL CONSIDERATIONS AND PROSPECTS OF HORMONOTHERAPY

For many years, the practice of hormone therapy in cancer management was mainly empirically based. At present, due to our improved knowledge regarding the role of hormones and hormone-like substances in the etiology and pathogenesis of cancer, hormone therapy is gaining a more important role in the treatment of many types of cancers (e.g., breast, prostatic, thyroid, endometrial, ovarian, and kidney cancers and lymphomas and leukemias). In many cases, hormonotherapy is replacing surgery, chemotherapy, and radiation therapy. Also, hormones and their analogs have recently been used in a variety of cancers (lung tumors, exocrine pancreatic cancer, melanomas, and colorectal carcinomas), which are not hormone-dependent cancers but are somewhat hormone-responsive cancers.

A few years after the role of hormones in the induction and development of cancer was demonstrated, it was also proved that hormones are important factors in the regression and extinction of cancers. Thus, human cancers can be controlled by endocrinologic methods.[1,2] Extinction of experimental DMBA-induced mammary carcinoma in rats was reported following estradiol-17β and progesterone administration.[3]

In addition, uterine and ovarian cancers, lymphomas and lymphosarcomas, lung tumors, liver tumors, and fibrosarcomas induced by estrogens in guinea pigs, were prevented or inhibited by a concomitant administration of progesterone, cortisone, androgens, or thymic hormones.[4-6] Long ago, before the endocrine concept was established, it was shown by empirical observations that removal of ovaries (ovariectomy) and thyroid extract exerts a beneficial therapeutic effect in women with advanced breast cancer.[7] Thus, ablative endocrine therapy (castration) has an important therapeutic role in cancer treatment, namely, those of hormone-dependent cancers. Breast cancer is an estrogen-dependent cancer, and prostatic cancer is androgen-dependent cancer. Endometrial cancer is somewhat estrogen and progesterone dependent, while kidney cancer is estrogen dependent. Ovarian cancer is estrogen dependent in premenopausal women and becomes more androgen dependent in postmenopausal women. There is considerable experimental and clinical evidence that hormones exert an important role in etiopathogenesis of various types of cancers, and they are potential therapeutic agents with dramatic beneficial therapeutic advantages in cancer treatment.

In addition to their direct therapeutic role in hormone-dependent cancers, hormones are important adjuvants or therapeutic factors (modifiers), and in combination with other agents, such as cytotoxic agents or radiation, they can enhance the therapeutic effects. At present, hormones are used as, (1) direct and potential therapeutic agents in hormonotherapy, and (2) adjuvant therapeutic agents or modifiers of other anticancer drugs, enhancing their original effect (hormonochemotherapy, hormonoradiation, and hormonoimmunotherapy). Hormones are also used as palliative therapeutic agents in several types of cancers in order to alleviate the general symptoms, such as pain, edema, cachexia, and secondary inflammatory diseases, and play an important role in palliation therapy. Hence, hormones presently are used on a large scale in adjuvant systemic therapy, in many cases replacing the conventional therapeutic methods (surgery, chemotherapy, radiation) providing more advantageous and less toxic effects, and they are also used in palliative therapy improving the general status of patients. Over the last two decades, hormonal therapy emerged as an important therapeutic method for cancer management due to a number of factors, such as: (1) the introduction of several new hormonal agents, (2) an increased knowledge of pharmacologic actions of hormones,

(3) the development of more accurate hormone receptor assays, and the use of tumor markers to better predict the hormonal responsiveness and the selection of patients for hormonal therapy, (4) new information relating to dosage, schedule and route of administration of hormonal agent, (5) the development of new hormone antagonists that can antagonize the hormonal action at cellular and molecular levels by a competitive hormone-receptor mechanism, and (6) the apparent plateau in efficacy of chemotherapy.

The clinical oncologist is particularly interested in hormonal therapy because it is less toxic and generally has lower morbidity as compared to chemotherapeutic agents. This is also true for the surgical ablative procedures, where the hormone antagonists have been and continue to be studied as a substitute for the surgery. In addition, regimens consisting of multiple hormones (multivalent hormonal therapy) have been examined, thus, evaluating a combination hormonal therapy or combination with cytotoxic agents.[8]

The commonly used hormonal therapies are based on the following principles:

1. Deficiency or deprivation of hormones — produced by removing or ablating the endocrine gland, which is the main hormonal source, (ablative hormone therapy), as in ovariectomy, orchiectomy, adrenalectomy, or hypophysectomy
2. Hormone interference — achieved by using large or pharmacologic doses of hormones, namely, the opposite or antagonistic hormones, e.g., estrogens, androgens, and progestins (additive hormone therapy)
3. Inhibitive hormone therapy — administered by using blocking hormonal effects, such as aminoglutethimide, danazol, and gonadotropic hormone-releasing hormone analogs
4. Competitive inhibition of hormones — produced by using inhibitors of estrogens or antiestrogens (tamoxifen)
5. Cytotoxic effects — obtained by using large doses of hormones, such as adrenocorticotropic hormone (ACTH) and cortisone in experimental lymphomas and leukemias in mice, where dramatic and apparently complete cures are produced[9]

Also, ACTH and cortisone resulted in temporary regression in human lymphatic leukemia and Hodgkin's disease.[10] Thus, large doses of hormones may exert specific cytotoxic effects or lethal effects only for cancer cells and leave the normal cells undamaged.

It is important to distinguish between the therapeutic role of hormones in: (1) hormone-dependent cancers, where the role of hormones for cell growth and cell differentiation is critical; without hormones cells cannot grow, will shrink, and will finally die; (2) hormone-responsive cancers, where cell growth and proliferation will only be delayed or slowed down for months or several years, but not eradicated; and (3) hormone-independent or autonomous, where hormones do not exert any influence on cancer development and do not exert any therapeutic effects.

It is interesting that a hormone-dependent cancer can lose its hormone dependency and become hormone independent during or following hormone therapy. The cancer cells escape hormonal control. The mechanism of hormonal escape and hormone resistance is complex and not yet fully understood. A hormone-independent tumor can originate from an apparently hormone-dependent tumor by different pathways. First, it may arise due to the selective growth of preexisting hormone-independent cells from a heterogenous tumor, or the development of a resistant mutation during hormone therapy. The response to hormonal treatment depends on both cell populations, namely, the ratio between hormone-dependent and hormone-independent cells. A second possibility is the loss of hormone receptors. Receptor changes during hormonal treatment, such as decrease in receptor number, loss of receptor function, defective hormone receptors, and post-receptor defects lead to hormone resistance. A third possibility is the increased production of growth factors, which can interfere with hormone action at the cellular level by autocrine and paracrine mechanisms. A fourth possibility is the level of the host; the pharmacokinetics of the hormonal agent and its metabolism and excretion, as well as the host immune defense and detoxification mechanisms, can also influence the hormone response.

Administration of hormones to hormone responsive cancer cells is associated with increases in several growth-related enzymes, proteolytic enzymes, and intracellular proteins of unknown function. It has been proposed that estrogens might interact with target cells by the synthesis and secretion of new factors called estromedins, which promote the growth of distant target cells.[11] Recently, it also has been proposed that tumors produce their own locally active or autocrine growth factors, allowing them to escape normal control mechanisms.[12] Breast cancer cells in culture have been found to secrete insulin-like growth factor 1 (IGF-I) and α-transforming growth factor (TGF-α).[13] Secretion of TGF-β has been associated with growth inhibition by tamoxifen. Epidermal growth factor (EGF) was reported to partially reverse the inhibitory effects of antiestrogens in T47D breast cancer cell lines.[14] Therefore, growth factors are of significant importance for the cellular response to steroid hormone and their antagonists. The presence of functional estrogen (ER) and progesterone (PR) receptors is necessary for breast cancer cells to respond to hormone therapy. From 50 to 60% of primary breast cancers are ER-positive; 30% of premenopausal patients and 60% of postmenopausal patients are ER-positive tumors. It was found that 50 to 60% of ER-positive and 75% of both ER- and PR-positive tumors will respond to hormonal treatment. Even a higher number, 80 to 90% of patients with prostate cancer respond clinically to hormonal manipulation (castration or estrogens).

In patients with endometrial cancer, 20 to 40% respond to progesterone therapy. As many as 89% of patients with PR-positive tumors responded, while only 17% of patients with PR-negative tumors responded to progestational therapy.[15-16] It is interesting to note that a small number (5 to 10%) of hormone receptor-negative tumors still respond to hormonal therapy. This suggests that additional factors are involved in the hormone responsiveness of cancers.

For selection of patients for hormone therapy, the medical oncologists have to use several criteria, such as receptor hormone estimation, DNA content, lymph node involvement, tumor markers, and oncogenic amplification in order to obtain a more accurate pattern. The use of only one criteria, such as hormone receptors or DNA content, can be misleading. Their diagnostic and prognostic value increase when they are used in concert.[16] Therefore, most neoplasms are composed of heterogenous cell populations and also have a hormone-receptor heterogeneity. Patients who responded to one hormonal manipulation and then failed had approximately a 50% chance of responding to a second hormonal treatment, whereas only 12% responded to secondary hormone therapy from those who failed to respond to primary endocrine therapy.[17]

Because of the cytotoxic effects of glucocorticoids on lymphoid cells, steroids are used in the lymphoproliferative disorders, including leukemia, lymphoma, and multiple myeloma. The presence of glucocorticoid receptors appears to be necessary, but not sufficient to produce the cytolytic effects of glucocorticoids. Recently, it has been found that glucocorticoid hormones elicit their cytotoxic effects on lymphatic cells by the presence of a glucocorticoid receptor-like molecule located in the plasma membrane of S-49 mouse lymphoma cells undergoing cytolysis while being treated with glucocorticoids.[18] Thus, the hormone therapies in cancer have been developed during the last three decades and now become a standard pattern in the treatment and management of certain neoplasms.[19-21]

Resistance to a single hormone administration does not preclude response to another hormone or combination of hormones with chemotherapy or radiation therapy. It is advisable that hormone therapy should be started first and then cytostatic agents or radiation therapy used.

It is essential that hormones or hormone antagonists act continuously for a sufficiently long time to allow the antitumor effect to occur and exert favorable effects. An inadequate dose or too short a duration of therapy, or both, decreases the effectiveness of endocrine therapy; tumor regression cannot be maintained and relapses occur. In the last decade, due to revolutionary changes that have taken place in endocrine physiology and pharmacology (the use of antiestrogens and the discovery of hormone receptors, growth factors, tumor markers, oncogenes, and LHRH agonists), hormone therapy has become a standard procedure for cancer treatment.

It seems that a golden age of hormonal therapy is taking place, mainly based on an improved understanding of tumor biology. Long before hormones were discovered, based on empirical observations, Schinzinger (1889) suggested that in "women who are still menstruating (surgeons) should first perform castration before operating for breast cancer in order to prevent it from spreading locally or to stop a rapid growth".[22] A few years later, Beatson[7] (1896) performed the first therapeutic bilateral ovariectomy for the treatment of advanced breast cancer in two out of three women and then placed the patients on thyroid tablets as "a powerful lymphatic stimulant". The patient was thought to have been cured and indeed she remained in remission for 46 months before the disease relapsed and she died. He believed that the ovary sent out influences "more subtle and more mysterious" than those from the nervous system and that there are grounds for the belief that the etiology of cancer lies in an ovarian stimulus.[7]

A. HORMONES AS POTENTIAL THERAPEUTIC AGENTS

At present there are at least 200 human hormones identified, and their role in experimental and human carcinogenesis is under current investigation. Most experimental investigations demonstrate that hormones play a crucial role in controlling the neoplastic cell growth and differentiation, which are the cornerstone of cancer development. Hormones may act as carcinogens, procarcinogens, and anticarcinogens.[21] Despite the fact there is no firm conclusion regarding the role of hormones as carcinogens, there is ample evidence indicating their role as procarcinogens in tumor progression, and their role as anticarcinogens in tumor regression. Recently, due to the discovery of hormone receptors and hormone antagonists, as well as the discovery of new hypothalamic-releasing hormones, a new exciting field of research regarding the potential therapeutic role of hormones in cancer management has just begun.

Since hormones control cell division and differentiation, they are important modifiers or modulators of cancers, thereby justifying their wide use in the treatment of cancer. The era of hormonotherapy began when Huggins found that testosterone administration on spontaneous dog prostate tumors stimulated tumor growth, whereas castration or injection of estradiol benzoate or stilbestrol induced a dramatic regression in dogs and in human prostatic cancers.[1,2] Diethylstilbestrol (DES), a synthetic estrogen discovered by Dodds et al.,[23] was the first anticancer drug.

At present, the eleven most commonly used hormones in cancer treatment are estrogens, antiestrogens, progestins, androgens, corticosteroids, aromatase inhibitors, danazol, LHRH-agonists, somatostatin, thyroxine, and melatonin. These hormones are used in different therapeutic approaches or hormone therapies, such as ablative hormone therapy, additive hormone therapy, inhibitive hormone therapy, and competitive hormone therapy.

1. Ablative Hormone Therapy

This is based on the removal by surgery or radiation of the endocrine gland (ovary, testis, adrenal gland, or pituitary), which is the main source of hormone synthesis, and usually induces a marked regression of hormone-dependent cancers. The commonly used procedures are castration (ovariectomy or orchiectomy), adrenalectomy, and hypophysectomy.

a. Castration (Ovariectomy or Oophorectomy and Orchiectomy)

Ovariectomy or oophorectomy in premenopausal women was one of the earliest forms of systemic therapy for advanced breast cancer used by Schinzinger in Germany and Beatson in England.[7,22] Ovariectomy produces no tumor regression in dogs or mice, but induces significant cancer regression in human and rat mammary cancers, which are hormone-dependent. Hormone determinations showed a sharp decrease in estrogen levels within 2 to 3 d after surgical castration; it takes 3 to 5 months to reach a comparable level after radiation castration, which can be achieved in 4 d by administration of relatively high doses (1200 to 1600 rad) to the ovaries. In unselected series, 30 to 40% of patients will respond, and the regression lasts 9 to 12 months. However, the results are considerably better (50 to 60%) in those with ER-positive tumors, even reaching 78% in those with ER-positive and PR-positive tumors. Ovariectomy should not be performed in women with less than 10% ER or ER-negative tumors. Prophylactic ovariectomy following mastectomy does not decrease the potential relapse rate or prolong the survival of those who relapse.

The metastatic sites likely to respond to ovariectomy include bone, soft tissue, lymph nodes, and lung. Metastases in liver and brain rarely respond. The rate of response following ovariectomy in premenopausal women is similar to that of tamoxifen.[24-26] From those who showed response to oophorectomy, the likelihood of subsequent response to another hormonal modality, either ablative or additive, is in the range of 40 to 50%. Tumor histology reveals distinctive cytologic changes, such as cytolysis and flattening of acinar epithelium in all tumors that diminish after ovariectomy. The marked effect of castration only in premenopausal women compared to postmenopausal women in which no effects can be seen, is similar to the observations made by Loeb.[27] He found that ovariectomy performed by the sixth week reduced to zero the incidence of mammary cancer in mice compared to ovariectomy performed after six months, when no changes were observed. Generally, the selection of patients for ovariectomy should be based on hormone receptor status (ER, PR) and histological differentiation.

Orchiectomy — A long time ago, orchiectomy was considered as the standard therapy for male breast cancer.[28] Remission after orchiectomy may be expected in 32 to 68% of the patients who show objective signs of tumor regression and clinical improvement after castration. The average duration of remission is approximately 30 months. Beneficial effects on bone metastases have also been reported. Subcapsular orchiectomy is the method of choice, but the removal of testicular tissue should be complete. Rationale of orchiectomy in male breast cancer is the fact that these tumors are androgen-dependent, and they quickly lose their hormone dependence and become more malignant than female breast cancer. Despite the fact that male breast cancer is a rare disease with an incidence only 1% of that in females, but a worse prognosis, there is a striking similarity in the natural history of breast cancer between men and women after initial treatment.[29]

Orchiectomy for prostate cancer — Orchiectomy (castration) is a relatively simple and effective means of hormonal therapy, and it is the standard one. After castration, the plasma testosterone levels are reduced to 10 to 15 μg/100 ml in virtually all patients. Castration is still an alternative approach to the administration of exogenous hormones in the treatment of prostatic carcinoma. Although both are beneficial for relief of pain, dysuria, and spread of metastases, there is no general consensus that orchiectomy is superior to estrogen therapy. However, given the side effects of exogenous estrogens, which include fluid retention, nausea and vomiting, gynecomastia, and a tendency toward both thromboembolic and cardiovascular complications, simple castration has many advantages and can be done in most medical centers under local anesthesia. For patients the major objection to orchiectomy appears to be the psychologic impact of castration, particularly in younger men.[30] Although total orchiectomy has the advantage of removing the whole source of androgens, it is difficult for patients to accept it because of the loss of libido and impotence, emptiness of the scrotum, and the occurrence of andropause. Subcapsular orchiectomy is therefore recommended more often, even though many Leydig cells remain that can multiply and provide an adequate androgen secretion that still responds to interstitial cell-stimulating hormone (ICSH). It is generally believed that orchiectomy and estrogens, e.g., diethylstilbestrol at a dose of 3 mg/d, are equally effective in rate and duration of response, and there is no evidence that the combination of orchiectomy and DES is superior to either used alone.[31] Debate continues between those advocating surgery as a first therapeutic approach and endocrinologists recommending estrogen therapy.[32] This depends on the androgen receptor status, histologic differentiation, and stage of disease, and finally, on the degree of hormone-dependency. If the tumor is well localized and encapsulated, surgery (prostatectomy and orchiectomy) or radiation therapy are first recommended. Conversely, when the tumor has spread widely with bone metastases, endocrine therapy is recommended. Recently, the use of analogs of luteinizing hormone-releasing hormone (LHRH) has attracted considerable attention because it decreases the testosterone levels close to that of castration.

b. Adrenalectomy

The rational basis for this procedure is the removal of the adrenal source of androgens. Adrenalectomy is performed by surgical or chemical methods (medical adrenalectomy). It is mostly recommended supplementary to castration. Adrenalectomy has a general response rate of 30 to 40% in most patients.[33]

Patients who respond well to castration or those with ER+ tumors will also respond well (59%) to adrenalectomy, whereas only 8% with ER− respond to adrenalectomy. Adrenalectomy became popular in the 1950s for treatment of metastatic breast cancer in postmenopausal women or in premenopausal women who had previously responded to ovariectomy. Adrenalectomy is mostly recommended in postmenopausal women with advanced breast cancer; for these women, beneficial effects can rise from 30 to 50%. Responses to adrenalectomy are seen primarily in patients with bone and soft tissue metastases, although a single visceral site, such as lung or pleura, is also likely to respond with equal frequency (30% to 40%). Multiple visceral metastases have a response rate between 20% and 30%. The disease-free interval >2.5 years generally is associated with a higher response rate (50%) as opposed to 30% for those <2.5 years. There is no advantage to premenopausal women being treated by adrenalectomy-ovariectomy as a single combined procedure over the sequence of ovariectomy followed by adrenalectomy.[34] In premenopausal women, ovariectomy is the first choice; only if tumor growth resumes, should adrenalectomy be performed. Adrenalectomy always should be bilateral. Regression of the primary tumor has an average duration between 18 and 26 months.

Contraindications to adrenalectomy include metastatic disease to the liver and central nervous system (CNS), and advanced lymphangitic pulmonary metastases. For patients who have had an adrenalectomy, replacement therapy is 50 to 70 mg/d of cortisol given orally, along with 0.1 mg of fluorohydrocortisone; this therapy is for life. Although 30 to 40% of previously castrated women respond to surgical adrenalectomy, this is still associated with morbidity, mortality, and permanent dependence on hormone replacement. At present, surgical adrenalectomy is replaced by chemical or medical adrenalectomy with the use of aminoglutethimide, which suppresses adrenal steroidogenesis and provides the same results.

c. Hypophysectomy

Hypophysectomy is the ablative procedure used as an alternative to adrenalectomy. The rational basis for hypophysectomy is the removal of all pituitary tropic hormones (ACTH, TSH, GH, prolactin, and FSH) that influence the growth and tumor progression in target tissues. Despite the fact that in most experimental carcinomas (mammary carcinomas, thyroid carcinomas) the inhibitory rate induced by hypophysectomy is high, attaining 87% in some cases, its effectiveness in human cancers is still less effective. The response by way of the transsphenoidal approach is about 40% rising to 60% in patients with ER-positive tumors. In the postmenopausal women, the response is higher in those who are 10 years or more from menopause. Replacement therapy, consisting of 25 mg of cortisone twice a day and 120 μg of thyroxine, is required. Transfrontal hypophysectomy appears to offer a more complete hormonal ablation, but not greater antitumor effect than the transsphenoidal approach. Hypophysectomy proved to be effective in 40% of patients who had become refractory to previous antiestrogen therapy.

Recently, radiotherapeutic hypophysectomy by implantation of [90]yttrium, cryohypophysectomy, or ultrasonic hypophysectomy has been used, but their effectiveness is not higher than that of previous methods. Effectiveness depends mainly on the presence or absence of hormone receptors. The duration of tumor regression is 1 to $1^1/_2$ years and depends on the tumor size, presence of metastases, and completeness of pituitary ablation. The completeness of hypophysectomy can be assessed by measurements of pituitary hormones (ACTH, TSH, prolactin). Incomplete ablation of pituitary does not preclude an antitumor response. A comparison of transsphenoidal hypophysectomy with medical adrenalectomy following aminoglutethimide demonstrated a superiority of the latter.[35] Thus, at present, hypophysectomy and surgical adrenalectomy are less recommended.

In conclusion, ablative endocrine therapy is an appropriate and important method in managing advanced and metastatic cancers. It is always less toxic than other procedures (e.g., chemotherapy and radiation therapy), but sometimes causes psychologic disturbances and difficult postsurgical management. Selection of patients should be carefully made, weighing advantages and disadvantages compared to additive hormone therapy or hormone antagonists (tamoxifen and aminoglutethimide), which can produce medical castration and medical adrenalectomy and have similar effects to surgical ablation. In most cases, ablation of an endocrine gland produces a dramatic effect on tumor regression, prolongation of life, and relief of pain. The hormone responsiveness largely depends on the presence or absence of functional hormone receptors, the histological stage of tumor evolution, and the general health status of the patient. In some patients the ablative endocrine therapy produces psychologic and emotional problems for the patient's life and his family; thus, this therapy is less safe compared to hormone administration (additive hormone therapy), which is less dramatic but safer. Hypophysectomy and adrenalectomy should not be recommended for terminally ill patients or for patients whose tumors are deficient in hormone receptors.

2. Additive Hormone Therapy — Hormone Administration

The use of hormones in large (pharmacologic) doses has long been tried alone or in combination with other methods (chemotherapy, ablative endocrine therapy, and radiation therapy) for treatment of cancers. Therefore, additive hormone therapy is an important part of endocrine manipulation or endocrine control of malignant disease. Steroid therapy (estrogens, androgens, progestins, or corticosteroids) is commonly used in the treatment of cancers, especially when ablative therapy (ovariectomy, adrenalectomy, or hypophysectomy) failed to control tumor growth and progression. Selection of one of these hormone therapies depends on the developmental stage of the tumor, its hormone responsiveness, the general health status of the patient, and the judgment of the physician. Estrogens, androgens, and progestational agents have been used to treat advanced breast cancer in postmenopausal women and prostatic cancer since 1950.

a. Estrogens

The most commonly used hormones in the treatment of cancers, mainly in breast cancers and prostate cancers, are the estrogens. However, their use is more cautious and limited in postmenopausal women because of the development of uterine adenocarcinoma; it has also been implicated as a cause of rare vaginal adenomas in daughters of estrogen-treated pregnant patients. Experimental investigations demonstrated the extinction of DMBA-induced mammary rat carcinomas, following combined administration of estradiol-17β with progesterone; 52% of the rats treated with this hormonal combination were cancer-free after 6 months.[3] Similar beneficial therapeutic effects were reported in human breast cancers following the same combined hormone therapy (50 mg of progesterone and 5 mg of estradiol benzoate injected i.m. daily) mostly in patients in whom castration or adrenalectomy failed to control the growth and progression of cancer. About 30% of unselected postmenopausal patients may show an objective response lasting 12 to 14 months.[19] The presence of ER predicts a response in up to 50% of cases. The antitumor response to estrogens usually is quite slow, requiring several weeks, and is confined primarily to metastatic disease in the skin, lymph nodes, breast, and bone lesions.

The mechanism by which estrogens act on cancer cells is still unknown. At low physiologic doses, estrogens may stimulate tumor growth; at higher doses they may suppress tumor growth by binding to intracellular ER receptors and consequently releasing differentiation-promoting substances that might cause the tumor to mature, differentiate, and stop proliferating. Thus, high doses of estrogens prove to be cytotoxic, killing mainly the neoplastic cells.

The most commonly used estrogen is diethylstilbestrol (DES) (see Figure 1) because it is less toxic, less expensive, and longer-lasting compared to natural estrogens. DES is used in a dose of 5 mg t.i.d. Higher doses than the standard dose of 15 mg/d are more toxic and are associated with anorexia, nausea and vomiting, and an increased risk of death from cardiovascular disease. Thus, higher doses should be reserved for patients with slowly growing tumors that have failed to respond to the standard estrogen dose. After absorption, DES is metabolized by the liver. In carcinoma of the prostate, DES is mainly used in a dose of 3 mg/d, which has recently proved to be more effective regarding the complete suppression of testosterone than a dose of 1 mg/d.[36] The hormonal treatment with DES in prostate cancer provides response rates as high as 60 to 80% and a median duration of response of 18+ months in most series.[37]

The effects of estrogens on mammary and prostatic cancer cells are multiple. They inhibit the release of the luteinizing hormone (LH) from the pituitary, and may inhibit the prolactin secretion from the pituitary. They increase the sex steroid-binding globulin, decreasing the circulating concentration of testosterone; they also inhibit conversion of testosterone to dihydrotestosterone (DHT) by inhibiting the enzyme 5α-reductase, which interferes with the binding of DHT to its receptors.[38] Estrogen in high doses may exert a cytotoxic action on prostate and breast cancer cells.

In addition to DES, other estradiol esters have also been used in the treatment of prostate and breast cancers. They are Estinyl (3 mg/d) and conjugated estrogens, such as Premarin (10 mg t.i.d.). High doses of DES diphosphate (fosfestrol), which must be administered i.v., also alleviate patients with prostate cancer. Chlorotrianisene (TACE), which suppresses pituitary LH and decreases modestly the serum testosterone level, is also effective in the treatment of prostatic carcinoma. TACE has little advantage over DES in prostatic carcinoma. Estramustine phosphate (Emcyt) links nitrogen mustard and estradiol in a single molecule. Response rates to estramustine in patients previously untreated are equal to those of estrogen therapy.[39]

The short-term undesirable side effects of estrogen treatment are mainly dose related. They may include nausea and vomiting; sodium and water retention in patients with cardiac, liver, or renal disease; changes in libido in women and impotence in men; aggravation of chronic cystic mastitis, uterine fibroids, migraine, and endometriosis; a very low risk of thrombophlebitis, embolism, and hypertension; and liver dysfunction with high doses and hypercalcemia in women with breast cancer. With the exception of hypercalcemia, these

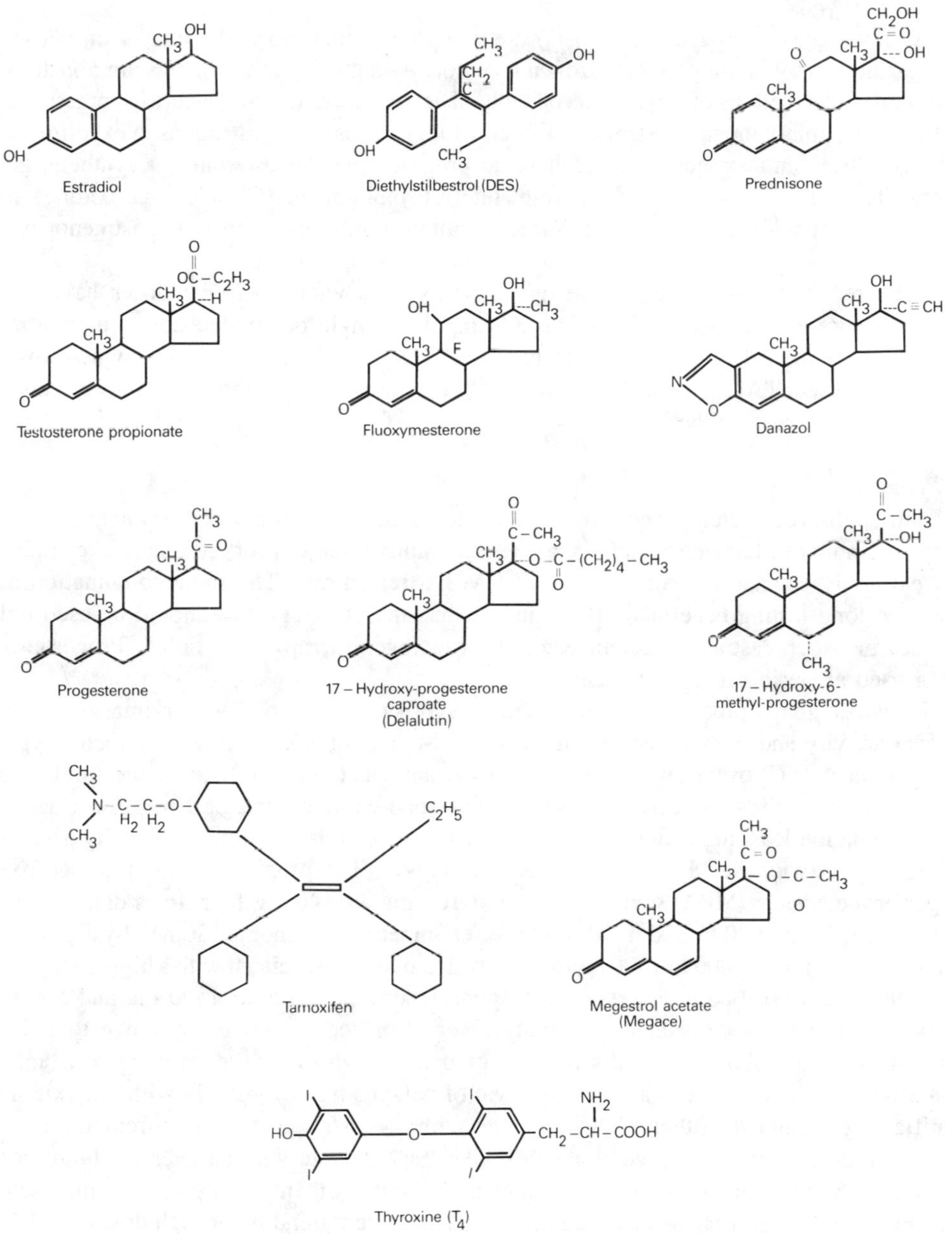

FIGURE 1. Chemical structures of commonly used hormones in cancer treatment.

side effects do not generally require the cessation of treatment. In men, gynecomastia may develop. Most of these toxic effects appear after large doses and they are dose-related. Nipple pigmentation is very common following estrogen therapy.

Estrogen rebound regression — This is an interesting phenomenon which occurs in up to 32% of estrogen responders. Patients who show a rebound response have a significant longer disease-free interval than those who do not.[40]

In male breast cancer, which is mainly androgen-dependent, estrogen therapy is preferred if castration fails. Occurrence of hypercalcemia may indicate that the tumor has retained its hormone responsiveness and often heralds a response to continued hormonal treatment.[41]

b. Antiestrogens

Antiestrogens (estrogen antagonists) are compounds that block the uptake of estrogen in target tissues by binding to the estrogen receptor. As a group, antiestrogens are nonsteroid amino-ether derivatives of polycyclic phenols. The structural resemblance to synthetic stilbestrol may explain the mild estrogenic effects of high doses of antiestrogens in experimental animals. These antiestrogens are unrelated to progesterone, testosterone, or synthetic gestagens. Three members of this class are of interest: clomiphene (Clomid), nafoxidine, and tamoxifen (Nolvadex) (see Figure 1); all three result in antitumor responses in postmenopausal women.

All three of the antiestrogens are given orally, and widely varying doses have been effective: Clomiphene (Clomid), 100 to 300 mg/d in single or divided doses; nafoxidine, 90 to 240 mg/d in divided doses; and tamoxifen (TAM), 10 to 80 mg in divided doses. Most trials used TAM 20 mg b.i.d. Lack of responses at one dose level rarely can be improved by increasing the dose.

c. Progestins

Although progesterone used alone accelerates the incidence and development of mammary carcinoma in female rats, a concomitant administration of progesterone and estradiol-17β extinguishes cancer in almost 52% of DMBA-treated rats. The same combination has produced long-lasting beneficial effects in human cancers. Progestins should be used only in cases in which castration, adrenalectomy, or estrogen therapy have failed. Progesterone is not used alone in cancer treatment.

However, many progestins are available as synthetic derivatives with primarily progestational activity and minimal androgenic and fluid-retaining effects, including medroxyprogesterone acetate (Provera), hydroxyprogesterone caproate (Delalutin), and megestrol acetate (Megace). From these, injected hydroxyprogesterone caproate and oral megestrol acetate appear to be the least toxic and most widely useful progestins. Delalutin is usually given in a dose of 1 g twice weekly or as much as 5 g weekly. The usual preparation is medroxyprogesterone acetate (MPA) given in a dose of 160 mg/d or 40 mg four times daily (q.i.d.) in breast cancer and 40 to 320 mg/d orally for endometrial carcinoma. Some physicians use a high-dose regimen, 1000 to 1500 mg/d i.m., which may be associated with a higher response rate. Others did not find a difference in responses between doses of 1500 mg and 500 mg of medroxyprogesterone acetate i.m. daily. Megestrol acetate has been shown to induce remissions lasting about 7 months in 30% of patients who relapsed or were resistant to tamoxifen. However, the disease-free survival of patients treated initially with tamoxifen is significantly greater than that of those treated with megestrol acetate. In carcinoma of the uterus, progestins commonly yield a 30 to 35% response rate with an average duration of 27 months. Such treatment is widely accepted as the primary therapy for patients with disease beyond control by surgery or radiation therapy. The current trend is for high doses of MPA. In premenopausal women with metastatic breast cancer, it was used orally in a dose of 1 g/d for a period of time up to 18 months. Only 19 to 20% responded with a median time approximately 27 months. The major adverse effects were increasing dyspnea in 24% of patients and edema. Nausea, vomiting, depression and alopecia were less common side effects. This drug cannot be recommended for use in end-stage of breast cancer and in patients with respiratory symptoms.[42]

In addition to the treatment of breast and endometrial carcinomas, progestins have been used in the treatment of hypernephroma with controversial results; preliminary reports suggest that progestins may be active as cyproterone acetate in the treatment of prostatic carcinomas. Also, progestins used alone or in combination with low doses of estrogens may be useful in the prevention of uterine bleeding in thrombocytopenic females, especially in patients with acute leukemia. Comparative clinical trials using megestrol acetate vs. tamoxifen or megestrol acetate combined with aminoglutethimide showed some slight therapeutic advantages of progestins. Thus, in patients with advanced breast cancer when megestrol acetate was used as a dose of 40 mg orally four times daily or tamoxifen 10 mg orally twice daily, 23% of patients responded to megestrol acetate and only 22% responded to tamoxifen after being crossed over from megestrol acetate. There was no association between PR levels and the response for either tamoxifen or megestrol acetate.[43] Combination hormone therapy using megestrol acetate and aminoglutethimide in metastatic breast cancer showed an overall response rate of 34% with a 5-month median duration of response; patients with soft tissue, visceral, and bone metastases responded while 72% of patients have progressed or relapsed. The median survival time was 15 months.[44]

The precise mechanism of action of progestins is unknown; however, it has been shown that progestins will compete for androgen and progestational receptor sites on cell membranes. Regression is noted more frequently in tumors containing large amounts of androgen receptors.[45] When they occur, responses can last for about 12 to 14 months. Progestins appear to have a direct cytotoxic action on human breast cancer cells in long-term tissue culture.[46] Progestins are also antiestrogenic and exhibit a general inhibitory effect on estrogen-induced proteins synthesis. Thus, progestins are capable of influencing estrogen-dependent tumor proliferation by: (1) lowering the ER content; (2) lowering LH and FSH release, resulting in a diminished steroid synthesis; (3) slowing down testosterone catabolism; and (4) speeding up estradiol turnover into the less active estriol by catalyzing the activity of estradiol-17β-dehydrogenase in human breast cancer cells.[26] Progestins also may have direct and estrogen-independent mechanisms. They can inhibit the synthesis of an E_2-induced protein; they also inhibit the growth of a tamoxifen-resistant variant of MCF-7.[26] Progestins have minimal or no side effects; fluid retention and weight gain occur in some patients, but this is rarely a serious clinical problem. Hypercalcemic and pain flares have also been reported with megestrol acetate. As with tamoxifen flares, a megestrol flare may herald a response to treatment.[47]

d. Androgens

Androgens were the first additive agents to prove useful for the hormonal therapy of mammary cancer. Following the experimental research of Lacassagne and Raynaud, it became evident that testosterone could inhibit certain transplantable and spontaneously occurring neoplasms.[48] Immediately, several cases of women with breast tumors, who improved after they received androgens, were reported. Androgens are used mostly in cases of advanced breast cancer with bone metastases in postmenopausal women. Favorable responses appear, mainly in cases with estrogen receptors. In a study of 564 postmenopausal women with metastatic breast cancer treated with testosterone propionate, an overall objective regression rate of 21% was observed. The androgen chosen was testosterone propionate, given in a dose of 100 mg three times a week i.m. Based upon pre-ER data, the response of bone metastases to androgens is equivalent to that of estrogens, 25 to 30%, but the response rate of soft tissue metastases (breast, skin, nodes) to androgens, 20 to 25%, is significantly less than the 35 to 45% reported for estrogens.[49]

Because of the inferior response rate of visceral and soft tissue lesions, metastatic bone disease should be considered the primary indication for the use of androgens. When oral treatment is preferred, one may choose between fluoxymesterone, 10 mg orally b.i.d., and Δ-1-testolactone (Teslac). Testolactone may be given i.m. in a dose of 100 mg/d three times weekly, or orally in a dose of 250 mg q.i.d. Despite the increase of androgen levels in blood, the effects may not be apparent for 6 to 12 weeks. Up to 20% of unselected patients in the postmenopausal period respond to androgen therapy. The responses are confined generally to bone metastases and last 12 to 14 months. The response to both androgens and estrogens increases with years postmenopause up to 8 years. Most comparative trials revealed a superiority of estrogens in postmenopausal women (29>10%) especially for soft tissue metastases.

Testosterone and its esters are metabolized by the liver, with the metabolites appearing in the urine. Failure to respond to androgens does not preclude a response to estrogens, but failure to respond to estrogens precludes a response to androgens. Pharmacologic doses of androgens have produced a regression in 50 to 80% of DMBA-induced mammary carcinomas in rats[50] and in 15 to 30% of breast carcinomas in human subjects. A higher response rate from androgen therapy was found in patients with ER positive in the cytoplasm of the breast cancer cells. Moreover, at least some androgens affect estradiol metabolism, leading to a net decrease in the estrogenic potency of endogenous estrogens. Androgens exert their antiestrogenic effects by complex interactions with three receptors: ER, PR, and AR (androgen receptor). Androgens in high doses are stimulating to human breast cancer cells in tissue culture, and this effect is mediated via the ER.

However, at lower doses, androgens compete with estradiol for the ER and are antiestrogenic. Because the dosage of androgen required to give an antiestrogenic effect is in the range to saturate the AR, but is too low to saturate the ER, it is possible that the therapeutic effect is mediated via the AR.[51] Androgens also exert hematopoietic and anabolic effects. They may stimulate erythropoiesis, probably via erythropoietin, and give an increased sense of well-being, despite the progression of disease. Experimentally, they are also used in cases with hypernephroma and secondary anemia, and in debilitating patients as anabolic steroid therapy after chemotherapy or radiation.

The most frequent side effects of androgens include virilization of female patients with hirsutism, deepening of the voice, acne, clitoral hypertrophy and amenorrhea and less frequent plethora, increase in libido, and fluid retention. The virilizing effects are related to the androgen used, its dose, and the duration of treatment. They occur in more than 50% of patients treated with testosterone propionate, in 35 to 40% of patients treated with fluoxymesterone, and in none treated with testolactone.

The orally effective halogenated androgens rarely cause cholestatic jaundice, which may require discontinuation of the drug. Androgens may precipitate severe hypercalcemia in women with breast cancer and bone metastases; this occurs in as many as 10% of such patients and represents an oncologic emergency. Androgens with a 17α-methyl-substitution, such as fluoxymesterone and methyltestosterone, may cause reversible cholestatic jaundice, and rarely, a multifocal hepatocellular necrosis, called peliosis hepatis. Recently, cyproterone acetate (CPA), an antiandrogenic compound, was used with some therapeutic benefits in metastatic male breast cancer.[52] From all androgens, fluoxymesterone (Halotestin) has emerged as the androgen of choice because it is at least as potent as testosterone propionate, is less virilizing, and can be taken orally. The dosage is 20 to 30 mg/d taken orally.

e. Corticosteroids

Corticosteroids are used in cancer therapy due to their catabolic, anti-inflammatory and cytotoxic actions on cancer cells. One mechanism involves binding to their intracellular receptors, or glucocorticoid receptors (GR), followed by translocation to the nucleus. Other mechanisms are involved as well, since some of the biochemical effects of corticosteroids occur without entry into the cells. Corticosteroids cause a wide variety of biochemical, metabolic, and cytologic changes on neoplastic cells. Thus, they exert antitumor effects in a variety of experimental tumors, such as mammary carcinoma, lymphoid tumors, lung tumors, liver tumors, and squamous and basal cell carcinomas by inhibiting the DNA synthesis and inducing advanced cytolysis with cell membrane disruption.[6,21]

A variety of anti-inflammatory and immunosuppressive effects may also be seen with corticosteroid therapy. A principal mechanism by which steroids inhibit inflammation appears to be related to their ability to impede the access of neutrophils and monocytes to the inflammatory site. The lymphocytopenia that is seen following corticosteroids involves mostly suppressor T-lymphocytes derived from the thymus. Also, corticosteroids may directly kill lymphoid cells or interfere with essential lymphoid functions by inhibiting lymphoid growth factors. It is also possible that corticosteroids exert their antitumor effect by suppressing pituitary ACTH production. Thus, glucocorticoids should be used only: (1) in treatment of lymphomas, leukemia, Hodgkin's disease, and myelomas; (2) as supportive treatment for disease-related complications, such as central nervous system metastases or secondary inflammation; (3) in breast and prostatic cancers as palliative therapy; and (4) in tumor complications, such as hypercalcemia, dyspnea, pain, anorexia, and jaundice from hepatic metastases.

There are many synthetic corticosteroids now available, and we can separate the commonly used corticosteroids into two groups: (1) those with a relatively short duration of action and (2) those with a prolonged duration of action and great relative potency. Hydrocortisone and prednisone are relatively weak corticosteroids, with a short duration of action. After oral administration, their respective plasma half-lives are approximately 1.5 and 3.5 h. Dexamethasone, a more potent and longer acting synthetic derivative of cortisol, has a plasma $T^{1}/_{2}$ of 4.7 h. They have different potencies. In one study, the relative potencies of hydrocortisone (cortisol), prednisone, and dexamethasone (Decadron) at 0, 8, and 14 h after oral administration were as follows: hydrocortisone, 1, 1, 1; prednisone, 1.05, 3, 5.2; and dexamethasone, 17, 52, 154. Thus, the relative intrinsic biologic potency and relative rates of disappearance from plasma are critical factors in determining the duration and intensity of glucocorticoid action.[53]

Corticosteroids are commonly used either alone or in combination with other cytotoxic drugs in the treatment of malignant hematopoietic diseases, such as acute lymphoblastic leukemia (ALL), chronic lymphocytic leukemia, lymphomas, and multiple myeloma. Short, intensive courses of prednisone are usually employed alone or in combination with ACTH and produce dramatic effects in some cases. However, corticosteroids have only limited indications as single agents for metastatic breast cancer or prostate cancer. High doses of glucocorticoids equivalent to 200 to 300 mg/d of cortisol, result in a 10 to 18% response rate in metastatic breast cancer.[54] Remission is generally of short duration, but may be of rapid onset, making glucocorticoids useful in treatment of rapidly advancing disease. Specific tumor responses appear to be limited to premenopausal patients with a prior response to castration and to postmenopausal women with a prior response to other forms of hormone therapy. It is difficult to make dose recommendations because no dose-response data are available for breast cancer or prostate cancer. Objective tumor regression has followed cortisone acetate, 100 to 400 mg/d and prednisone, 30 to 250 mg/d. The lower doses may be as effective as the high doses. Euphoria can be produced by 20 to 40 mg/d of oral prednisone. For patients with edema of the brain or spinal cord, the potent, long-acting steroid prednisone is employed in a dose of 4 mg q.i.d.

The side effects of long-term corticosteroid administration are well known. Some complications may occur with short-term treatment, such as sodium and fluid retention, hypokalemia, psychosis, and exacerbation of diabetes mellitus, whereas other complications are more often seen with prolonged treatment. These may affect the musculoskeletal system (myopathy, osteoporosis, aseptic necrosis of bone); gastrointestinal tract (pancreatitis, peptic ulceration); central nervous system (pseudotumor cerebri); cardiovascular system (hypertension); metabolism (obesity, hyperlipidemia, hyperosmolar nonketotic coma); immune system (defects of cell-mediated immunity, immunosuppression with secondary infections); skin (striae, impaired wound healing); and endocrine system (amenorrhea, growth failure, and overt Cushing's syndrome). Several of these complications are due to the suppression of the hypothalamic-pituitary-adrenal axis and their mineral corticoid potency. As a consequence, if the corticosteroid treatment has been given to the patient for 2 weeks or less, it can be discontinued abruptly. Patients treated for longer periods should generally have steroid slowly withdrawn. If prolonged treatment is required, it is preferable to administer the corticosteroid on alternate days or, if that fails, as a single dose each morning. Patients who have been on corticosteroids for very long periods of time may suffer withdrawal symptoms and treatment should be progressively discontinued.

f. Aromatase Inhibitors

Aminoglutethimide (AG) was first used as an antiepileptic, and since 1973 it has been used as a compound capable of inhibiting adrenal steroid synthesis and subsequently to suppress adrenal function. Aminoglutethimide blocks the first step in steroid synthesis, the conversion of cholesterol to pregnenolone. However, the inhibition is less than complete for Δ-4 types of steroids such as testosterone, progesterone, 17-α-hydroxyprogesterone, dihydrotestosterone, and androstenedione. The last compound is especially important because the adrenal gland secretes no estrogens per se, but rather secretes androstenedione, which is converted in extra-adrenal tissues to estrone and estradiol (aromatization reaction). This is the principal source of estrogens in postmenopausal or castrated women, and is inhibited almost completely by aminoglutethimide.

Because aminoglutethimide results in adrenal suppression and a concomitant fall in cortisol level, leading to a rise in ACTH level which can overcome the adrenal blockade, the drug should be administered with cortisol, whose metabolism is not altered by aminoglutethimide, and leads to a therapeutic regimen that effectively suppresses adrenal function in most patients. Thus, aminoglutethimide combined with hydrocortisone is capable of producing declines in plasma estrone and estradiol levels similar to those seen after adrenalectomy; a randomized trial of aminoglutethimide (medical adrenalectomy) vs. surgical adrenalectomy showed that response rates and durations were equivalent. (The advantages of medical or chemical adrenalectomy will be described in Chapter 3 of this book.)

Maximal estrogen suppression requires that aminoglutethimide be given in a dose of 250 mg orally four times a day together with 40 mg hydrocortisone in divided dose (10 mg at 8 a.m., 10 mg at 5 p.m., and 20 mg at bedtime). In patients treated with aminoglutethimide-hydrocortisone, the urinary cortisol and plasma estrone, estradiol, fall significantly while on continuous therapy. As with most other endocrine therapies, the response rate in unselected patients is about 35%, with an increase of 40 to 50% in patients with ER-positive tumors, and a median duration of response in the 11- to 17-month range.[56] Aminoglutethimide (Cytadren) therapy can induce a second remission in patients relapsing after prior hormonal therapy. Approximately half of previous responses to antiestrogen therapy will have a second objective response to aminoglutethimide. The duration of secondary response averaged 10 to 12 months.[57] Aminoglutethimide can interact with other drugs, such as coumarin anticoagulants. Larger doses of coumarin are needed when given with aminoglutethimide.

In a recent study, aminoglutethimide (AG) was administered as palliative therapy in patients with metastatic breast cancer at a dose of 1000 mg/d or 500 mg/d. Objective regression was observed in 31% of patients with the duration of response ranging from 4 to 36 months (mean = 12 months). Response was observed in 35% of patients with soft tissue metastasis; 27% of patients with osseous metastases, and 36% with visceral metastasis. The side effects (skin rash, fever, somnolence, ataxia, dyspnea, headache) were fewer and less severe in patients treated with a lower dose of 500 mg/d as compared to those receiving 1000 mg/d, although the therapeutic effects were similar. It is possible that most of therapeutic effects at lower dose are due to inhibition of peripheral aromatization of androgens. Thus, aminoglutethimide supplemented by hydrocortisone is a valuable method in the treatment of metastatic breast cancer.[58]

In addition to adrenal suppression, aminoglutethimide can cause a variety of reversible dose-dependent side effects. A generalized macular, pruritic skin rash, sometimes associated with fever, has been noted within 10 d of treatment. If the rash continues or worsens,

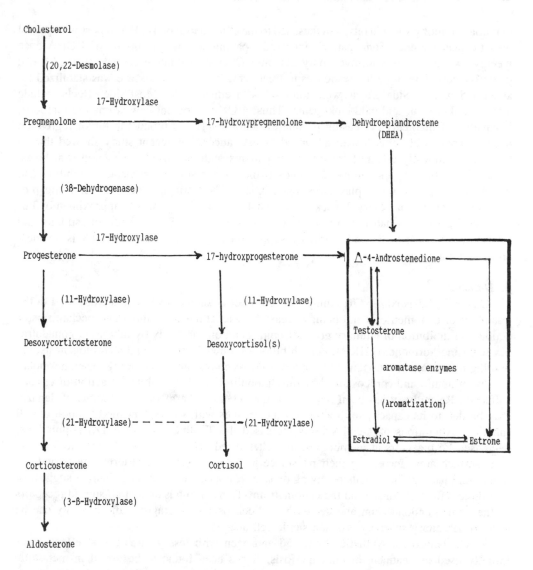

FIGURE 2. Steroid hormone synthesis and major enzymes involved in steroidogenesis and aromatization.

aminoglutethimide should be discontinued. Central nervous system reactions may also occur, including somnolence, dizziness, ataxia, nystagmus, or lethargy. These reactions generally disappear by lowering the dose of aminoglutethimide. The drug aminoglutethimide (Cytadren) is not usually marrow suppressive or immunosuppressive; however, marrow suppression may rarely occur, e.g., pancytopenia may occur in up to 4% of patients.[59] Postural hypotension and hyponatremia, mild hypothyroidism, and virilization can also rarely be seen. The ready reversibility of its metabolic effects is an obvious advantage of aminoglutethimide, as adrenal function returns to normal within 2 to 3 d after discontinuation of treatment. Another inhibitor of peripheral aromatization, 4-hydroxyandrostenedione (4-OHA), which is a less toxic but more potent inhibitor of aromatase *in vitro* than aminoglutethimide, has gone into clinical trials. It has been shown to inhibit ovarian estrogen synthesis in rats and peripheral aromatization in rhesus monkeys.[60] Aromatization is a chemical reaction, due to enzyme aromatase, by which Δ-4-androstenedione is converted to estrone and testosterone to estradiol (see Figure 2).

Previous observations revealed that 4-OHA inhibits the growth of estrogen-dependent mammary tumor growth in rats, and these led to the clinical trial of 4-OHA in postmenopausal breast cancer patients. Some patients received a parenteral dose of 500 mg of 4-OHA once weekly, whereas others received only 250 mg. Overall evaluation showed that 27% had objective complete or partial responses to treatment. In 19%, the disease was stabilized for at least 8 weeks. Side effects were minimal with either route. Most side effects include lethargy, skin rash, and mild leukopenia. Thus, 4-OHA, a potent new aromatase inhibitor, is capable of markedly decreasing plasma estradiol levels and producing tumor regression in postmenopausal patients with advanced breast cancer.[61] A recent study showed that 4-OHA is a clinically effective treatment for patients with advanced postmenopausal breast cancer by both p.o. and parenteral routes (i.m.) as a result of aromatase inhibition and consequent suppression of plasma estrogen levels. The optimal doses were 250 mg p.o. daily and 500 mg i.m. every 2 weeks. The half-life of 4-OHA p.o. was approximately 3 h, whereas the apparent half-life of injected drug was 5 to 10 d. Serum levels of estradiol and estrone were consistently and markedly suppressed (by 40%). Thus, 4-OHA is an ideal aromatase inhibitor.[62]

g. *Danazol*

Danazol (2,3-isoxazol-17α-ethinyl testosterone) is another synthetic steroid used in the treatment of endometriosis and benign breast disease. It has four important mechanisms of action: (1) inhibition of pituitary gonadotropin secretion, probably by inhibiting gonadotropin-releasing hormone, (LHRH), (2) inhibition of adrenal and gonadal steroidogenesis, (3) binding to androgen, estrogen, and progesterone receptors, and (4) binding to sex hormone-binding globulin and corticosteroid-binding globulin.[63] It also inhibits the action of estrone sulfatase. Recently, it has been shown that the versatile pharmacologic actions of danazol may be due to its capacity to modify cell membranes with subsequent modification of cell function. Alterations of T-cell subsets increased the T-helper/inducer (CD_4) populations, decreased Fc receptors in membranes, and altered red cell membranes directly to increase their surface area, increasing their resistance to osmotic lysis. Short-term effects and endometrial histology in patients receiving danazol revealed early atrophic changes suggestive of a direct effect of danazol on the endometrium. Danazol binds almost all steroid receptors of the human endometrium and decreases red cell osmolytic fragility and possibly can be used in hereditary spherocytosis and sickle cell anemia.

Thus, danazol, a synthetic attenuated androgen with less virilizing side effects, was initially used in treatment of endometriosis. It has been found to be useful in metastatic breast cancer, namely in postmenopausal women, cystic disease of the breast, hereditary angioneurotic edema, α1-antitrypsin deficiency, and Melkersson-Rosenthal syndrome (an autosomal dominant inherited granulomatous disorder).[64] Danazol also can be used in treatment of idiopathic thrombocytopenia purpura (ITP), autoimmune hemolytic anemia, and paroxysmal nocturnal hemoglobinuria (PNH). However, danazol and its metabolic ethisterone and 2-OH-methyltestosterone increases the percentage of unbound E_2 and unbound testosterone by displacing these hormones from sex hormone-binding globulin (SHBG) building sites.[26] Danazol exerts also an antitumorigenic activity. Thus, a 66% objective response rate to danazol in the treatment of DMBA-induced mammary cancers in rats has been reported. In doses of 100 to 200 mg three times daily (same as for treatment of chronic cystic mastopathy), objective responses in 7 of 37 postmenopausal patients treated with danazol have also been reported.

Recently, from 67 patients with metastatic breast cancer treated with danazol at doses between 300 mg/d to 600 mg/d, only 15% responded to therapy and a further 9% showed stabilization of disease. Concerning the effect of menopausal status, only one patient from 14 premenopausal patients responded compared to 9/53 postmenopausal patients. Thus, danazol does not seem sufficient enough to be used as first or second line therapy.[65] Mild adverse effects, such as androgenic effects and hypoestrogenic effects, hepatic dysfunction, thrombocytopenia, muscle cramps, and skin rash, were observed. Recently, a similar synthetic alternated androgen, called Stanozolol, with similar therapeutic properties, but which is less toxic, has been used.

h. Luteinizing Hormone-Releasing Hormone (LHRH) Agonists

We have known for more than 15 years that release of the pituitary gonadotropins (LH and FSH) is regulated by a decapeptide from the hypothalamus, called gonadotropin-releasing hormone (GnRH). The linear sequence of GnRH is: Glu^1-His^2-Trp^3-Ser^4-Tyr^5-Gly^5-Leu^7-Arg^8-Pro^9-Gly^{10}-amide. Naturally occurring LHRH is a decapeptide synthesized in the hypothalamus and released in brief pulses, in a pulsatile pattern, if the median basal nucleus is intact. If this nucleus is destroyed, pulsatile secretion is lost. GnRH stimulates luteinizing hormone (LH) and follicle-stimulating hormone (FSH) release from the pituitary gland. The concentration of anterior pituitary hormones in the peripheral blood are dependent not only on the amplitude of these pulses, but also on their frequency. The pauses between pulses are required to allow receptors time to recover their sensitivity, which is partially lost when they are stimulated. Binding to the plasma membrane, receptors appear to involve the 1 to 10 amino acids that are in close physical proximity at the lowest energy state of the molecule. Activation of the effector appears to involve the first three amino acids.

Present studies regarding the molecular basis of gonadotropin-releasing hormone revealed that GnRH is released episodically, in a pulsatile pattern, from the median eminence into hypophysial portal vessels; Ca^{2+} is a second messenger for GnRH and calmodulin, the multifunctional Ca^{2+} binding protein, appears to be an intracellular receptor for Ca^{2+} mobilized in response to GnRH. Calmodulin inhibitors, including naphthalene sulfonamides, inhibit GnRH-stimulated LH release with the same potency that they inhibit calmodulin. *In vivo* studies in primates indicated that continuous exposure to GnRH led to a refractory pituitary while intermittent delivery of GnRH restored responsiveness.[66] This observation explains why GnRH and its agonists can be administered to provoke or inhibit gonadal function and thus continuous exposure can evoke a functional castration. Agonist analogs of GnRH cause intense stimulation in the pituitary if given once, but then become inhibitory if given repeatedly. This occurs because they are resistant to degradation by pituitary enzymes and thus block the gonadotroph receptors in the pituitary and make it unresponsive after initial supraphysiologic stimulation.[67] Since studies in hypogonadal men undergoing testosterone replacement therapy suggested that FSH is concomitantly secreted with LH from the pituitary, in response to the same stimulus, we referred to GnRH as LHRH. There are many different such analogs, and they have been recently used to treat hormone-responsive cancers and have opened new doors in cancer treatment.[68]

LHRH agonists are synthetic analogs of LHRH in which the amino acids necessary for hormone-receptor binding and biological activity have been replaced by others that improved these properties. Thus, substitution of L-glycine at position 6 by a D-amino acid and replacement of the C-terminal glycinamide by ethylamide residue increases the potency of these compounds over LHRH by 50- to 200-fold. Continuous LHRH agonist treatments are sufficient to promote regression of ovary-dependent carcinogen-induced mammary tumors and Dunning prostate tumors in rodents; also they are recognized as "castration-like" and form the basis of the use of LHRH agonists in breast and prostate cancer patients.

In animals, chronic treatment with supraphysiologic doses of luteinizing hormone-releasing hormone (LHRH) agonists causes: (1) decreased gonadotrophin (FSH and LH) excretion, (2) decreased prolactin excretion, (3) decreased concentration of plasma sex steroid, (4) reduced weight of secondary sexual organs, and (5) inhibited actions of the sex steroids at their target organs. Recently, it has been demonstrated that there is a significant decrease in tumor weight and volume in mouse and rat mammary cancers treated with D-Trp^6-LH-

RH (decapeptyl).[67] Currently, the LHRH analogs, buserelin, decapeptyl, and leuprolide are in clinical trials.[26]

Furthermore, steroid hormones may modify the pulsatile pattern. When estrogen levels rise, the frequency of spontaneous LH pulses increases while their amplitude decreases, resulting in a fall in LH. Androgens have the opposite effect; they lower the frequency but increase the amplitude. In both instances, peripheral levels of gonadotropin fall. Although LHRH may serve as an extrahypothalamic neurotransmitter in amphibians and lower mammals, there is no evidence for such a role in humans. However, it is now recognized that the extrapituitary site of GnRH biosynthesis is the trophoblast of human placenta, where high concentrations of GnRH stimulate HCG synthesis and release *in vitro*. Recently, several LHRH analogs have been synthesized by introducing various substitutions in the original molecule, primarily at the 6th and 10th amino acid positions. Such structural changes have resulted in the synthesis of a series of analogs that proved to be several times more potent than the parent hormone in stimulating the release of LH and FSH. Therefore, these compounds are referred to as LHRH agonists or superagonists. The substitution of hydrophobic amino acids in certain positions of the LHRH molecule has led to the synthesis of a series of analogs that function as antagonists of LHRH. Four of these LHRH agonists are mainly used in hormone-dependent human cancers. Their chemical structure is shown below:

Native sequence of GnRH
pyroGlu-His-Trp-Tyr-Ser-Gly-Leu-Arg-Pro-Gly-amide

D-Lys⁶-GnRH
pyroGlu-His-Trp-Tyr-Ser-D-Lys-Leu-Arg-Pro-Gly-amide

Buserelin (superagonist)
pyroGlu-His-Trp-Tyr-Ser-D-ser(*tert* Butyl)-Leu-Arg-Pro-ethylamide

Leuprolide (superagonist)
pyroGlu-His-Trp-Tyr-Ser-D-Leu-Leu-Arg-Pro-ethylamide

Nafarelin (superagonist)
pyroGlu-His-Trp-Tyr-Ser-D-Nal(2)-Leu-Arg-Pro-Gly-amide

When administered acutely, LHRH analogs cause a prompt increase in plasma LH and FSH levels; however, long-term administration of LHRH analogs leads to a paradoxical inhibition of gonadotropins. Thus, these potent agonists cause down-regulation of receptors and eventual pituitary desensitization to the effect of further GnRH.[69] The major therapeutic applications of GnRH and GnRH agonist analogs are listed in Table 1.

Thus, induction of puberty, induction of ovulation, and induction of spermatogenesis can be therapeutically achieved by chronic pulsatile GnRH treatment.[66] However, GnRH has no place in the treatment of true cryptorchidism for which early surgery is indicated. We are focusing mainly on the therapeutic use of GnRH antagonists in hormone-dependent cancers (prostate cancer, breast cancer, and ovarian and endometrial cancer).

Long-term suppression of LH and testosterone with long-acting GnRH agonist analogs is now well established. There is abundant evidence that primary treatment of advanced prostate cancer with LHRH agonists is effective and produces initial clinical response rates of about 70%, which is similar to those achieved by orchiectomy or diethylstilbestrol (DES). Randomized prospective trials confirmed these initial results. One group randomized 199 patients with metastatic prostate cancer to receive either 3 mg DES or 1 mg/d of leuprolide; 46% of those treated with DES and 38% of those treated with leuprolide responded. Only

TABLE 1
Major Therapeutic Applications of LHRH and GnRH Agonist Analogs

Stimulation of pituitary-gonadal function LHRH
    Induction of puberty
    Ovulation induction
    Induction of spermatogenesis
Inhibition of gonadal function (LHRH analogs)
    Prostate cancer
    Premenopausal breast cancer, male breast cancer
    Endometrial cancer (?)
    Central precocious puberty
    Benign gynecological disease — endometriosis, fibroids, menorrhagia
    Ovarian cancer
    Premenstrual syndrome (PMS)
    Contraception (?)
    Erythropoietic protoporphyria (EPP)

10 of the 98 patients treated with leuprolide had cardiovascular side effects, compared with 33 of the 101 treated with DES.[70] In another randomized study, 41% of 70 patients treated by orchiectomy responded compared with 50% of those treated with the LHRH analog decapeptyl (D-Trp-6LHRH). The duration of the response seems to be the same with conventional treatments and with the analogs. In the leuprolide study, the duration of treatment failure was identical in the two groups (46 weeks), and median survival was 146 weeks in those treated with leuprolide and 136 weeks in those treated with DES. In the decapeptyl study, median survival was 16 months and 13 months in those treated by orchiectomy. LHRH analogs have minimal side effects as compared to orchiectomy, which produces appreciable psychological stress, and those of DES treatment with cardiovascular effects and gynecomastia. The fact that the analogs are stimulatory in the first few days of treatment indicates that they exacerbate the disease at first: about one third of patients had minor transient exacerbations (with flare in bone pain) and 1% had appreciable complications. LHRH analogs are contraindicated if the patient has neurological dysfunction or obstructive uropathy. Antiandrogens, such as cyproterone acetate or flutamide, may reduce these initial problems.

Of particular interest, are the data claiming that LHRH analog treatment combined with peripheral antiandrogen flutamide or "total androgen blockade" not only increase the initial clinical response rate (95 vs. 80% LHRH alone), but also produce survival (85 vs. 50% at 2 years).[71] Originally, this combined hormonal treatment was designed to block the production of adrenal androgens, mainly 5α-dihydrotestosterone, which can accumulate in the prostate, and then to stimulate the remaining androgen-dependent cell populations that escaped from the blockade by LHRH. These cells may undergo transformation into completely androgen-insensitive cells. Many urologists in Europe (EORTC-GU group) have conducted other studies using total androgen blockade with LHRH analog goserelin (Depot Zoladex) and flutamide vs. Depot Zoladex alone; they found no difference at all, and cannot confirm the original results of Labrie.[72] However, depot injections of LHRH analogs are better in elderly patients. Depot treatment is as effective as daily treatment and has two biochemical advantages: serum testosterone concentrations are lower and implants are not followed by transient rises in serum LH concentrations.

In breast cancer, the GnRH analogs might be effective since it has been shown that LHRH analogs inhibited the development of DMBA-induced mammary tumors in rats and that Buserelin had a dose-dependent growth-inhibitory effect when added to MCF-7 breast cancer cells in culture; thus, it is possible that LHRH may have a direct antitumor effect. Later, it was found that 14 of 45 premenopausal women with breast cancer responded partially to either daily subcutaneous or monthly depot injections with the analog goserelin. Patients without estrogen receptors did not respond, and tumor flare was not seen. Also, in a group of 25 premenopausal patients with advanced breast cancer, daily subcutaneous administration of 1 to 10 mg of leuprolide induced objective tumor regression in 44% with a median duration of 9 months. Profound suppression of gonadotropins, estradiol, and progesterone secretion occurred in all patients on chronic therapy. These effects on tumor growth and ovarian hormone levels are similar to those observed after surgical ovariectomy. Other LHRH analogs, such as Buserelin and Zoladex, have been found to have similar antitumor and hormonal effects, which are also comparable to those produced by surgical ovariectomy. The use of GnRH in postmenopausal women with advanced breast cancer is disappointing. Association with antiestrogens produced a complete blockade of estrogen action and could potentiate the antitumor effect.[69] Thus, LHRH analogs might prove useful in providing a "reversible" medical oophorectomy for premenopausal women with breast cancer.[73] Certainly, the recent identification of LHRH binding sites on human breast tumors, and the inhibitory effects of the LHRH agonist Buserelin on MCF-7 human breast cancer cells suggested that LHRH agonists are playing a central role in the development of breast cancer. In agreement with this is the fact that some authors reported responses in both premenopausal and postmenopausal women with advanced beast cancer, using decapeptyl.

Also, partial and sometimes complete regression of tumor growth and metastases were reported in metastatic carcinoma of the male breast cancer. Carcinoma of the male breast is rare with an incidence of only 1% of that in females. Nevertheless, the principles of the management of the disease in men are the same in women. Administration of Buserelin by nasal inhalation to an elderly man with metastatic carcinoma of the breast produced a complete regression of pulmonary metastases. Presumably, the mechanism whereby LHRH agonists would be effective in the treatment of male breast cancer is that it would inhibit testicular production of androgen, and consequently, decrease its conversion to estrogens. Because orchiectomy is an effective palliative procedure in some 60 to 70% of males with breast cancer, long-term LHRH analog treatment might be considered a more acceptable way of inducing castration in the management of male breast cancer.

There is clear evidence of benefit from long-acting GnRH agonists in benign gynecological diseases (endometriosis, fibroids, and menorrhagia), though symptoms of hypoestrogenism occur frequently, and the possibility of effects of bone mineral content may limit their long-term use for these diseases. Cyclical attacks of acute intermittent porphyria can be prevented with LHRH analogs presumably because they are precipitated by estrogens. Also, premenstrual syndrome (PMS) can be alleviated by GnRH agonists.

Gonadotropin hormone releasing analogs have been used in ovarian cancer. The first patient was report in 1985 and responded for one year. Since then, 6 out of 36 patients have responded to a depot preparation of decapeptyl. Their mechanism of action consists mainly of reducing the concentration of LHRH receptors in the pituitary by a process of down-regulation.[74]

i. Somatostatin

Somatostatin (somatotropin-release inhibitory factor) was detected first in the rat hypothalamus and shown to inhibit the release of growth hormone from the pituitary.[75] It is a 14-amino acid-containing peptide (tetradecapeptide) bridged by a sulfur bond and designated as somatostatin 14; later other mammalian somatostatins were isolated, such as somatostatin 28. Several other larger prohormones (somatostatin-like peptides) from early vertebrates were also found and closely similar. It has been shown that somatostatin is also secreted by the D-cells of the islets of Langerhans. Considerable amounts of somatostatin were also extracted from the gut and the antrum, and nerve fibers that produce somatostatin have now been found in the genitourinary system, heart, eye, thyroid, thymus, and skin. Somatostatin secreted into the gut lumen modifies acid and gastric secretion and it is classified as a "lumone".[76] Somatostatin has been identified in the salivary gland (saliva contains somatostatin), and this peptide decreases salivary flow after systemic injection. Some of the parafollicular cells (C cells) of the human thyroid also contain somatostatin, whereas others contain only calcitonin. Somatostatin is synthesized by medullary-thyroid-carcinoma cells and secreted by certain endocrine tumors (somatostatinomas), including small cell carcinomas of the lung, VIPomas, and pancreatic endocrine tumors. A somatostatinoma syndrome has been described with weight loss, malabsorption, diabetes, gallstones, and hypochlorhydria. Catecholamines may interact with somatostatin in cell regulation. Intracerebroventricular injection of somatostatin inhibits ACTH secretion and adrenal epinephrine and prevents hyperglycemia in response to certain stimuli. It also interferes with ADH and inhibits calcitonin and renin secretion. Somatostatin is secreted in the urine.

There are differences in function for different forms of somatostatin. For example, somatostatin 28 is more potent than somatostatin 14 in suppression of insulin secretion and also is a more potent neuromodulator than is somatostatin 14. Somatostatin is synthesized as a preprohormone on the endoplasmic reticulum and translocated to the Golgi system, where it is further processed within secretory granules to form somatostatin 14 and somatostatin 28. It is postulated that somatostatin is released from the cell and diffuses into the interstitial space, where it comes into contact with somatostatin receptors on the cell membrane. This is called "autocrine regulation."[76] Specific receptors for somatostatin are identified in many sites, but the intracellular mechanism of action is unknown. It may be related to Ca^{2+} influx, suppression of intracellular cyclic adenosine monophosphate (cAMP), and stimulation of potassium permeability. Cortical concentrations of somatostatin are dramatically reduced in Alzheimer's disease, but the cause and consequence of this reduction are unknown.[77]

Physiological functions of somatostatin vary from tissue to tissue and are highly diverse. It was found to inhibit the secretion of growth hormone (GH), thyrotropin (TSH), prolactin, and adrenocorticotropin (ACTH), but has no effect on gonadotropins (FSH, LH). Somatostatin inhibits insulin and glucagon release, and pentagastrin-induced gastric secretion. Somatostatin also inhibits cholecystokinin, kallikrein, serotonin and other growth factors such as epidermal growth factor (EGF) and transforming growth factor-β (TGF-β). Somatostatin analogs possess significant antitumor activity in experimental tumors, including rat prostate carcinoma.[78] Somatostatin has a short duration of action (half-life in the circulation is about 3 min). Blood levels of somatostatin widely varying from 40 to 88 and even 675 pg (picograms) per ml. In patients with somatostatinoma, plasma levels of 3000 to 25,000 ng (nanograms) per ml have been reported. Due to its short half-life, the initial therapeutic effects were disappointing and new long-acting peptides, or somatostatin analogs had to be developed.

Such a somatostatin analog, SMS201-995 (Sandostatin), was developed by Sandoz Company and has been widely tested clinically. Sandostatin is an octapeptide that differs in its action from native somatostatin in four ways: (1) it inhibits GH hormone secretion in preference to insulin secretion, (2) it can be administered subcutaneously (s.c.) or even orally, (3) it is long-acting (half-life after s.c. administration is 113 min), and (4) there is no rebound hypersecretion of hormones when the effect of the analog recedes.[79] Somatostatin analogs have been shown to inhibit the growth of a variety of tumors in different animal models, such as chondrosarcomas, osteosarcomas, mammary and pancreatic adenocarcinomas, insulinomas, and prostatic carcinomas.[79] Most endocrine pancreatic tumors, carcinoids, VIPomas, and pituitary tumors acromegaly resistant to radiotherapy respond sometimes dramatically to Sandostatin. Somatostatin receptors are found in a variety of cancers, such as meningiomas, astrocytomas, and breast carcinomas; and most endocrine pancreatic tumors contain somatostatin receptors with high affinity for Sandostatin, such as gastrinomas, VIPomas, and insulinomas.

Thus, Sandostatin therapy must be aimed at controlling the clinical symptoms of endocrine pancreatic tumors and carcinoids, such as improvement of electrolyte and water disorders, and peptic ulcerations and hypoglycemia. A special place for Sandostatin is in the acute treatment of life-threatening complications, e.g., dehydration and hypokalemic acidosis in patients with metastatic vasoactive intestinal polypeptide tumors (VIPomas), and severe diarrhea, severe hypoglycemia in insulinomas, and acute hypertension in carcinoid crisis. Diarrhea caused by the carcinoid syndrome and glucagonomas has also been successfully treated with somatostatin. Somatostatin has been used in treatment of patients with bleeding due to gastric ulcer and hemorrhagic pancreatitis due to a local "cytoprotective" effect. The usual therapeutic dose has been a bolus i.v. dose of 250 μg/h. Sandostatin is a synthetic compound and it is used as optimal dose of 200 to 300 μg/d in two or three s.c. injections and is well tolerated. Even very high doses up to 1500 μg/day are well tolerated. No problems of allergy and no local reactions were observed even during long-term therapy. Sometimes mild gastrointestinal reactions, such as abdominal pains, diarrhea, and a slight impairment of postprandial glucose tolerance may occur. Sandostatin is also used in the metabolic control of Type I diabetes mellitus and nesidioblastosis (hyperplasia of islets of Langerhans) of the newborn, especially acute hypoglycemia in children with nesidioblastosis. It was also reported that Sandostatin might be beneficial in the long-term management of patients with portal hypertension by inducing a liver cytoprotection.

Somatostatin, called "endocrine cyanide" because it inhibits several peptide hormones, and its long-acting analogs are dramatically successful in the treatment of endocrine pancreatic tumors, VIPomas, carcinoids, and pituitary tumors as well as their life-threatening conditions.[80] They exert an important antitumor activity and are able to improve the quality of life in most of these patients.[81]

j. Thyroxine

The thyroid hormone does not appear to be essential for breast development or lactation, although both processes may be adversely affected in states of hyperthyroidism or hypothyroidism. Experimental studies show that thyroxine enhances the development of mammary rat carcinoma, lung adenocarcinoma in guinea pigs, squamous cell carcinomas in mice, and basal cell carcinomas in rats. Although thyroid extracts have been used as an adjuvant therapy in advanced metastatic breast cancer since the end of last century, their role in breast cancer treatment is mainly palliative.

In thyroid carcinoma, there have been no trials of treatment with thyroid hormones as primary therapy. Instead, the therapy is used following surgery (thyroidectomy) and radioiodine. In most instances, the administration of thyroid hormones is regarded as an adjuvant to prevent tumor recurrence, tumor progression, and long-term survival. Since thyroid-stimulating hormone (TSH) has proven to be an important growth factor for thyroid follicular cells, the use of thyroid hormones to suppress TSH secretion after resection of differentiated thyroid cancers (follicular and papillary thyroid carcinomas) has been practiced for many years, and in a few cases, metastatic thyroid carcinoma has decreased markedly following treatment with thyroid hormones. In patients with tumors larger than 1.5 cm that were multicentric, locally invasive or metastatic to lymphatic nodes, it was found that the tumor recurred significantly more often (17.2 vs. 34.4%) when thyroid hormone was not given postoperatively.[82]

However, not all authors were able to demonstrate such an effect of thyroid hormones on survival. These observations are consistent with the concept that thyroid hormones are generally palliative but not tumoricidal. The preparation of choice is sodium levothyroxine because the serum concentrations of thyroxine (T_4) and triiodothyronine (T_3) are more stable in patients treated with thyroxine. The use of desiccated thyroid or triiodothyronine is less physiologic because at 2 to 6 h after administration of these preparations, there are large supraphysiologic peaks of serum T_3 concentrations. These fall to lower levels over the next 24 h, thus making therapy with these preparations less physiologic. The determination of TSH concentration is not sufficiently sensitive to demonstrate the response to treatment. For this reason, the suppression of the TSH response to thyrotropin-releasing hormone (TRH) may be a more helpful test in the followup of patients with thyroid cancer.

The recommended dose of thyroxine is about 220 µg in patients with thyroid carcinoma (or 3.1 µg/kg/d) and 175 to 200 µg in patients with benign goiter. In patients older than 60 years, the dose is lower (1.5 to 1.8 µg/kg/d). The dose should be adjusted for each patient. Excessive doses of thyroxine, desiccated thyroid, or triiodothyronine confer no advantage and should be avoided because they may produce symptoms of thyrotoxicosis, exert deleterious effects on the cardiovascular system, e.g., arrhythmia and angina pectoris; and cause demineralization of bones.

The use of liothyronine sodium (Cytomel) as replacement therapy is less advantageous than sodium L-thyroxine (Synthroid) in patients with thyroid cancer in regard to the tumor recurrence and survival. Almost 70 to 75% of human thyroid cancers (papillary carcinoma and follicular carcinoma) and 40% of undifferentiated thyroid carcinomas are responsive to thyroid hormones (thyroxine) therapy as demonstrated by tumor regression and survival for 10 years. The effects of thyroid hormones are less beneficial in metastatic thyroid cancers (autonomous tumors) with lung, bone, and brain tumors. Use of thyroid hormones in breast cancer is based on experimental observations that mammary tumorigenesis is increased in T_3-treated mice, as well as clinical observations that hyperthyroid patients develop less mammary carcinoma than euthyroid subjects. Thus, in a study of 14 patients, after mastectomy and use of thyroid hormones, 13 patients remained cancer-free at a 4-year followup.[21] It is likely that the hypothalamic-pituitary-thyroid-ovarian axis may play an important role in pathogenesis of breast cancer.

k. Melatonin — A New Antitumor Hormone

Melatonin (5-metoxy-N-acetyltryptamine) is a lipid-soluble derivative of 5-hydroxytryptamine, which is produced via the pineal gland under the influence of sympathetic neural tone governed by diurnal variation in light exposure. Melatonin secretion is maximal with the onset of darkness and it controls diurnal rhythms, reproductive behavior, and pigmentation. Melatonin may have primary immunologic modulating action, suggesting a possible role in the immunologic control of malignancy. Most important to hormonal control of tumor growth, it has been found that melatonin increases the cytoplasmic estrogen receptor in vitro in hamsters; similar effects have been observed in ER-binding activity in human breast cancer cells.[83]

Reviewing the medical literature, it appears that melatonin: (1) may exert therapeutic effects in breast cancer, notably ER + tumors, alone or combined with estrogen and antiestrogenic agents; (2) may affect prolactin and TSH production in breast cancer; (3) has effects on prostatic cancer and benign prostatic hypertrophy (BPH); (4) may exert beneficial effects on the treatment of sarcoma alone, or in combination with standard treatment; (5) has effects on hematopoiesis, platelets, and immune response; (6) can be used therapeutically as a prime chronobiologic regulator to enhance the effects of chemotherapy and radiotherapy; (7) exerts sedative, antiepileptic, and narcotic effects; and (8) may affect cell proliferation in vitro and in vivo. The wide range of melatonin physiologic effects suggests that melatonin acts as a ''buffer neurohormone'' or as a biologic transducer and modulator.

Melatonin administered orally or intravenously to animals or healthy subjects has proved to be clinically safe. Even in high doses of 3 to 6 g of melatonin given orally daily for 1 month, only minimal side effects (abdominal cramps and tranquilization), which are reversible, were observed. Additionally, a positive correlation exists between the nocturnal melatonin peak and progesterone and androgen receptor concentrations in primary tumors, indicating a direct involvement of melatonin in the growth control of breast cancer. It was concluded that changes of serum melatonin in primary breast cancer affect perhaps the immune system, and it may be a vital part of the host-tumor interaction. Thus, due to its wide-ranging immunologic, analgesic, sedative, and possibly cytostatic effects, melatonin may be used as an antitumor or supportive drug alone or combined with conventional therapy.

Hormones are now used as single agents (see Table 2) or combined with other systemic agents in order to inhibit or delay tumor growth and its metastases or to relieve symptoms of incurable malignant disease (as palliative therapy). In patients who do not respond to single hormonal therapy, the addition of a second or third hormonal procedure should be tried in order to achieve improvement. Multiple hormonotherapy (multivalent hormone therapy) can be recommended by using two to three hormone preparations concomitantly or alternately. First, one hormone should be tried; if patients do not respond or exhibit a low response, then it is better to recommend an additional, second, or third hormonal preparation, and cytostatic agents or radiation therapy (chemohormonotherapy, radiation-hormonotherapy) in order to enhance the responsiveness of a primary tumor or its metastases. These hormone therapies, as well as the introduction of new synthetic hormone antagonists, may replace the major endocrine ablation (oophorectomy, orchiectomy, adrenalectomy, hypophysectomy) or fit them as a second or third additive procedure.

3. Treatment of Hormone-Dependent Cancers
a. Breast Cancer

Breast cancer is an extremely common disease, with almost 110,000 to 120,000 cases diagnosed annually in the U.S. It is also the most frequent killer among women with cancer (about 40,000 deaths annually). Despite the fact that fewer than 10% of women will present with advanced cancer initially, still 40% of patients will develop metastatic cancer, and virtually all patients with metastatic breast cancer ultimately die of their disease. Since Beatson's original description of bilateral oophorectomy as treatment for premenopausal women with breast cancer, a variety of hormone therapies have been examined.

Hormone therapy for breast cancer largely depends on the menopausal status, presence of estrogen receptors and progesterone receptors, tumor stage, and histologic differentiation. Hormonal therapy is an effective form of treatment for patients with primary and metastatic breast cancer.

In 1985, the NCI (National Cancer Institute) Consensus Conference provided the guidelines for treatment of patients with breast cancer according to their menopausal status and lymph node involvement.[84]

Premenopausal

Node positive: combination chemotherapy, or combination hormone therapy (oophorectomy and tamoxifen, tamoxifen alone)

Node negative: adjuvant therapy not generally recommended; adjuvant chemotherapy or hormonotherapy should be considered only for high risk patients

Postmenopausal

Node positive: hormone receptors (ER, PR) positive: tamoxifen, (Nolvadex)

Node positive: hormone receptors (ER, PR) negative: combination chemotherapy or hormonotherapy should be considered, but not recommended as standard practice

Node negative: no indication for routine adjuvant therapy; for high risk patients, adjuvant therapy may be considered

More recently, NCI reviewed its previous guidelines and now recommends chemotherapy for all node-negative breast cancer patients regardless of their status (high risk), which stirs

TABLE 2
Hormones and Hormone Antagonists Commonly Used in Cancer Treatment

Drug (synonyms)	Dose, route, schedule (when used as single agent)	Side-effects (toxicity)
Androgens		
Fluoxymesterone (Halotestin)	10—40 mg/d p.o.	Virilization, hirsutism, voice change, clitoral hypertrophy, amenorrhea, edema; increased appetite and weight gain; hypercalcemia, especially those with bone metastases; cholestatic jaundice and rarely peliosis hepatis; dosage reduction required for hepatic dysfunction; gynecomastia
Testosterone propioniate (Oreton)	50—100 mg i.m., t.i.w.	Androgen therapy should be carefully monitored and dosage reduced in patients with renal, hepatic, and cardiovascular impairments; injectable products are poorly soluble and patients may become sensitized to oil carriers
Testosterone enantheate (Delatestryl)	600—1200 mg i.m., q.w.	
Testolactone (Teslac)	250 mg q.i.d., p.o. or 100 mg i.m., t.i.w.	
Calusterone (Methosarb)	40 mg q.i.d., p.o.	
Methyltestosterone (Metandren)	100—200 mg/d p.o.	
Dromostanolone propionate (Drolban)	100 mg i.m., t.i.w.	
Antiandrogens		
Cyproterone acetate (CPA)	100 mg t.i.d.	Few side effects (gynecomastia, impotence)
Flutamide (Eulexin)	750—1500 mg/d p.o.	
Anandron	200—300 mg/d p.o.	Gynecomastia
Ketoconazole	200—400 mg t.i.d., p.o.	Nausea, asthma, hepatotoxicity
Estrogens		
Diethylstilbestrol (DES, stilbesteron)	1—3 mg/d p.o. (prostate cancer); 5 mg t.i.d. (breast cancer)	Feminization, gynecomastia, endometrial hypertrophy, uterine bleeding; hypercalcemia and thromboembolic complications; nipple pigmentation; nausea, vomiting, and liver dysfunction (with high doses); most serious hypercalcemia in patients with metastatic bone cancer; most of these side effects are dose-related
Fosfestrol (Diethylstilbestrol diphosphate, Honvan)	50—200 mg t.i.d., p.o.; 500—1000 mg i.v. × 5 d, then 250—1000 mg i.v. q. wk	
Chlorotrianisene (TACE)	12—25 mg p.o., t.i.d.	
Conjugated equine estrogenic compound (Premarin)	1—10 mg t.i.d., p.o.	
Ethinyl Estradiol (Estinyl)	0.5—1 mg t.i.d., p.o.	
Antiestrogens		
Tamoxifen citrate (Nolvadex)	10—80 mg q.d., p.o. (divided doses); (20—40 mg for breast cancer)	Hypercalcemia; transient "flare" in bone metastases; mild estrogenic activity, vaginal discharge, corneal opacity, and retinopathy with high dose >240 mg/d 1 year
4-hydroxytamoxifen (Nafoxidine)	90—240 mg q.d., p.o.	
Progestins		
Hydroxyprogesterone caproate (Delalutin)	1—2.5 g i.m., b.i.w. or 5 g/q. wk.	Generally well tolerated; mild edema, nausea, vomiting, occasionally hypercalcemia, dyspnea, thromboembolism; use with care in patients with liver dysfunction, allergy to oil carrier

TABLE 2 (continued)
Hormones and Hormone Antagonists Commonly Used in Cancer Treatment

Drug (synonyms)	Dose, route, schedule (when used as single agent)	Side-effects (toxicity)
Medroxyprogesterone acetate (Provera) (p.o.)	20—200 mg q.d., p.o. or 1000—1500 mg i.m./d	
Depo-Provera (i.m.)	200—800 mg i.m., b.i.w.	
Megestrol acetate (Megace)	40—320 mg q.d., p.o. (160 mg q.d. for breast cancer)	
Danazol (Danocrine)	300—800 mg q.d., p.o.	Mild androgenic effects (acne, hirsutism, change in voice); hypoestrogenic effects; hepatic dysfunction; vomiting, muscle cramps, and skin rash
Aromatase inhibitors		
Aminoglutethimide (Cytadren)	250 mg q.i.d., p.o.	Lethargy, dizziness, orthostatic hypotension, hypothyroidism and virilization; skin rash, mild androgenic effects, nausea, vomiting
4-Hydroxyandrostenedione (4-OHA)	250 mg q.d., p.o. 500 mg b.i. wk. i.m.	
Trilostane	240—900 mg/d	
Corticosteroids		
Hydrocortisone (Hydrocortone; Cortef)	20—240 mg/q.d., p.o. 15—240 mg/q.d. i.m. or i.v.	Edema, hypertension, hypokalemia, sodium and fluid retention; emotional lability, euphoria, psychosis
Sodium succinate (Solu-Cortef)	100—500 mg q.d., i.v. or i.m.	
Prednisone (Deltasone)	40—80 mg q.d., p.o.	Sodium and fluid retention; gastrointestinal irritation and bleeding; should be administered with antacids
Prednisolone	40—80 mg q.d., p.o.	
Methylprednisolone (Medrol)	10—25 mg i.v. or i.m.	Immunosuppression and risk of infection
Sodium succinate (Solu-Medrol)	10—40 mg i.v. or i.m.; large doses: 30 mg/kg i.v.	Edema, hypertension, hypokalemic alkalosis, myalgia, arthralgia, osteoporosis, GI bleeding, peptic ulcer
Acetate (Depo-Medrol)	50—100 mg i.v. or i.m., q.d.	Hyperglycemia, diabetes mellitus, hyperlipidemia
Dexamethasone (Decadron)	0.5—12 mg/q.d., p.o. or i.m.; i.v.	Cushingoid symptoms; acne, osteoporosis, aseptic necrosis; glaucoma, cataracts
LHRH agonists		
Leuprolide (Lupron)	1 mg q.d., s.c. or monthly depot	Hot flashes, occasionally gynecomastia, nausea, vomiting; transient flare in prostate cancer; should be contraindicated in patients with spinal cord compression or bilateral hydronephrosis
Buserelin (Receptal)	300—500 μg/q.d., s.c. up to 1 month; then 1200 μg intranasally i.n., q.d.	
Goserelin (Zoladex)	250 μg/q.d., s.c. or depot 3.6 mg/month	
Nafarelin	100 μg/q.d., s.c. or 600 μg/q.d., i.n.	
Tryptorelin (Decapeptyl)	500—1000 μg/q.d./7 d; then 250 μg/q.d., s.c.	
Somatostatin (Sandostatin)	200—300 μg/q.d., s.c.; high doses: 450—1500 μg/q.d., s.c.	No allergic reactions, gastrointestinal reactions, abdominal cramps, diarrhea and steatorrhea; may impair postprandial glucose tolerance, cholelithiasis
L-Thyroxine (T_4) sodium (Synthroid)	200—350 μg/q.d., p.o.; i.v. for suppression therapy: 1.56 μg/kg body weight for 7 d	Headache, irritability, tachycardia, menstrual disorders; may induce or aggravate: angina pectoris arrhythmia, congestive heart failure, and diabetes mellitus

TABLE 2 (continued)
Hormones and Hormone Antagonists Commonly Used in Cancer Treatment

Drug (synonyms)	Dose, route, schedule (when used as single agent)	Side-effects (toxicity)
L-triiodothyronine (T₃) sodium (Cytomel)	25—100 µg/q.d., p.o.	
L-thyroxine sodium αL- L-triiodothyromnine sodium (Thyrolar)	6.25—75 µg/q.d., p.o.	
Antiprolactins		
Bromocriptine Mesylate (Parlodel)	2.5 mg b.i.d.	Hypertension, severe headaches, seizures

a lot of controversies among practicing physicians due to the toxic effect of chemotherapy. Further studies are clearly indicated to resolve this dilemma. However, early results from a number of controlled clinical trials, such as the Nolvadex adjuvant trial (NATO), the Scottish trial, and North American National Surgical American Breast Project, reported similar therapeutic results in both premenopausal and postmenopausal patients following adjuvant hormone therapy. These are (1) most women with node-negative breast cancer will not relapse, (2) those women at higher risk for early relapse can be predicted by currently available prognostic markers, and (3) adjuvant hormonal or chemotherapy can prevent or delay some of the relapses seen in this high-risk group. It is noted that almost 20 to 30% of unselected and randomized patients will respond to endocrine therapy, and approximately 50 to 60% may respond in women with ER-positive tumors, and almost 70 to 80% in women with both ER and PR positive tumors. It is also clear that patients who respond to one hormonal agent have a higher likelihood of responding to subsequent hormone therapy than do nonresponders. However, both the duration and response rate tend to decrease with each successive trial.[41]

Thus, the method of choice for premenopausal women with node-positive tumors is ablative hormone therapy (bilateral oophorectomy or castration). The overall response rate in unselected cases is about 25 to 35% in premenopausal women to either surgical or irradiation-induced castration; the median duration of response is 9 to 12 months, but responses lasting 25 years have also been reported. As mentioned previously, the response rate can be increased to 55% by performing oophorectomy to patients with ER-positive receptor only, and to 78% by restricting oophorectomy to ER-positive and PR-positive patients.[25] The response rate is low, less than 10% in ER-negative women. Also, in perimenopausal and postmenopausal women, the regression rate is lower than that seen in women with ovarian function. Surgical castration is generally preferred, as ovarian radiation gives similar results, but can require 2 months to several months to be effective, and residual ovarian function due to incomplete destruction may be observed. The metastatic sites likely to respond to oophorectomy as well as to other hormone therapies include bone, soft tissue, lymph nodes, and lung. Brain and liver metastases rarely respond. Contraindications to surgical castration are uncontrolled central nervous system metastases, massive hepatic metastases, uncontrolled hypercalcemia, myelophthisic anemia, more than 1 year postmenopausal, hemorrhagic pleural effusion, and ER-negative receptor status.

Until recently, oophorectomy was the treatment of choice for premenopausal women, but now is challenged by the antiestrogen tamoxifen. Recently, tamoxifen has been used in treating premenopausal women with recurrent breast cancer, and its efficacy has been proven to be equal to that of oophorectomy. In comparative trials, tamoxifen has been as effective as alternative endocrine treatments, and has greatly reduced toxicity with no irreversible side effects.[85] Thus, tamoxifen should be used as primary therapy and oophorectomy restricted to those patients who have not previously responded to tamoxifen. Premenopausal women with positive axillary nodes and postmenopausal women with positive and negative axillary nodes were randomized either to an untreated control group or to receive 10 mg of tamoxifen twice daily for 2 years. The Nolvadex Adjuvant Trial Organization was able to report a significant improvement in the disease-free interval in the tamoxifen-treated group and a significant improvement was reported in absolute survival.[86] There were 34% fewer deaths in the tamoxifen-treated group than in the untreated controls. The benefit seemed to be independent of menopausal, nodal, or ER status. Other trials also showed a response rate of about 30%, comparable with that seen with oophorectomy in this patient population. It has also been shown that those women who progressed after a response to tamoxifen had a relatively high likelihood of response to subsequent oophorectomy compared to nonresponders. Other randomized trials of tamoxifen and oophorectomy in premenopausal women yielded similar response and overall survival rates with the two modes of therapy.

The initial hormone therapy with tamoxifen for metastatic breast cancer in 85 premenopausal patients revealed a 27% complete (CR) and partial response (PR) or 43% including patients who remained stable (ST) (CR + PR + ST). Serial FSH, prolactin, and estradiol level determination suggested that tamoxifen does not act by changing prolactin levels in premenopausal patients. Tamoxifen is a nonsteroidal antiestrogen that binds to estrogen receptors and forms an inert complex, thus blocking estradiol effects on the target organs. The usual dose of tamoxifen ranges from 20 to 40 mg/d, and has an excellent tolerance. No dose-response relationship has been identified. The drug is available as a monocitrate salt (Nolvadex). A dose of 10 to 20 mg, twice daily, is usually used and is now considered as a standard dose. Its pharmacokinetics, mechanism of action, and therapeutic effects will be discussed later. Despite the fact that tamoxifen is as effective as oophorectomy for frequency of response and the duration of disease control, the drug does not block completely the effects of circulating estrogens, even used up to a dose of 40 mg/d. Consequently, these patients should be treated with tamoxifen and then have bilateral oophorectomy. The response to bilateral oophorectomy in premenopausal women that respond to tamoxifen is significantly higher (50 to 60%) compared with a response rate of 15 to 20% in patients who did not respond to the drug.[85]

Chemotherapy should be preferred only in patients with rapidly progressive disease or extensive visceral metastases. Trials using combined chemotherapy and tamoxifen or chemohormonotherapy are now underway and initially reveal that the effectiveness of this combination is related to the quantitative levels of both ER and PR. However, in women younger than 50 years old, no difference was seen, regardless of receptor concentration. The rationale for the use of the combination is based on the facts that: (1) tumors are heterogenous (breast cancers are composed of different proportions of receptor positive and receptor negative cells); (2) there is a differential response between receptor positive and receptor negative cells to cytotoxic chemotherapy and hormone therapy; and (3) neither hormonal therapy nor chemotherapy interferes with the action of the other form of treatment. There is a well-documented differential response between ER + and ER − cells to hormonal therapy, but it is not sure if there is also a differential response to chemotherapy or if cytotoxic chemotherapy kills ER + and ER − cells indiscriminately. Thus, the standard hormonal approach to the patient with metastatic breast cancer in the premenopausal status and positive hormone receptors (ER +, PR +) is oophorectomy, followed by tamoxifen or aminoglutethimide, and later megestrol or fluoxymesterone. If there is no response to oophorectomy or tamoxifen alone or combined, then cytotoxic chemotherapy should be administered.[25] Megestrol acetate, 160 mg/d or fluoxymesterone (Halotestin), 10 to 30 mg/d given orally, also may be useful in this situation. Aminoglutethimide (AG) appears to be equally effective in suppression of estrogen synthesis in premenopausal women who had a prior oophorectomy. The recommended dosage of AG is 250 mg b.i.d. for 14 d, to be increased to four times a day; plus 100 mg of Cortisol (20 mg in the morning, 20 mg at 5 p.m., and 60 mg at bedtime).

However, due to its more toxic side effects than those of tamoxifen, Megace or oophorectomy, AG assumes a tertiary role in hormonal therapy. To date, there are no convincing data that the simple addition of tamoxifen to a chemotherapeutic regimen, such as CMF (cyclophosphamide, methotrexate, and 5-fluorouracil) or CAF (cyclophosphamide, Adriamycin, and 5-fluorouracil), has increased the response rate or duration of response over that of either regimen alone.[25] In premenopausal women with metastatic breast cancer and negative hormonal status (ER −, PR −), combination chemotherapy is the method of choice. Also, if the disease is potentially life-threatening, such as lymphangitic lung metastasis and massive hepatic metastases, the patient should be directly treated with cytotoxic chemotherapy because of its more rapid onset of action, regardless of the receptor status.

Until recently, in premenopausal patients with node negative, the adjuvant therapy was not generally recommended; only for high risk patients, adjuvant chemotherapy or hormonotherapy should be recommended. The group of high-risk patients includes women with: (1) negative hormone receptors (ER −, PR −), (2) a larger primary tumor size (≥2.5 cm), (3) a poor nuclear grade and poorly differentiated tumor, (4) aneuploidy, diploidy with a high S-phase and high oncogene amplification, (HER-2/neu), and (5) a family history of breast cancer. More recently, the National Cancer Institute has recommended adjuvant chemotherapy or hormonal therapy for all patients, regardless of lymph node status, the exact treatment being based on estrogen- and progesterone-receptor status.

Adjuvant chemotherapy has been an integral part of the treatment of breast cancer since 1974, and several reports have confirmed the benefits of adjuvant medical treatment with either chemotherapy or hormonal therapy.[49] However, the therapeutic benefits of adjuvant therapy for premenopausal women with node-negative tumors is not well established, since 20 to 30% of patients with negative nodes will relapse and die within 10 years after diagnosis. Thus far, no single prognostic factor or constellation of factors can reliably distinguish these patients from the larger group of patients who are cured without adjuvant therapy.[87] The most commonly used adjuvant chemotherapy is CMF and CAF. Additional benefits of the use of doxorubicin, vincristine, prednisone, CMFVP, or higher doses of chemotherapy do not provide more therapeutic benefits, but merely increase the toxic effects. Combination chemotherapy in sequence with hormonal therapy achieves a greater effect. Thus, combination of chemotherapy and oophorectomy provided a longer duration of disease control of 53 weeks compared to 17 weeks for oophorectomy alone.[24]

Surgery remains an integral part of the treatment of primary breast cancer, for local control ranging from excisional biopsy to mastectomy. The Halsted radical mastectomy has been replaced by the modified radical mastectomy, and more recently by segmental mastectomy. At present, surgical ablative endocrine therapy has largely given way to medical castration.

The treatment of choice for postmenopausal patients with node-positive tumors and positive hormone receptors (ER, PR) is tamoxifen. Tamoxifen has been extremely valuable in the management of postmenopausal breast cancer where the overall response rate is about 40% in the unselected cases and reaches a 75% response rate in ER-positive patients. Soft tissue and bone metastases are more likely to respond, requiring several weeks before becoming apparent.

A comprehensive review of 45 studies on tamoxifen treatment in 2889 patients showed that the overall response rate was 34%, with less than 7% achieving a complete response. Response rate ranged from 14 to 57%, depending on patient selection and prognostic variables in determining treatment outcome. Previously untreated patients had a response rate of 43%. Those who had responded to prior hormone therapy responded in nearly 60% of the cases, while hormone nonresponders had only a 21% response rate. The response rate was not affected by previous chemotherapy and 41% of patients chemotherapeutically treated responded to tamoxifen.[88] Because of its efficacy and lack of toxicity, tamoxifen is the agent of choice for endocrine therapy in postmenopausal patients. Only minor side effects, including nausea, vomiting, leukopenia, and thrombocytopenia, occurred in 10 to 15% of patients, and dose modification was rarely required. Retinitis and hypercalcemia may occur, especially in patients with extensive bone disease or following high doses, and careful monitoring of these patients is required. Thus, antiestrogen therapy with tamoxifen has replaced additive hormone therapy as well as adrenalectomy and hypophysectomy as the first-line hormonal treatment in postmenopausal women, and it may replace oophorectomy in premenopausal women. Antiestrogens are also being studied in the treatment of a variety of hormone-responsive tumors, such as prostate carcinoma, endometrium, and kidney cancers.

The standard dose of tamoxifen is usually 20 mg (10 mg b.i.d. or 20 mg q.d.) and no dose-response relationship has been identified; doses up to 90 mg have no advantage.[85] A randomized trial of diethylstilbestrol (DES) and tamoxifen showed response rates of 41% and 33%, respectively; however 12% of DES-treated patients stopped therapy because of adverse reactions, whereas no patients in the tamoxifen-treated group stopped therapy because of toxicity.[8] Trials comparing aminoglutethimide (AG) with tamoxifen showed a response rate of 30 to 36% for AG as compared to 30 to 38% for tamoxifen, again with greater toxicity in the AG-treated patients.

Studies comparing tamoxifen with high-dose progestational agents, particularly megestrol acetate (Megace), also document equivalent response rates of nearly 30%, and toxicity for both drugs is similar, suggesting that progestins may be acceptable first-line agents as well. However, the need to be administered four times daily (q.i.d.), makes them less convenient than tamoxifen, which can be administered once a day (q.d.). Also a major metabolite of tamoxifen, 4-hydroxytamoxifen, is at least ten times as potent as tamoxifen, has a relative affinity to that of estradiol, and can antagonize the effect of plasma estrogens, even in premenopausal women. A recent trial with tamoxifen alone in operable breast cancer was used as an adjuvant therapy in 433 patients with stage I, II, or III (T3a), or in combination with cyclophosphamide, methotrexate, and fluorouracil (CMF). Thus, 308 premenopausal node-negative and postmenopausal node-negative or node-positive patients were randomized and received either tamoxifen in doses of 30 mg for 2 years or no therapy; 125 premenopausal node-positive patients were randomized to receive either CMF plus tamoxifen, or CMF alone. After a median followup of 63 months, tamoxifen reduced significantly the incidence of relapses and deaths compared with no therapy.

Despite intense study, tamoxifen's mechanism of action is unclear. Pharmacokinetic studies using radiolabeled tamoxifen have shown that ^{3}H-estradiol is displaced from the estrogen receptor sites. Because the action of tamoxifen requires binding with ER, it is ineffective in ER-negative cases. The complex of ER and tamoxifen is then translocated to the nuclear chromatin (DNA) where the biochemical effects of estrogen action are inhibited by mechanisms still not elucidated. Distinct antiestrogen binding sites have been described. These sites have limited affinity for estrogens and do not translocate from cytoplasm to nucleus. *In vitro* studies regarding the effect of tamoxifen on cancer cell lines from patients with hormone-dependent breast cancer have shown that the effect depends on the drug concentration. At low concentrations, tamoxifen exerts a cytostatic effect, by which ER-positive cells are blocked by the drug in the early G_1 phase of the cell cycle. At higher concentrations of tamoxifen (more than 4 μg) it has cytotoxic effects characterized by cell death of both ER-positive and ER-negative cells, and this effect is not reversed by estrogens.[89] Interestingly, tamoxifen has mild estrogenic effects at low concentrations. Some premenopausal women continue to have normal menstrual cycles throughout therapy, concurrent with objective tumor regression; sometimes a "flare" of tumor growth, occasionally leading to hypercalcemia, can be seen. This curious phenomenon, characterized by increased bone or soft pain and occasionally hypercalcemia, occurs in approximately 10% of cases. When a tamoxifen flare occurs, it develops in the first few weeks of therapy and generally heralds a response to treatment. Flares should be treated with analgesics or other symptomatic therapy, and the full dose tamoxifen should be continued.

In postmenopausal patients with node-positive tumors, but negative hormone receptors (ER−, PR−), chemotherapy or chemohormonotherapy should be considered, but not recommended as standard procedures. In addition to antiestrogens (tamoxifen), other additive hormone therapies with estrogens, androgens, progestins, corticosteroids, Danazol, LHRH agonists, and somatostatin should be considered.

i. Estrogens

Prior to the introduction of tamoxifen, diethylstilbestrol (DES), a synthetic estrogen, and conjugated estrogen (Premarin) were the hormonal treatments of choice in postmenopausal women with advanced breast cancer. Now, ethinyl estradiol (Estinyl) is included in this group.

The overall random response to estrogens is 36%, and the overall response rate to DES in ER-positive tumors is 63%. In general, the median duration of response to estrogen is 12 to 18 months, but responses longer than 5 years have been seen. Remission rates are less than 10% in patients who underwent adrenalectomy or hypophysectomy. The antitumor response to estrogens is quite slow, requiring several weeks, and is primarily confined to metastases in the skin, lymph nodes, breast, and bone lesions. The most commonly used preparations are DES, premarin, and estinyl. DES remains the most commonly used, in the dosage of 5 mg t.i.d. Other preparations are Premarin 10 mg t.i.d. and Estinyl, 3 mg/d (1 mg t.i.d.). In breast cancer, the effects of estrogen appear to be dose dependent. Recently, a sequential cyclic hormonal therapy consisting of 50 μg of ethinyl estradiol given orally and daily for 7 d, followed by 400 mg of medroxyprogesterone acetate given orally for 21 d, followed by 7 d of rest, was used in postmenopausal patients with metastatic breast cancer. From 30 patients, 17 patients had either a complete response (CR, 6 patients) or a partial response (PR, 11 patients). Median remission duration was 22 months. Thus, cyclic sequential therapy was effective and well tolerated.[90]

The mechanism of action of high-dose estrogens is unknown. It is possible to decrease the prolactin secretions, but there is evidence that suggests a direct effect of the high-dose estrogens on the cancer cells. Numerous toxicities have been reported. Nausea is the most common early side effect of DES. Vomiting, anorexia, and even diarrhea may occur, but usually subside within two weeks. Increased nipple, areolar and axillary pigmentation is frequent. Fluid retention and edema occur in one third of cases and may aggravate or even precipitate congestive heart failure. The use of high doses of estrogens may be associated with thromboembolic phenomena. Vaginal and uterine bleeding may occur in 40% of patients and can be controlled by administration of progestins. Persistent uterine bleeding may signal the presence of endometrial carcinoma. Hypercalcemia may occur in 10 to 25% of women with metastatic breast cancer, especially with widespread bone metastases, and may herald a higher response rate because the tumor retained its endocrine responsiveness. Patients who respond to estrogen therapy and who later escape from the therapeutic effect with progression of metastatic disease may respond to the sudden withdrawal of estrogens with another period of tumor regression (estrogen rebound regression). The duration of rebound regression is usually 3 to 10 months, but duration of regression in excess of 18 months was also reported.

ii. Androgens

Androgens have been used in the treatment of metastatic breast cancer for over 30 years. Several cases with metastatic breast cancer who responded favorably with tumor regression following androgen treatment were reported at about the same time in different countries (England, France, Argentina, and the U.S.). The androgen chosen is testosterone propionate given i.m. in a dose of 100 mg three times a week (Oreton, Neo-Hombreol). When oral treatment is preferred, one may choose between fluoxymesterone (Halotestin) as 10 to 40 mg/d in divided doses, and testolactone (Teslac) given i.m. in a dose of 100 mg/d, three times weekly, or orally in a dose of 250 mg q.i.d. (four times daily). Their effects may not be apparent for 6 to 12 weeks. Androgens display their antitumor effect in receptor-positive patients with breast cancer by: (1) blocking the pituitary gonadotropin release and consequently the estrogen secretion, and (2) producing an antiestrogenic effect. Testolactone (Teslac) blocks the peripheral conversion of androgenic precursors to estrogens (aromatization). The response rate to androgens is lower than that seen with other endocrine therapies, e.g., 21% in one study of testosterone propionate administered to 521 women. It was less than 10% in perimenopausal patients and highest in postmenopausal women. The median duration of remission was about 8 months. The response of bone metastases to androgen is equivalent to that for estrogens (25 to 30%), but the response rate of soft tissue metastases (breast, skin, nodes) to androgens (20 to 25%) is significantly less than that of estrogens (35 to 40%).[49] Thus, metastatic bone disease should be considered the primary indication for the use of androgens. The most undesirable and frequent effects of androgen therapy are virilization of female patients, including hirsutism, acne, change of voice, hypertrophy of clitoris, amenorrhea, fluid retention, and increased libido. They occur in more than 50% of patients treated with testosterone propionate, in 35 to 40% of patients treated with fluoxymesterone, and in none treated with testolactone. Androgens may precipitate acute and severe hypercalcemia in patients with breast cancer and bone metastases; in approximately 10% of these patients this represents an oncologic emergency. In addition to discontinuation of therapy, a rigorous hydration is required. Three androgens, testolactone, stanozolol, and danazol, cause minimal virilization.[91] Methylated androgens have been associated with peliosis hepatis, hepatic adenomas, and very rarely hepatomas. Most comparative trials reveal a superiority of estrogens in postmenopausal women (29>10%) especially for soft tissue metastases. Despite their adverse effects, the subjective, hematopoietic, and anabolic effects of androgens are notable. Androgens stimulate erythropoiesis probably via erythropoietin. Patients treated with androgens may experience euphoria, pain relief, increased appetite, and weight gain, despite progression of disease.

iii. Progestins

The progestins have emerged as the clear second choice, after tamoxifen, in the additive hormonal therapy of endocrine responsive breast cancer in postmenopausal women. Although the response rates in ER+, PR+ patients appear to be equivalent to those for tamoxifen, the disease-free survival of patients treated initially with tamoxifen is significantly greater than those treated with megestrol acetate (Megace). The side effects of progestins are minimal, and they have an improved efficacy in high doses.

It is possible that progestational agents exert an antitumor effect by binding to progesterone receptor, interfering with estrogen receptor, and causing synthesis and effects on the immune system. Progestins appear to have a direct cytotoxic effect on human breast cancer cells in long-term tissue culture. Progestins exert their antiestrogenic effects by decreasing ER concentrations. They are more active in PR positive patients. It has also been shown that progestins will compete for androgen receptors and progesterone receptors sites on cell membranes. Regressions are seen more frequently in tumors containing large amounts of AR.[45] Progestins are largely catabolized in the liver, and their metabolites are excreted in the urine. The usual preparations are medroxyprogesterone acetate (MPA) and megestrol acetate (Megace). MPA is given in doses of 100 mg, three times weekly i.m. or in high-dose regimen of 1000 to 1500 mg/d i.m., which may be associated with higher response rate. Using a schedule of 1 g MPA i.m. for 10 d and an oral maintenance treatment of 200 mg/d three times/d, the median survival time was significantly longer for responders (19.9 months). Although a higher proportion of postmenopausal patients responded, the remission duration in premenopausal women was remarkably long. Favorable sites of response were soft tissue, lymph nodes, and bone lesions. The dose of Megace is 40 mg q.i.d., although a single oral dose of 160 mg daily appears to be well tolerated and to have comparable therapeutic effects. Progestins may exhibit a dose-response curve.

Response rates of 20 to 30% have been observed and may be seen in patients previously treated with other hormones. Responses, when they occur, can last for about 12 to 14 months. Improvement is most marked in patients with soft tissue metastases; bone metastases rarely regress. Megestrol acetate (Megace), is an orally active synthetic progestational steroid which exerts important anticancer activity and is active in other diseases as well.[92]

Tumors	Other disease
Malignant melanoma	Benigh prostatic hypertrophy (BPH)
Endometrial carcinoma	Cachexia and anorexia
Breast cancer	Endometrial hyperplasia
Ovarian cancer	Contraception
Prostate cancer	Euphoria, gain in weight
Renal cancer (hypernephroma)	

Progestins have no side effects, or they are minimal. Fluid retention and weight gain occur in some patients. Hypercalcemic and pain flares have also been reported with megestrol acetate and may herald a response to treatment.[47,92]

iv. Corticosteroids (Glucocorticoids)

There are only limited indications for the use of glucocorticoids as primary agents for metastatic breast cancer. High doses of corticosteroids equivalent to 200 to 300 mg of cortisol/d induce a 10 to 15% response rate in metastatic breast cancer. Specific tumor responses appear to be limited to premenopausal women patients with prior response to castration or to postmenopausal women with a prior response to other additive hormone therapies. Corticoids are often used in combination with cytotoxic agents, but this combination chemotherapy remains questionable. Large doses of corticosteroid should not be used in the routine treatment of metastatic breast cancer due to their toxicity. Because of the low response rate and numerous side effects of chronic therapy, corticoids should be used only as: (1) supportive treatment for acute hypercalcemia medical management, brain or spinal cord metastases, increased intracranial pressure (a dose of dexamethasone, 8 mg i.v., followed by 4 mg i.v. or orally q.i.d.), jaundice from hepatic metastases, and dyspnea from pulmonary involvement; (2) treatment in conjunction with chemotherapy; or (3) treatment of fast-growing tumors for a short time only. It is possible that corticosteroids exert their action by binding to intracellular receptors. Corticosteroid may be useful as palliative therapy in terminally ill patients.

Side effects of chronic corticosteroid therapy are numerous. They cause leukocytosis, reduction in circulating eosinophils, and lymphocytes. They inhibit inflammation and are immunosuppressive. Glucocorticoids can induce fluid and electrolyte imbalances (edema and hypokalemia) and steroid myopathies and osteoporosis. Psychosis and exacerbation of diabetes mellitus and hypertension may also occur. A small percent (1.8%) may develop peptic ulcers while on corticosteroids. Patients receiving a short-term therapy can be discontinued abruptly; however, patients who have been on corticosteroids for a long time should be progressively withdrawn because they may subsequently suffer unusual withdrawal symptoms.

v. Danazol

Danazol is a relatively nontoxic synthetic steroid used in the treatment of endometriosis and benign breast disease (chronic cystic mastopathy). Its mode of action is partly due to inhibition of gonadotropin secretion, but it can also bind to the progesterone and androgen receptors. It also inhibits steroid synthesis[63,65] and the action of estrone sulfatase. In premenopausal women, danazol causes amenorrhea. It has been reported that there is a 66% objective response rate to danazol in the treatment of DMBA-induced mammary cancers in rats, in the same doses of 100 to 200 mg t.i.d. (the same range as treatment of chronic cystic mastopathy). From 67 patients treated with danazol at doses between 30 mg/d and 600 mg/d, only 15% responded to therapy, and a further 9% showed stabilization of disease. From 14 premenopausal patients, only one responded compared to 9 from 53 postmenopausal women. Therefore, danazol doses not seem sufficiently good to be used as first- or second-line therapy.[20,65,91]

vi. LHRH Agonists

Since the LHRH analogs act directly or indirectly on the pituitary, the gonads, and the target organs of the sex steroids, it has been demonstrated that there is a significant decrease in tumor weight and volume of mouse and rat mammary cancers treated with decapeptyl (D-Trp^6-LH-RH).[67] Leuprolide was first used in premenopausal women with advanced breast cancer, and objective responses were reported in 11 of 25 cases treated with leuprolide; sometimes leuprolide or zoladex (depot), a long-acting analog, did indeed induce a complete "medical castration".[69] This indicates that ovarian suppression by the analogs is the mechanism whereby they cause tumor regression in premenopausal women with breast cancer.

Preliminary data from different studies using Buserelin as a nasal spray in premenopausal and postmenopausal women with breast cancer have been favorable. Eight of seventeen premenopausal women had an objective response to Buserelin alone or in combination with tamoxifen. Also, a collected series from the literature indicates an overall objective response rate of 11% in 84 postmenopausal women. Encouraging results by using depot preparation (Zoladex) in doses of 3.6 mg/month in 4/10 premenopausal women have been seen. Buserelin (Receptal), which is a substituted decapeptide D-Ser[TBU]^6-LHRH, Ethylamide, is given in a dose of 1200 μg/d intranasally or 300 to 500 μg/d s.c. In some studies, leuprolide, 1 mg/d, resulted in a 44% response rate in a group of 25 premenopausal women patients with metastatic breast cancer.[69] Intranasal spray may cause incomplete suppression of the pituitary-gonadal axis. Also, LHRH agonist would be effective in the treatment of male breast cancer because it inhibits testicular production of androgens and thus, less of this hormone to be converted to estrogens. Hence, long-term LHRH analog treatment must be considered as being more acceptable to orchiectomy.

vii. Somatostatin

Somatostatin analogs possess significant antitumor activity in experimental tumors, including rat DMBA mammary carcinomas. Clinical trials of somatostatin analogues in human breast cancer are now initiated.[93]

Male breast cancer—This is a rare disease in men, accounting for less than 1% of all breast carcinomas and less than 1.5% of all malignant tumors in men. There are predisposing familial factors, altered estrogen metabolism, idiopathic gynecomastia, and Klinefelter's syndrome.[94] Several reports have confirmed a high frequency of ER and PR in male breast cancer tissue. The disease is similar to female in the histologic pattern, clinical prevention, and tendency to metastasize to bone. Therapeutic considerations are also similar. Castration (orchiectomy) is the method of choice.[28] The disease may also respond to diethylstilbestrol (DES), tamoxifen, androgens, LHRH agonists, adrenalectomy, and hypophysectomy. Thus, males with breast cancer should be managed in a similar manner to female breast cancer.

Patients with ER and PR positive (ER + , PR +) tumors and slowly growing disease limited to lymph nodes, bones, and soft tissues should be initially treated with radical mastectomy and endocrine therapy. This usually includes orchiectomy, or DES and tamoxifen are reasonable alternatives. Second-line endocrine therapies would include "medical" adrenalectomy with aminoglutethimide. If these procedures are not sufficient, then chemohormonotherapy or combination chemotherapy as used in female breast cancer should be instituted.

Recent advances in treatment of breast cancer, especially those with node-negative tumors have been reported. In breast cancer, studies indicate that both hormonal therapy and chemotherapy can delay tumor recurrence in that large group of patients with localized disease and negative axillary lymph nodes at the time of initial surgery. Although these women have traditionally been considered to have a relatively favorable prognosis, there are from 67,000 to 81,000 new node-negative patients every year, and approximately 30% will eventually have recurrent disease. Thus, in a recent double-blind manner study, 2644 women with ER-positive and node-negative breast cancer were randomized to receive either tamoxifen or placebo. After a 4-year median followup, disease-free survival was observed in 83% of women who received tamoxifen compared with 77% in women who received placebo. In a second National Surgical Adjuvant Breast and Bowel Project (NSABP) study, ER-negative and node-negative patients were randomly assigned to receive either chemotherapy or observation. The chemotherapy consisted to sequential methotrexate and fluorouracil with leucovorin rescue and treatment began between 2 weeks and 35 d after mastectomy. With a median followup of 4 years, 80% of 368 women in the chemotherapy group were alive and free of disease compared with 71% of 373 women in the control group. In both NSABP studies, the benefits from therapy were apparent in both premenopausal and postmenopausal patients. These studies indicate that adjuvant hormonal therapy or chemotherapy can have a meaningful impact on the natural history of certain node-negative breast cancers. However, these studies did not include women with preinvasive or carcinoma *in situ*, and adjuvant therapy is not considered necessary for these noninvasive cancers. Also, only few patients with small (<1 cm) invasive cancers were included, and consequently there are not sufficient data to indicate whether adjuvant therapy is clearly beneficial for these patients.

b. Prostate Cancer

Prostate cancer is the second most common form of cancer in American men over the age of 50; approximately 99,000 new cases were diagnosed in 1988, and nearly 28,000 deaths from prostate cancer occur annually.[32] It can be estimated that 750,000 males living in the world today will have prostate cancer. The prostate carcinoma is higher among blacks and lower in certain oriental populations. The most common histologic tumor type is adenocarcinoma. The etiology remains unknown at present. No toxic or environmental agents have been implicated. Studies that have focused on the role of viral infection, sexual activity, diet, and occupational exposure have been inconclusive, and the specific cause of prostate cancer remains unknown.[95,96] However, several experimental studies strongly suggest that hormones (androgens, pituitary hormones, and estrogens) play an important role in induction and extinction of prostate carcinoma. Also, recent epidemiologic studies indicate that certain vitamins (A and E) may increase the incidence of prostate cancer.

This cancer is usually discovered by rectal examination or incidentally found on histologic sections of a prostate removed for urinary obstructive symptoms. Approximately 50% of patients have clinically localized disease at presentation. Prostate cancer is a hormone-dependent (androgen-dependent) cancer, and in 75 to 80% of the cases, respond to hormonal therapy. Although benign prostate hyperplasia also increases in incidence with age, there is no indication that it is a necessary step or a proximal cause in the development of prostate cancer.[97] The extent of tumor involvement (stage) is described by a classification system, mainly based on clinical findings, and the system used by the American Urological Association consists of A, B, C, and D stages. One widely accepted classification is the Gleason system, which is based on histologic differentiation of the tumor and its relationship to the prostate stroma. Tumors are assigned to Gleason grades 1 to 5 on the basis of histologic differentiation. The commonly used staging system in the U.S. is A, B, C, and D, or American Urological system: stage A—no palpable lesion; stage B—tumor confined to prostate; stage C— tumor localized to periprostatic area; stage D — metastatic disease present. The TNM (tumor-nodes-metastases) system was developed and usually parallels the A, B, C, and D. Both are based on the digital rectal examination. The treatment and management of prostate cancer is different in: (1) clinically localized prostate cancer, and (2) advanced metastatic prostate cancer.

i. Treatment of Clinically Localized Prostate Cancer

About 50% of patients have clinically localized lesions at presentation. According to a NIH (National Institutes of Health) consensus statement, patients with disease limited to the prostate (stages A_2 and B) are treated with either radical prostatectomy or radiation therapy.[98] Radical prostatectomy is the method of choice and consists of the total excision of the prostate gland with its capsule, seminal vesicles, and ampulla of the vasa deferentia, followed by anastomosis of the bladder neck to the membranous urethra. Recently, the surgical technique has been refined to preserve the nerves essential for potency. Radical prostatectomy may cause a higher incidence of urinary incontinence, but this should not preclude the intervention. The long-term disease-free survival is 90% and the disease-specific mortality is 1% for stage A_2 and 51% with a 15-year disease-free survival for stage B patients. For most patients with stage A_1, no further therapy is generally indicated. Radiation therapy is another form of definitive treatment and is usually given by means of high-energy, externalbeam photons (X-rays) with linear accelerators. Comparison across studies suggest comparable 10-year survival rates with either form of management.

Diagnosis of localized prostate cancer is very important, since the patient with prostate cancer may be asymptomatic at the time of diagnosis. In addition to rectal examination, which is one of the most reliable screening tests, but still misses 20% of tumors that are elsewhere in the prostate other than in the peripheral zone (the zone palpated on rectal examination), other more sensitive imaging methods, such as transrectal ultrasound and computerized axial tomography (CAT), should be used. However, the sensitivity of ultrasound is only between 62% and 65% and cannot be used for screening. CAT scan has a poor resolution and cannot differentiate between malignant and normal prostate; its value is mainly in staging and detecting the presence of lymph node, soft tissue, and bone metastases.

ii. Treatment of Advanced Metastatic Prostate Cancer

Some 80 to 85% of men at diagnosis have regional or distant metastatic disease that is incurable by local treatment with surgery or radiation therapy. For these advanced stages (C and D), hormonotherapy is an effective means of treatment and palliation. Chemohormonotherapy is recommended in patients with poor or mild responses and chemotherapy generally has been used in the patients with advanced hormone-refractory disease. Hormone therapy in the management of early disease is under renewed investigation as an adjuvant to definitive therapy of the primary tumor.[98] Hormonal therapy is the mainstay of treatment of advanced prostatic carcinoma. All hormonal treatments in prostate cancer seek: (1) to reduce androgenic stimulation of prostate carcinoma by ablation of androgen source, (2) to suppress pituitary gonadotropin release, (3) to inhibit androgenic synthesis, and (4) to interfere with androgen action (in target tissues).

The main goal of hormonal therapy in prostate cancer is to deprive the prostate of androgenic stimulation. Removal of circulating androgens by bilateral orchiectomy to eliminate testicular androgens and by adrenalectomy or hypophysectomy to eliminate adrenal androgens was one of the first hormonal manipulations. At present, about 70 to 80% of patients show definite clinical improvement of symptoms of variable duration.[95] The principal circulating androgens secreted by the testes are testosterone and androsterone, while androstenedione and dihydro-3-epiandrosterone are synthesized by the adrenal gland. About 95% of circulating plasma testosterone is produced by the Leydig cells of the testes under the influence of pituitary luteinizing hormone (LH). Testosterone is converted peripherally by 5α-reductase (present in nuclear membrane and endoplasmic reticulum) to dihydrotestosterone (DHT) or by aromatization to estradiol. Over 95% of testosterone and DHT is bound with high affinity to a plasma B-globulin, as sex hormone-binding globulin (SHBG), and only 5% is unbound or free testosterone, which is the active form.

Since 90 to 95% of circulating testosterone is produced by the testes, the usual method to remove it is bilateral orchiectomy, which produces a fall in serum testosterone levels from about 500 to 50 ng/ml. Bilateral orchiectomy is relatively simple and safely accomplished and can be done under local anesthesia. Some prefer subcapsular orchiectomy, which leaves the testicular capsule and epididymis behind, thus lessening the psychologic side effects to the patient. The loss of libido and potency, which usually accompanies castration, is an important factor that affects the life of the patient and his family; this must be taken into account in the physician's decision and timing for hormonal ablative therapy. However, given the side effects of exogenous estrogens, which include fluid retention, nausea and vomiting, gynecomastia, and a tendency toward thromboembolic and cardiovascular complications, simple castration has many advantages. Using objective response criteria in patients with metastatic cancer, it was found that bilateral orchiectomy produced similar effects to estrogens, e.g., diethylstilbestrol (DES); 41% of patients had complete or partial responses in both treatments and an additional 40% of patients had disease stabilization for 12 weeks or more. Pain relief and general status improved in 70% of patients.

Since 1950, it has been conclusively demonstrated that a 5-year control of prostatic cancer is most effectively obtained by the combination of orchiectomy and DES in patients who are free from metastases. When metastases are present, bilateral orchiectomy is significantly more effective than DES. The combination of orchiectomy and DES does not appear to offer any advantage over orchiectomy alone in this group of patients. Thus, it is generally believed that orchiectomy and DES at 3 mg/d are equally effective in rate and duration of response, and there is no conclusive evidence that the combination of orchiectomy and DES is superior to either used alone.

iii. Adrenalectomy

This was introduced in patients who had relapsed following castration or estrogen therapy. The rationale for adrenalectomy was that adrenal androgen secretion increased following orchiectomy, and it is responsible for reactivation of prostatic carcinoma. However, there is considerable evidence to suggest that adrenal androgens do not play a significant role in reactivation of prostatic cancer and that adrenalectomy provides few, if any, therapeutic benefits. Hypophysectomy also produces similarly disappointing results. The rationale for hypophysectomy is removal of the source of ACTH, which stimulates the secretion of adrenal androgens; only a mean survival of 11 months has been reported, and in conclusion, hypophysectomy in the treatment of relapsing prostate cancer is not warranted.

iv. Inhibition of LH-Release Estrogens

Estrogens exert their major effect of prostatic cancer by inhibiting the release of LH from the pituitary, thus, blocking testicular synthesis of testosterone and decreasing testosterone synthesis in the testes. Other effects include a stimulation of TEBG (testosterone-binding globulin); a decrease in pituitary prolactin secretion, which enhances the use of androgens by the prostate; and in very high concentrations, a decrease of DNA synthesis in the prostate. It is possible that estrogens exert a direct cytotoxic effect on prostatic cancer cells. Low levels of estrogen receptors have been identified in the prostate. DES is the estrogen most frequently used in the treatment of prostatic cancer. A dose of 1 mg/d will suppress plasma testosterone to castration levels in about 70% of men, while a dose of 3 mg/d will suppress testosterone to castration levels in all men. Higher doses have no additional effect. Studies by the Veterans' Administration Cooperative Urologic Research Group (VA-CURG) have shown that cardiovascular side effects of DES are dose-related and probably somewhat higher at the 3 mg/d dosage. A history of significant cardiac disease could be a general contraindication to estrogen therapy.

Other estrogen preparations that have been used include chlorotrianisene (TACE), a dose of 12 to 25 mg three times daily (t.i.d.) orally; conjugated equine estrogenic compound (Premarin), a dose of 1 to 10 mg t.i.d. orally; and ethinyl estradiol (Estinyl), 0.5 to 1 mg t.i.d. orally. Estramustine (Estracyt) is a combination of an estrogen with nitrogen mustard and is used solely in patients with advanced prostate cancer refractory to estrogens. A dosage of two 140 mg capsules t.i.d. is usually used for a 60-kg man. This drug is more expensive than DES. Diethylstilbestrol diphosphate (fosfestrol) is a water-soluble estrogen that can be given by intravenous infusion in high doses of 500 to 2000 mg over 1 to 4 h. The rationale for its use is that the phosphate groups are cleaved in prostatic tissue by acid phosphatase, thus exposing the prostate cells directly to high concentrations of estrogens. The results with fosfestrol (Honvan) are controversial. The side effects of estrogens are numerous. Immediate side effects include nausea, vomiting, and fluid retention. More significant long-term side effects include gynecomastia, loss of libido and feminization, hypertension, and the most serious cardiovascular complications including edema, thrombophlebitis, and myocardial infarction.

Megestrol acetate (Megace) is a progestin that inhibits pituitary LH release. It also acts as an antiandrogen by blocking 5α-reductase activity in the prostate, thus inhibiting the conversion of testosterone to DHT, and also by binding to the DHT receptor. The usual doses are 40 to 320 mg/d orally. Megace does not cause fluid retention or increased cardiovascular side effects.

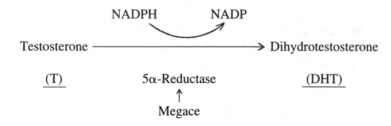

v. LHRH Analogs

Recently, use of the analogs of luteinizing hormone-releasing hormone (LHRH) has attracted considerable attention as an alternate form of endocrine manipulation. The action of LHRH analogs is paradoxical; short administration causes increased release of pituitary LH and subsequently results in a concomitant increase in serum testosterone, whereas a chronic administration of LHRH analogs causes a complete depression of LH and reduces serum testosterone to castrate levels. The mechanism by which LHRH agonists sharply decrease the testosterone level is not clear, but appears to involve: (1) changes in the central feedback control of LH release, (2) desensitization of the testes to LH by reduction in testicular receptor sites, and (3) direct inhibition of testicular androgen synthesis.[99] The most widely applied analogs agonists are Buserelin (D-Ser(TBU)[6] Pro[9] Net LHRH), decapeptyl (D-Trp[6]-LHRH), leuprolide (D-Leu[6]Pro[9] Net LHRH) and Zoladex (D-Ser(TBU)[6]-Aza-Gly[10] LHRH). These agents appear to be as effective as surgical castration (orchiectomy) or conventional treatment with 3 mg of DES, but have a reduced cardiovascular and thromboembolic toxicity. However, other side effects become more troublesome than those with DES (e.g., hot flashes). Gynecomastia does not occur, although loss of libido and impotence are seen as frequently as with DES or castration. Leuprolide (Lupron) has been most extensively used in the U.S. at doses of 1 mg/d or monthly depot. Buserelin (Receptal) given s.c. and i.m. in doses of 300 to 500 μg/d is poorly absorbed; it is used both in the U.S. and Europe. Long-acting preparations, such as Zoladex (250 μg/d given s.c.) or Depot (3.6 mg/month) are also used. A recent study using long-term therapy with Zoladex Depot (optimal dose of 3.6 mg s.c.) in 191 patients with advanced prostatic carcinoma (stages T_3 and T_4) shows overall objective and subjective responses similar to those obtained by castration or estrogen therapy because it maintains long-term castrate levels of testosterone in all patients.[100]

Recently, reports published by Labrie and associates attracted much attention. Patients with advanced prostate cancer (stages C or D) were treated with an LHRH agonist (HOE-766) to achieve surgical castration (by blocking testicular androgens) in combination with a pure antiandrogen (flutamide or its analog anandron) to block the residual prostatic DHT derived from adrenal circulating androgens (5 to 10%). This procedure was called "complete or total androgen blockade" or better-termed, "combined androgen blockade". Positive responses, determined by bone scan and/or prostatic acid phosphatase (PAP) were reported in 97% of previously untreated patients, but only 25% of previously castrated patients showed similar responses with this treatment. Also, with the data available thus far, the death rate at 1 $^1/_2$ years for patients with metastatic prostate cancer and treated with DES or orchiectomy (24 to 37%) is seven to nine times higher than for patients treated by the new approach of complete androgen blockade (3.3%). According to Labrie, complete androgen blockade should be initiated immediately after diagnosis in order to obtain remission in a greater proportion, and to minimize the appearance of androgen-resistant cell clones. Recent studies reviewing the "total androgen blockade" in the treatment of advanced prostatic cancer could not reproduce initial results and do not establish the benefit of total androgen blockade. Thus, the addition of a pure antiandrogen to LHRH analogs or castration in relapsing patients does not bring a very substantial benefit.[72] Others suggest an alternative to the total androgen blockade with LHRH and flutamide by using megestrol acetate and a low-dose of estrogen, which also provides blockade of adrenal as well as testicular androgens, but at lower cost and with greater ease of administration.

vi. Inhibitors of Androgen Synthesis

There are several agents that inhibit the androgen synthesis from cholesterol by inhibiting the five enzymes involved in the synthesis of testosterone from cholesterol and they are listed in Table 3.

Aminoglutethimide (AG) blocks the enzyme 20,21-desmolase, thus inhibiting the side-chain cleavage of cholesterol to pregnenolone and subsequent hydroxylation. This drug blocks not only the androgen synthesis, but that of cortisol and aldosterone as well. The usual dose is 250 mg 4 times a day. Overall responses in patients treated with AG range from 20 to 40%, but sustained objective responses are rare. Chemical adrenalectomy induced by Ag-produced responses is used in patients in whom primary hormonal therapy with orchiectomy or DES has failed. It is better that AG should be administered with hydrocortisone. However, treatment with AG can be toxic, causing orthostatic hypotension, skin rash, hypothyroidism, nausea, lethargy, and dizziness. Cyproterone acetate (CPA), in doses of 100 to 200 mg t.i.d., has multiple actions eliciting both progestational and antiandrogenic effects. In addition to inhibiting gonadotropin release, it acts by inhibiting the binding of DHT to its receptors. A large number of trials, particularly in Europe and the U.S., have been performed and have demonstrated clinical activity when the CPA is used as the first

TABLE 3
Inhibitors of Androgen Synthesis

Drug	Enzyme
Aminoglutethimide	20,21-desmolase
Spironolactone	17,20-desmolase
Ketoconazole	17,20-desmolase
	P-450-dependent
Cyanoketone	3β-hydroxysteroid dehydrogenase
Cyproterone acetate	3β-hydroxysteroid dehydrogenase
17β-Estradiol	an isomerase complex
Hydroxymethylene	3β-hydroxysteroid dehydrogenase
Medrogesterone	an isomerase complex

treatment of metastatic cancer. It has also been used in patients in whom initial hormonal therapy fails.

Flutamide is another antiandrogen drug, recently approved by FDA as Eulexin in the treatment of metastatic prostatic cancer. It is usually administered orally in doses of approximately 750 to 1500 mg/d. Response rates in initial trials appear to be equal to those with DES or orchiectomy, although long-term followup is missing in these trials. Flutamide acts mainly by competing for androgen receptor sites and therefore blocks the dihydrotestosterone-androgen (DHT-AR) complex. The relatively limited side effects of flutamide make it a potentially attractive drug.

Ketoconazole is a nonestrogenic antifungal drug and inhibits several enzymes of androgen synthesis (both testicular and adrenal). In high doses it diminishes serum testosterone levels, and has much less effect on cortisol production. It has also been suggested that a major effect of Ketoconazole is partial inhibition of 17 to 20 desmolase, in the conversion of the C_{21} steroids to C_{19} steroids. Administration of 400 mg Ketoconazole orally t.i.d. caused serum testosterone to fall to castrate level within 24 h. The patients have been followed for 3 to 10 months without relapse and with few side effects (asthenia, dry skin, and very rarely, hepatotoxicity). Since Ketoconazole produces a much more rapid decrease in plasma testosterone than does DES, it is useful in previously untreated patients for urgent relief of skeletal pain or impending spinal cord compression and for those who are not candidates for orchiectomy. Spironolactone, an antimineralocorticoid, has also been successfully used in small groups of patients for treatment of hormonally refractory prostatic carcinoma, and the effect presumably results from inhibition of steroidogenesis.[32] Although 80% of patients are initially sensitive to the suppression of testicular androgens, 10% of patients die within 6 months, 50% die within 3 years, and only 10% survive 10 years.

This phenomenon of hormonal escape reflects the selection of hormonoresistant clones. When hormonal escape occurs, changing the modalities of androgenic suppression or escalation of the hormone therapy are generally of very limited value. Even the use of chemotherapy, with or without androgens, has not been shown to be significantly more effective than symptomatic treatment. Thus, in patients with prostate adenocarcinoma, 20% are at the beginning hormonoresistant and 80% are hormonosensitive. Recent comparative trials with complete androgen blockade (orchiectomy and Flutamide) vs. androgen blockade with cytostatics (orchiectomy and Estramustin) in the previous untreated patients with prostate cancers, showed no significant difference either in the response rate or the progression rate between the two groups.[101]

An important debate still persists about when hormone therapy should be started, or early vs. delayed therapy. Does the early introduction of hormonal therapy in any way delay progression of the disease or increase survival time? For those patients who present with severe bone pain or compromised lower urinary tract due to compression by a tumor, hormonal therapy has proven extremely effective. For those patients with metastatic disease who are asymptomatic at presentation, the timing of hormonal therapy remains controversial. Initial studies of patient survival before and after the introduction of hormonal therapy suggested that this treatment indeed prolongs life. Thus, Nesbit and Baum[102] compared the survival of 263 patients treated with hormonal therapy with the untreated group of the same authors and found that at 36 months, the treated group had a 34% survival rate compared with 11% for the untreated group; at 5 years, the treatment group had a 17% survival rate as compared with 6% in the control groups. Therefore, it was concluded that hormonal therapy significantly prolonged survival and should be instituted at the time of diagnosis.[102]

Although there is no evidence to support the development of prostate carcinoma from benign prostatic hyperplasia (BPH), prostatic hyperplasia is also dependent on the presence of androgens and probably of high-molecular-weight growth factors recently identified in prostatic tissue. Based on examination of autopsy specimens, a 30% incidence of BPH was noted in prostates of men aged 60 to 69, and a 100% incidence from men over 90. Because androgen must be present for prostatic enlargement to occur, and prostatic enlargement does not occur in individuals genetically deficient in testosterone 5α-reductase, androgen antagonists have been used.

c. Endometrial Cancer

Cancers of the cervix and uterus occur in approximately 50,000 women (14,000 carcinoma of the cervix and 36,000 endometrial cancer) each year in the U.S. As a group these cancers represent the sixth most common cancer overall, and are second only to breast cancer. The overall death rate from these two cancers has decreased more than 70% in the last 40 years due to the effective techniques for early diagnosis and the careful application of established treatment approaches (surgery, radiation therapy, hormonal treatment, and combination chemotherapy).[103-105] The conventional cytologic smear (Pap smear) is considered 90% accurate for cervical cancer, but is only 50% accurate for cancer of the endometrium.

The role of hormones in development of endometrial cancer has been the subject of investigation for many years. Recent studies revealed that factors which increase the exposure of the uterus to unopposed estrogens, either exogenous or endogenous, are associated with increased risk of endometrial carcinoma. Administration of progesterone can reverse endometrial hyperplasia and protect against the development of endometrial cancer. Exogenous estrogens used in the last decades to relieve menopausal symptoms showed a dramatic increase (four- to eightfold) in the risk to endometrial cancer compared to control studies. Oral contraceptives containing both estrogen and progestogen have the lowest incidence of endometrial cancer. Women at highest risk for developing endometrial cancer are those with: (1) obesity, (2) infertility, (3) tendency toward diabetes, (4) failure of ovulation, (5) dysfunctional uterine bleeding, (6) adenomatous hyperplasia, and (7) estrogens taken for a prolonged period of time.

The mechanisms of antiestrogenic effects of progestogens include changes in steroid receptors (ER and PR) and enzyme activity in endometrial tissue. Progesterone is also able to increase the aromatase activity in ER + and PR + tumors, namely human uterine sarcomas that are sensitive to steroid hormone; thus progesterone may be potentially beneficial for treatment of certain uterine sarcomas. The modern staging formula used by the Federation of International Gynecologists and Obstetricians (FIGO) shows the magnitude of clinical virulence and allows individualization of treatment for surgery, radiation, and hormone therapy. There are four stages: stage I — confinement to corpus; stage II — involvement of corpus and cervix; stage III — extension outside the uterus, but not outside the true pelvis; and stage IV — involvement of the bladder, rectum, or distant metastasis.

Surgical or combined treatment by surgery and adjuvant irradiation in endometrial carcinoma is well tolerated. In endometrial carcinoma stage I and randomly assigned patients for treatment, hysterectomy alone produces a 64%, 5-year survival; preoperative radiation and hysterectomy produces a 76%, 5-year survival; and hysterectomy and postoperative radiation produces an 81%, 5-year survival. In stage II, radiation therapy and surgery (hysterectomy) produced variable results at 5-year survival, ranging from 44 to 65% and 85%. Radiation therapy includes radium only or radium and external.

i. Hormonal therapy

Synthetic progestational agents have been the next commonly used as systemic treatment of recurrent endometrial carcinoma, with response rates ranging from 30 to 37%. Responses to systemic progestogen therapy are associated with prolonged survival. Median survival of responders ranges from 23 to 29 months, compared to 6 months for patients who fail to respond. In general, well-differentiated tumors respond more commonly than poorly differentiated. About one third of the patients with lung metastasis can be palliated by this method. Also, metastasis in the vagina, lymph nodes, and soft tissue and bone and hepatic metastasis are more likely to respond to hormone therapy. Multiple studies now document the correlation between progesterone receptors and response to progesterone therapy.[103-105] Thus, 89% of progesterone responsive tumors were PR+ and 94% of patients failing progesterone therapy were PR− tumors (progesterone receptor negative). Although progestogens have been widely used for more than 25 years, there is no evidence that a particular hormone preparation is preferred. The most commonly used has been hydroxyprogesterone caproate (Delalutin) at a dosage of 500 mg, three times a week i.m., which is the most effective, or medroxyprogesterone (Depo-Provera). Oral megestrol acetate (Megace) appears to produce similar results. The usual dose is 1000 to 3000 mg/week i.m. for the initial dose, followed by a maintenance dose of 400 to 800 mg/week until recurrence or distant metastasis develops. Alternative endocrine therapy has been investigated, including tamoxifen and danazol, and both appear to have some activity. A response rate of 30 to 39% for tamoxifen and well-differentiated tumors was found. However, use of progestogen therapy as prophylaxis in the early stage of endometrial carcinoma remains controversial. A recent study using progesterone therapy with surgical stage I endometrial adenocarcinoma and malignant peritoneal cytologic washings showed that 95% of patients at second-look laparoscopy had no evidence of recurrent endometrial carcinoma and all (100%) patients remain clinically free of disease from 12 to 64 months after discontinuation of therapy.[105]

Recently, 49 patients with advanced/recurrent endometrial carcinoma were treated with tamoxifen (20 mg, twice daily) and had a 20% response rate. The median survival of responders was 34 months compared to 6 months in nonresponders. Thus, the results of this study confirm the value of tamoxifen as second-line hormonal therapy in patients with advanced endometrial carcinoma and in whom progesterone therapy has failed. Tamoxifen flare (as acute abdominal pain) can be seen also in patients with advanced endometrial carcinoma. Danazol has been shown to be effective in the treatment of endometriosis, benign breast disease, angioderma, and precocious puberty. Due to its multiple physiologic effects previously described, danazol, by inhibiting follicular function through hypothalamic-pituitary and ovarian mechanisms, produces a hypoestrogenic-hypoprogestational state and produces atrophy of the endometriotic implants. Danazol is used mainly in a dose of 800 mg/d for an average duration of 4 to 6 months and relieves clinical symptoms and laparoscopic findings in 72 to 95% of treated patients. Therefore, Danazol is an effective drug in treatment of endometriosis. Therapy should be initiated during menstruation and in nonpregnant women and should be started as a dose of 400 mg/d, which produces relief in most patients. In those patients who do not respond to 400 mg/d, the dose can be increased to 600 or 800 mg/d. Side effects include edema, acne, hirsutism, hot flashes, changes in libido, and muscle cramps. Only relatively few contraindications to Danazol therapy exists, such as hepatic dysfunction or patients with severe hypertension, congestive heart failure, and borderline renal function. However, the use of the synthetic steroid danazol has significantly advanced the medical management of endometriosis.[63]

d. Ovarian Cancer

Ovarian cancer is the leading cause of death from pelvic gynecologic malignancy among American women. Each year in the U.S. approximately 18,000 new cases of ovarian cancer are diagnosed and approximately 11,000 women die of this disease. Only 5 to 15% of the patients with advanced disease (stage III and IV) survive 5 years or longer. The 5-year survival rates are higher for stage II (45%) and stage I (72%). Since most of patients are in stage III or IV at the time of diagnosis, the overall survival rate for ovarian cancer is low. Ovarian neoplasms can originate from the surface epithelium, the germ cells, and the ovarian stroma; the vast majority of ovarian cancers are of the common epithelial type and include the papillary serous cystadenocarcinoma, mucinous, endometroid, and the rare benign Brenner tumor.

Recent experimental animal studies and epidemiologic studies suggest that ovarian cancer is an endocrine-related disease. Thus, chronic administration of estrogens has been shown to produce ovarian cancer in animal studies.[106] High levels of gonadotropins have also been correlated with ovarian neoplasms in animal experiments. Epidemiologic studies revealed an increased incidence of ovarian cancer in women whose ovulations were not suppressed by pregnancy or oral contraceptives, and this supports the hypothesis that ovarian cancer is an endocrine-related tumor. Recent investigations demonstrated the presence of estrogen, progestin, and androgen receptors, and emphasized the presence of AR in ovarian cancers, suggesting that the tumor may be androgen-dependent, particularly in postmenopausal women.[106] Recent studies showed that high levels of PR were associated with better survival. Thus, patients with advanced ovarian cancer and PR-positive tumors have better survival than those with advanced disease and PR-negative tumors. Patients in which ER and AR were absent or in which PR and AR were absent, had poor survival. Thus, receptor status, especially of PR, may be of prognostic value and receptor status and aromatase activity may be useful in selecting ovarian cancer patients for hormone therapy. Tumor markers, especially carcinoembryonic antigen (CEA) might be useful for the diagnosis and monitoring of the ovarian cancer, during and after treatment. Elevated levels of CEA are noted in patients with ovarian cancer (46%), carcinoma of the cervix (53%), carcinoma of endometrium (37%), and in healthy volunteers (11%).[106] Early detection is the most difficult. Pap smears are unreliable. Palpation and ultrasound should be performed in women with vague abdominal pain or enlarged ovaries.

i. Endocrine Therapy

The fact that the ovary is not only the main source of estrogens and progesterone, but also a target organ for these and other hormones, supports the use of hormonotherapy in ovarian cancer. The most used are progestogen agents, but a true objective response was reported in only 10 to 15% of the patients, with an additional 10% of patients with stabilization of disease. It has been shown that i.m. administration of medroxyprogesterone acetate (MPA) is more effective than an oral administration dosage of 500 mg/d i.m. for 4 weeks, and a maintenance dosage of 1000 mg of MPA weekly and also high-dose megestrol acetate (Megace) were recommended. In a study of 33 patients with advanced endometroid ovarian cancer treated with MPA, 55% response rates were observed. Overall, the survival of patients who responded to treatment was significantly longer than for nonresponders. Progestins have also been used in combination with other agents. Thus, patients with ovarian carcinoma refractory to chemotherapy received a sequential combination of ethinylestradiol (EE), in a dose of 100 µg/d and medroxyprogesterone acetate in a dose of 50 mg b.i.d.; from 65 patients, 9 (14%) responded to treatment and 13 (20%) had stable disease. Vascular complications occurred in 3 patients.[107] Recently, tamoxifen was used as a loading dose schedule of 100 mg m^{-2} in four divided doses/d, followed by a maintenance dose of 20 mg b.i.d., administered continuously; it was concluded that the true activity of this treatment is minimal. The LHRH agonists, namely Decapeptyl (D-Trp-6-LHRH) has also been used in the treatment of ovarian cancer. In a study of ten women in whom LHRH agonist treatment was started after the failure of chemotherapy, tumor stabilization or shrinkage was seen in 50% of the cases.[106] The rationale for this treatment is the down regulation of gonadotropins, and thus, the minimization of the steroid output of the ovarian carcinoma. Also, leuprolide acetate (Lupron) was administered s.c. at a 1-mg dose for at least 8 weeks to 23 patients with refractory epithelial ovarian cancer. Four patients (17%) had a partial response with a median duration of 52 weeks in a Grade I ovarian cancer. Therefore, leuprolide acetate shows evidence of antitumor activity against refractory Grade I epithelial adenocarcinoma of the ovary. Hence, hormonal therapy for ovarian cancer has resulted in uneven responses.

e. Thyroid Carcinoma

Thyroid cancer is estimated to comprise approximately 1.1% of all new malignancies diagnosed annually in the U.S. but accounts for only 0.2% of all cancer deaths. Among persons under age 45, thyroid cancer is a more common disease accounting for over 6% of all cancers. Roughly 70% of all thyroid cancers observed today are papillary thyroid carcinomas, including almost all radiation-induced thyroid cancer. There is considerable experimental and clinical evidence demonstrating that thyroid tumors are TSH-dependent. Administration of thyroid-stimulating hormone (TSH) or thyrotropin stimulates development and propagation of these tumors, whereas its suppression by thyroid hormones (thyroxine, triiodothyronine) induces regression of thyroid carcinomas.

Thyroid suppression therapy was used for a long time in the treatment of cancers. Desiccated thyroid, thyroxine (T$_4$), or triiodothyronine (T$_3$) were mostly used to treat papillary and follicular carcinoma. The response rate to thyroid suppressive therapy largely depends on early detection, histologic differentiation, and the presence of TSH receptors. Most of differentiated thyroid carcinomas have TSH receptors. Serum thyroglobulin (Tg) levels increase in response to rising endogenous TSH levels, suggesting that TSH tumor receptors are biologically active.[82] Thus, thyroglobulin (Tg), carcinogenic embryonic activity (CEA), and calcitonin (CT) are accurate tumor biologic markers in determining the prognosis as well as the response to therapy of well-differentiated tumors (papillary and follicular cancers) and medullary thyroid carcinoma. However, they have to be collaborated with determination of DNA content, oncogene amplification (ras oncogenes), ^{131}I uptake, ultrasound and ultrastructural, autoradiography, and cell surface studies of thyroid tumor cells.

Since the overall survival and response rates of patients largely depend on early diagnosis of thyroid cancer, use of more accurate and sensitive methods are critical in achieving an early detection and followup of patients with thyroid carcinoma.

The two main endocrine therapies used in thyroid cancer management are (1) ablative endocrine therapy (surgery, ^{131}I radiation) and (2) additive endocrine therapy. The first, surgical removal of thyroid gland, includes hemithyroidectomy and total thyroidectomy. Hemithyroidectomy is mainly recommended in both papillary and follicular cancer, which is well-differentiated, has small tumors (0.1 to 2.5 cm in diameter), is confined to one lobe, and has no local lymph node or distant metastases. Total thyroidectomy is preferred when the tumor is more than 2 cm in diameter. Temporary cord damage and transient hypoparathyroidism occurred in 0.8% and 1.9% of all patients. Recommendation for ^{131}I ablation is based on the following criteria: functional activity of the tumor, age of the patient, size of the metastases (micrometastases have a better response than macrometastases), and histologic type (well-differentiated tumors do take up more ^{131}I than less differentiated subtypes). There is general agreement that ^{131}I treatment following thyroidectomy more often cures micrometastases and is often only palliative for patients with macrometastases. It should be given to all patients with follicular carcinoma and also to patients with advanced papillary cancer.

Temporary side effects of ablative ^{131}I therapy are nausea, vomiting, occasional parotitis, and decrease in leukocytes and platelet counts. Permanent side effects (which are rare) include aplastic anemia, pulmonary fibrosis, amenorrhea, leukemia, and prolonged leukocytes and platelet depression. Replacement therapy should be recommended to all patients following surgical or ^{131}I ablation at a dose of 150 to 200 μg/d of L-thyroxine (Synthroid).

The second main therapy, additive endocrine therapy, using desiccated thyroid, L-thyroxine (T_4), or L-triiodothyronine (T_3), is widely used as thyroid suppressive therapy at a dose of L-thyroxine (sodium levo-thyroxine) 200 to 350 μg/d orally (or 1.5 to 2.8 μg/kg/d). There is no advantage by giving toxic doses. Sodium L-triiodothyronine (Cytomel) is also effective in lower doses of 25 to 100 μg/d orally or in a combination of both L-thyroxine and L-triiodothyronine (Thyrolar) as a dose of 6.25 to 75 μg/d orally. The response rates are favorable in almost 75% of patients with papillary thyroid cancer and in 40% of undifferentiated carcinomas. Thyroid suppression therapy is mainly used as an adjuvant therapy following surgery or radiation ^{131}I therapy, and it was found that disease recurrence is more often (34 vs. 17%) when thyroid hormones were not given postoperatively.[82] Additive thyroid therapy provides favorable results in many cases of papillary and follicular adenomas or carcinomas (53 to 70%), and it is widely used following hemi- or total thyroidectomy to prevent recurrence of disease or spread of metastases to the bone, lung, or brain. Temporary side effects of thyroid therapy are nervousness, palpitations, arrhythmia, or angina pectoris. They also can aggravate hypertension, congestive heart failure, and diabetes mellitus. Thyroid hormones are not tumoricidal per se, but exert mainly a palliative effect. The only treatment for medullary thyroid carcinoma (MTC) is the total thyroidectomy and followed by excision or medical management of possible adrenal medullary disease. Followup by estimation of calcitonin (CT) levels, is required since lymph node metastases occur frequently in this disease.

f. Renal Carcinoma

The basis for the hormonal therapy of human renal adenocarcinoma was found in animal experiments, namely in the estrogen-induced renal carcinoma in the male golden Syrian hamsters. Kidney tumor induction can be almost completely inhibited by simultaneous administration of testosterone, progesterone, and desoxycorticosterone, and thus, the concept that renal adenocarcinoma is a hormone-dependent tumor. However, no conclusive evidence supports the beneficial effects of hormone therapy in human renal cell carcinoma (RCC). Androgen receptors have been found in both malignant and normal tissue. A vast number of clinical studies, using progestins, namely medroxyprogesterone acetate (MPA), found only small and occasional responses. A randomized multicenter trial using a combination of MPA and recombinant interferon-α found that overall response rate in 93 evaluable patients was 5.4% and the median survival was 7 months. The low response rate of IFN is not increased by addition of MPA to IFN. Thus, the response rates in metastatic renal cell cancer after chemotherapy, hormonal treatment, or immunotherapy rarely exceeds 15%.

g. Leukemias and Lymphoid Tumors

Corticosteroids were used for a long time in the treatment of chronic lymphatic leukemia and Hodgkin's disease due to their cytolytic effects on lymphoid cells, especially when they are used in pharmacologic doses. Their use was based on experimental investigation that showed a dramatic remission of transplanted lymphosarcomas in mice following cortisone administration.[9,10] Temporary remission of human lymphatic leukemia and Hodgkin's disease were previously reported by administration of cortisone and ACTH.[10] The beneficial therapeutic effects can be explained by the presence of glucocorticoid receptors (GR) and cytolytic effects on lymphocytes. These GRs are intracellular receptors, and the steroid hormones interact with the receptor of soluble cytosol and form a complex H + GR, which is later translocated into the nucleus. Some human cancer lines contain GR and consequently are responsive to corticoid therapy, whereas others lack these receptors and are hormone resistant. Because of the cytotoxic effects of corticoids on lymphoid cells, steroids are used in the treatment of lymphoproliferative disorders, including leukemia, lymphoma, and multiple myeloma. The presence of GR appears to be necessary, but not sufficient, to produce the cytolytic effects of glucocorticoids. Measurement of GR has not proven to be useful in predicting response. Sometimes, the GR number is normal, but lytic effects do not occur due to a postreceptor defect. Commonly used hormones are cortisol, prednisone, prednisolone, methylprednisolone, and dexamethasone. Standard dosage varies for cortisol, 20 to 100 mg; prednisone, 40 to 80 mg/ orally; methylprednisolone (Medrol), 10 to 25 mg/d i.v. or i.m./d; and dexamethasone, 5 to 10 mg/d orally (see Table 2). Corticosteroids can be used as single agents or in combination with chemotherapy or radiation. Thus, dexamethasone or prednisone can be used combined with leukeran (chlorambucil) in chronic lymphatic leukemia (CLL), acute lymphatic leukemia (ALL), malignant lymphoma, Hodgkin's disease, and multiple myelomas; the response rate varies between 60 to 70%. Corticosteroid can enhance the responsiveness to chemotherapy and radiation therapy.

h. Carcinoma of the Exocrine Pancreas

Pancreatic carcinoma remains a disease difficult to diagnose and also difficult to treat. Most patients die within 6 months of diagnosis, and over 90% are dead within 1 year. A possible new approach to treatment, hormone therapy, was recently suggested, when high concentrations of ER, PR, and AR were demonstrated in both the cytoplasm and nucleus, in human pancreatic tumors, and in experimentally induced tumors in rats.[108] Also, enzymes which are distributed in androgen and estrogen target tissues, such as uterus, prostate, and breast cancers, are now found in pancreatic carcinoma (aromatase, 5α-reductase). These studies strongly suggest that pancreatic cancer should be considered as a hormone-sensitive neoplasm, and that hormone therapy may offer a new approach to the treatment of pancreatic carcinoma. Clinical studies are now in progress. Two Phase II studies, using tamoxifen (Nolvadex) in patients with unresectable pancreatic carcinoma, have shown an increase in median survival and also an increased number of patients with long survival. There has been encouraging preliminary reports of the use of an analog of LHRH in animal models of pancreatic carcinoma and in five patients with stage IV tumor and liver metastases, and all showed clinical and subjective improvement. Another trial, using tamoxifen vs. cyproterone acetate (CPA) and vs. an untreated group, revealed that CPA showed no difference in survival when compared with the control group, whereas 8 of 37 patients treated with tamoxifen survived more than 1 year. Other hormonal therapies should now be investigated, including progestogens, antiandrogens, orchiectomy, and aminoglutethimide.[108]

i. Uterine Fibroids

Fibroids (fibromyomata) are common benign tumors of the uterus producing menstrual problems, iron deficiency anemia, pelvic discomfort, infertility, and miscarriage. Recently, regression of uterine fibroids has been reported after administration of LHRH analogs. These agents suppress ovarian activity due to down regulation of the pituitary. The agonists may be given intranasally or subcutaneously; however, the ovarian suppression is variable when the drugs are given intranasally. There is a considerable demand for medical treatment of fibroids, especially in young women who like to preserve the uterus. At present, many prefer subcutaneously depot given every month, and this usually results in shrinkage of fibroids and amenorrhea. Treatment of fibroids with LHRH agonists should be limited to women close to natural menopause and those with medical contraindications to surgery. The mechanism of action is still unclear. It is possible to reduce concentrations of ER and PR, and to achieve reduction in the binding of epidermal growth factor (EGF) to myometrium and fibroid tissue. This binding was significantly reduced in women treated with goserelin (Zoladex) before surgery, suggesting that EGF may mediate the effect of estrogens on the growth of fibroids.

4. Possible Mechanisms by Which Hormones Exert Their Therapeutic Effects

Despite intense effort and growing interest in the last decade regarding the hormone effects at cellular and molecular levels, the exact mechanisms(s) of action of hormones on cancer cells is still undetermined. It is likely that hormones act on cancer cell biology, namely, cell division and cell differentiation by several mechanisms. Recent investigations revealed a strong relationship between hormones, hormone receptors, growth factors, and oncogenes. There is strong evidence that hormones modulate the synthesis of growth factors; also, growth factors can interfere with hormone action on cancer cells, stimulating their growth without the need of hormones, thus, becoming more hormone independent and growing autonomously.

Hence, recent advances in tumor cytokinetics and endocrine pharmacology suggest that hormones control neoplastic cell growth not only by changing the "hormonal milieu" or endocrine mechanisms, but also by autocrine and paracrine mechanisms. These complex and not yet fully understood mechanisms can explain the hormone dependence and the success of hormonotherapy as well as the failure of hormone therapy, or hormonoindependence. It is postulated that cell division is mainly under the control of hormones, whereas cell proliferation is under the control of growth factors. A link between hormone receptors, protooncogenes, and oncogenes has also been demonstrated. It has also been shown that most steroid hormones regulate not only cell proliferation, but also cancer cell death.

Estrogens and antiestrogen (tamoxifen) can regulate the human estrogen receptor gene, epidermal growth factor (EGF), and gene and oncogenes (myc, ras, and fos) in MCF-human breast cancer cells. Secretion of TGF-β has been associated with growth inhibition by tamoxifen. It has been found that antiestrogen resistant cells produced a decreased amount of TGF-β and failed to increase the amount of TGF-β produced in response to tamoxifen. Recognition that hormones and growth factor actions are regulated by oncogene expression suggest new strategies for cancer therapy at cellular and molecular level.[109]

From a comprehensive review of published reports as well as from personal findings, it is postulated that hormones act on cancer cells and exert their therapeutic effects by different mechanisms: (1) hormones act mainly as cytostatics, not as tumoricidal agents; (2) hormones act on cell metabolism; (3) hormones act on the cell cycle, as cell cycle specific (CCS) agents; (4) hormones act on receptor status (by blocking the hormone-receptor complexes); (5) they act on immune defense system; (6) they exert antiinflammatory activity; (7) they block the hypothalamo-pituitary axis; (8) they interfere with growth factors and their receptors on the target cells; (9) hormones act on precancerous cell populations and their transformation into cancerous cells; and (10) hormones act on tumor heterogenic subpopulations, stimulating the growth of hormone-sensitive cell lines over hormone-independent or hormone-resistant cells.

Hormones act on cell metabolism by reacting with the membrane-bound nucleotide cyclase system to stimulate the conversion of adenosine triphosphate (ATP) to the corresponding 3'5'-monophosphate, or cyclic adenosine monosphosphate (cAMP), which acts as a "second messenger". Studies using autoradiographic methods with [^{3}H]-thymidine revealed that in most tumors there are two different cell compartments: (1) a smaller, or proliferative compartment, which is represented by cells that proliferate at any time (or "growth fraction"); and (2) a large compartment of dormant or silent cells, which can remain for years in this stage. Most hormones and growth factors act on this rapidly proliferating pool.

Hormones act on cell cycle and its phases. Cell cycle is divided in at least five phases. First is the G_0-phase (resting phase or dormant cells). This phase is represented by cells which are going in this "out-of-cycle" stage and remain dormant or silent for long periods of time (months or years). Go cells can be stimulated by hormones to reenter the cell cycle into the G_1-phase. The shift of G_1 and G_0 populations is of crucial importance in controlling the proliferation rate of cancer cells and the therapeutic use of hormones and anticancer drugs. Second is the G_1-phase (period of RNA and protein synthesis). The length of the G_1-phase is highly variable (10 to 20 h, even 2 to 5 d); it is very short (2 to 3 h) or practically absent in rapidly proliferating erythropoietic stem cells or in ascites tumor cells). G_1 is a vital control period in the cell cycle. Cells with a shorter G_1-phase are rapidly dividing cells and cells with a longer G_1-phase are slowly growing population cells. Third is the S-phase (period of DNA synthesis) or the period during which DNA replication takes place and the number of chromosomes are doubled. The length of the S-phase is remarkably constant (approximately 7 to 8 h) in normal cells. However, neoplastic cells often have a longer S-phase than that of normal cells. Cancer cells heavily incorporate [^{3}H]-thymidine and are numerically increased in tumors and can be stimulated by mitogenic factors (hormones, growth factors, and nutrients), or arrested by chemotherapeutic agents. The G_2-phase (post-DNA synthesis) is the period of assembly by the mitotic spindle apparatus and is usually a short period (approximately 2 to 4 h), with few exceptions (e.g., mouse ear epidermis, mouse ascites tumors, and spermatogonia) in which the G_2 phase is longer (6 to 9 h). The M phase (mitosis) is a short period and varies in different tissues from 30 min to 2.5 h with an average of 1 h for most mammalian cells. Mitosis has four phases: prophase, metaphase, anaphase, and telophase.

The duration of the cell cycle is approximately 20 to 30 h. The length of the cell cycle in cancer cells differs from that of normal cells, only by the length of the G_1-phase. Dormant (silent) cells (G_0-phase) can be brought into the cycle at any time by appropriate stimuli, such as hormones, growth factors, vitamins, or nutrients. Whereas the G_0-phase represents only a small fraction of normal cells, dormant cells can reach a significant proportion in several neoplasms. Hormones, growth factors, and vitamins play an important role in controlling the cell cycle and its phases. Through the use of hormones, we can manipulate a cell to get "into the cycle" or get "out of the cycle" and stay in a dormant stage for several months or years. Thus, we can modulate the proliferative state or "growth fraction", which is extremely important in making therapeutic decisions (see Figure 3A).

Most anticancer drugs, including hormones, vitamins, and cytostatics, are classified as cell cycle specific (CCS) drugs, which can act during any phase of the cell cycle, although most act selectively on the S-phase, or transition between G_1-S phase. These include certain hormones (estrogens, corticosteroids, androgens), antiestrogens (tamoxifen), growth factors, prostaglandins, Vitamins A, E, D, and some chemotherapeutic agents (cytarabine, methotrexate, fluorouracil (5-FU), Vincristine, Thiotepa, and Chlorambucil) (see Figure 3B).

A second major group of cytostatic agents are classified as cell cycle nonspecific (CCNS) agents; they act by complexing with cellular DNA and are capable of doing this whether cells are proliferating or not. Examples are alkylating agents, such as cyclophosphamide, carmustine (BCNU), Cisplatin, and antibiotics, such as doxorubicin and mitomycin. These are mainly used in the treatment of solid tumors with slowly dividing cells. Hormones act on the hormone receptor status by blocking the binding of the hormone to its receptor and thus, inhibit the formation of hormone-receptor complexes (H + R ↔ HR) and their translocation into the nucleus. Hence, the presence of hormone receptors and receptor activation or transformation is very important in eliciting cellular responses, and consequently, the effectiveness of hormonotherapy. Hormone antagonists, such as tamoxifen, antiandrogens, or LHRH agonists, compete with estradiol, testosterone, or LHRH for the same receptors, which is translocated to the cell nucleus, failing to stimulate a full estrogenic,

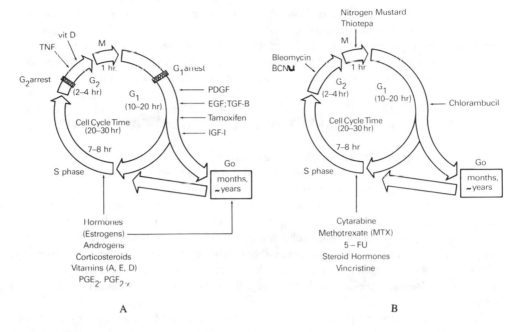

FIGURE 3. (A) Hormones, growth factors, and vitamins in the cell cycle; IGF-I (insulin growth factor-I). (B) Cytostatic drugs in the cell cycle 5-FU (Fluorouracil); BCNU (carmustine) bischloroethylnitrosourea).

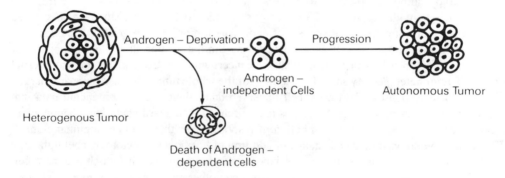

FIGURE 4. Progression of a hormone-dependent tumor (heterogenous tumor) into a hormone-independent or autonomous tumor.

androgenic, or LH response. Hormones may also act by inhibiting or delaying the rate of transformation of precancer cells toward cancer cells. Research regarding the role of hormones on precancer cell metabolism will enlighten the role of hormones in cancer treatment. Hormones also act on the immune system by increasing the host immune defenses; they interfere with antibody production, lymphokine, and cytokine formation. Hormones may exert anti-inflammatory and antiedematous effects on stromal cells surrounding the tumor.

Hormones also act by blocking the hypothalamo-pituitary axis and consequently, the effect of the feedback mechanism. Recent investigations revealed that tumors are composed of a mixture or mosaic of multiple, clonal, tumor cell subpopulations. This tumor heterogeneity also showed the coexistence of both hormone-sensitive and hormone-independent cells. Cell heterogeneity is found within tumors in the early stage, and prior to exposure to any treatment. During hormonal treatment, many originally hormone-dependent cancers acquired hormone independence and tumor autonomy because the hormone-independent cell lines are growing faster and finally predominate over hormone-sensitive cells. Experimental studies showed that ablative hormone therapy (castration) aided the growth of hormone independent cell subpopulations. Thus, castration of male rats with Dunning R-3327-H prostate carcinoma which originally contained both androgen-sensitive and androgen-insensitive cells, results in the relapsing of a more androgen-independent tumor (autonomous tumors) (see Figure 4).

B. HORMONES AS ADJUVANT THERAPEUTIC AGENTS (PALLIATIVE THERAPY)

Palliative therapy represents a change in the focus of treatment from control of disease to control of effects of disease. The rationale for the use of combination therapy with cytotoxic drugs (chemohormonal therapy), radiation therapy, and immunotherapy is based upon three assumptions: (1) tumors are heterogenous (composed of various proportions of receptor-positive and receptor-negative cells); (2) there is a differential response between receptor-positive and receptor-negative cells to chemotherapy and hormonotherapy (some of hormone-independent cells can be killed by chemotherapeutic agents); (3) neither chemotherapy, radiation, nor hormonotherapy interferes with the action of the other form of treatment, so that the response rates for combined therapy will be additive (immunoaugmentation) and not antagonists.

To date, reports in the predictive value of ER for response to chemotherapy have been contradictory. It can be concluded that, at least in the case of ER+ cells, chemotherapy and hormonal therapy are competing for the same cell population. A report including 240 patients confirmed that hormone nonresponders have an equivalent response to combination chemotherapy, although hormone responders tended to have a longer survival time from the initiation of chemotherapy (18 to 23 months vs. 13 months). Clinical studies also showed heterogeneity in hormone-sensitive cells of endocrine tumors. Heterogeneity has been seen within primary tumors as well as in metastases. Similar results have been reported for androgen receptors (AR) in human prostatic cancer, and for ER and PR in endometrial cancer. Tumor heterogeneity should be studied for the whole tumor because there are marked differences in responses of different cell lines. To date, there are no convincing data that the addition of a hormonal agent, such as tamoxifen, to a standard chemotherapeutic agent has increased the response rate or duration of response over that of either regimen alone.[25] The failure to demonstrate an advantage of addition of hormones to cytotoxic chemotherapy does not rule out the possibility that the kinetic effects of tamoxifen (which acts as a cell cycle inhibitor) might increase effectiveness of chemotherapy. Preliminary reports demonstrate that tumor cell synchronization by tamoxifen and then recruitment by equine estrogens (Premarin priming) may well enhance the response to chemotherapy.[110] The same unclear results were produced by the combination of a hormone (estradiol) and a cytotoxic drug (nitrogen mustard) in estramustine phosphate sodium (Emcyt). This drug has been used for the palliative treatment of metastatic prostatic cancer, and produced a stable disease in approximately 20% of cases. Adverse effects of estramustine are similar to those of DES and include gynecomastia, thrombophlebitis, stroke, myocardial infarction, and nausea and vomiting, which may be severe enough to require discontinuance of treatment.

In summary, trials published so far suggest that no survival benefit is achieved using hormones in combination. In addition, side effects are increased and the chances of second hormone therapy are lost. Sequential single-hormone therapy is to be preferred. There is no evidence that high-dose treatment is more effective than standard doses for either hormone therapy or chemotherapy. Prolonged maintenance chemotherapy for more than 6 months appears to offer no survival benefit and merely increases toxicity. Endocrine therapy should be tried first and then chemotherapy. The main exception to this sequence is the patient with rapidly progressive visceral metastases who should receive chemotherapy first. Cyclic sequential hormonochemotherapy was recently proposed. First, estrogen at physiologic doses was used to bring stem cells out of the resting phase and to stimulate cell division into partial synchrony; then high doses of progesterone were given, which enhanced their susceptibility to the subsequent chemotherapy. It has been proposed that corticosteroids may be helpful as adjuvants in the treatment of jaundice, due to hepatic metastases, and restricted lung function, due to lymphangitic pulmonary metastases. Adrenal corticoids are also helpful in the medical management of brain and spinal cord metastases.

A recent study showed that glucocorticoids are administered to virtually all patients with symptomatic brain metastases or epidural spinal cord compression. The rationale for steroid administration is to improve neurologic function presumably by reducing brain or spinal cord edema.[111] A starting dose of 16 mg/d of dexamethasone in divided doses of 4 mg every 6 h, is still considered "standard" initial treatment for patients with brain edema or epidural metastases. Patients with progressive neurologic deficits can receive higher doses to a maximum of 100 mg/d. In patients with epidural metastases, therapy should be based on the degree of myelographic block. Patients with >80% block should receive 100 mg i.v. of dexamethasone followed by 24 mg/d in four divided doses. Patients with <80% block received 16 mg/d in four divided doses. Adrenal corticoids are useful as adjuvant or palliative agents in the management of pain, causing euphoria and increasing the appetite in advanced or preterminally ill cancer patients. Subjective improvement occurs in as many as 75% of treated patients. This was in a randomized, double-blind, crossover trial using 800 mg Megace/d orally against placebo, in terminally ill cancer patients for 144 d; significant decrease of pain, decrease in depression, and increase in appetite and weight, compared to placebo-treated patients, was found. It was concluded that Megace increases the comfort of terminally ill cancer patients.[112] In a recent study of 37 patients with advanced prostatic cancer with bone metastases who were treated with low doses of prednisone (7.5 to 8 mg/d) an evaluation of pain and quality of life were used as pragmatic indices of response. After 1 month, a relief of pain (38%) was found and was maintained in an average duration of 4 months. In patients with severe and diffuse pain due to widespread bone metastases, neurosurgical procedures, such as chemical hypophysectomy, should be used. This involves the injection of alcohol into the sella turcica under radiologic supervision, and a dramatic pain relief in 60% was reported.[113] The mechanism of analgesia may be related in part to the disruption by alcohol of the hypothalamic endorphinergic pain pathways. Hormones may be helpful as anti-inflammatory and antiedematous agents by acting on the surrounding stromal cells of the tumor. Corticosterioids are also used in the antiemetic (nausea, vomiting) management of chemotherapy, and in the treatment of hypercalcemia during and following radiation.

Therapeutic use of calcitonin in high doses (Miacalcic) produced a marked relief of pain with a simultaneous improvement in the quality of life in 65.5% of patients with cancer. The pain-killing effect of calcitonin may be due to: (1) partial inhibition of algogenous peptides; (2) its possible cytostatic effect may inhibit the local cell proliferation; and (3) its conversion into β-endorphins, exerting its effect centrally. Thus, high doses of calcitonin are an important method for pain treatment in cancer patients.[114]

Important analgesic action of somatostatin in high doses by spinal injection is also occasionally used in relief of acute and chronic pain. This analgesic effect of somatostatin may be due to the presence of somatostatin receptors in many areas of the central nervous system, and not to blocking the opiate receptors.[115] A possible treatment for anorexia, weight loss, and cachexia was recently achieved by using high doses or oral megestrol acetate (480 to 1600 mg/d). Significant weight gain and improving quality of life occurred regardless of the extent of metastases. Thus, megestrol acetate provides an important relief of anorexia and cachexia in cancer patients.[112] Androgens in massive doses stimulate the erythropoiesis in animals and in man. Androgens are used sometimes in the treatment of anemia and myelosuppression or myelofibrosis following cytotoxic chemotherapy or long-term radiation therapy. Therefore, androgens should be considered in the treatment and management of anemia, thrombocytopenia, and especially myelofibrosis. However, the erythropoietic and hematopoietic effects require several weeks.[19]

II. COMMENTS AND CONCLUSIONS

Endocrine therapy is a well-established approach to the treatment of cancer disease. Recently, advances in endocrine pharmacology and tumor biology have greatly clarified the role of hormones and have provided working models for hormonotherapy. Before introduction of hormone receptors, in the so-called pre-receptor era, there were no objective criteria for patient selection, response rate, and overall survival rate. These were done largely on clinical basis, such as: (1) the number and sites of metastases, and (2) the disease-free interval. The response rates were only 20 to 30% and required up to 6 to 8 weeks for the response to occur. After the use of modern diagnostic methods, the response rates dramatically increased to 65 to 80%, with an increase in overall survival and decrease in recurrence of disease.

It is important to emphasize that response rates and response duration to both additive and ablative hormonal therapy are essentially the same: 75 to 80% in ER +, PR +; 33% in ER +, PR −; less than 10% in ER −, PR −; and 45% in ER −, PR +. The significant differences between the additive and ablative hormone therapy lie only in the side effects and the morbidity of the treatment. Also the response rate of primary tumor and metastatic disease (except brain metastases) in positive hormone receptor (ER +, PR +) patients to various forms of hormone therapy, are almost equivalent.

The concept of differential hormone and drug effectiveness during specific phases of the cell cycle of cancer cells appears to be important. However, the distinction between the cell cycle specific (CCS) and cell cycle nonspecific (CCNS) drugs is relative rather than absolute. The response to primary hormone therapy increases the response rate to a second form of hormone therapy. Thus, when there is a response to primary hormone therapy, the chance of responding to secondary therapy is approximately 55%. However, as many as 30% of patients with failure to respond to initial therapy will still respond to subsequent hormone therapy. There is no conclusive evidence that combined hormonal therapy is more effective than sequential hormonal therapy. However, the effects of combined hormones and cytotoxic drugs (chemohormonotherapy) are superior to that of chemotherapy alone. Generally, patients with negative hormone receptors (ER −, PR −) should not be treated with hormonotherapy since the response rates are consistently less than 10%. Therefore, hormonotherapy should be mainly recommended in patients with hormonosensitive tumors, whereas hormonochemotherapy, in mixed responsive tumors and chemotherapy, only in hormone nonresponsive (autonomous) neoplasms (see Figure 5). The use of hormone antagonists, such as tamoxifen, aminoglutethimide (AG), and LHRH agonists, on a large scale in cancer therapy produce beneficial therapeutic results identical to surgical ablative therapy, but with less toxic effects. Hormonotherapy is a systemic adjuvant therapy and should be tried as a primary therapy in all hormone-dependent cancers and a palliative therapy in other types of cancers. Hormonotherapy provides in all hormone-sensitive tumors prolongation of life and remission of tumor growth and can be tried again after recurrence.

Even half a century ago when hormone therapy was in its empirical stage (mainly as glandular therapy or opotherapy), this method was judged to be superior to surgery or radiation therapy. The use of hormonotherapy is mainly based on the studies and progress made in the last four decades that reveal that cancer is not always autonomous, self-perpetuating, and fatal; it is not a curable but a controllable disease.[1,2]

A critical appraisal showed that hormonotherapy produced equally beneficial therapeutic

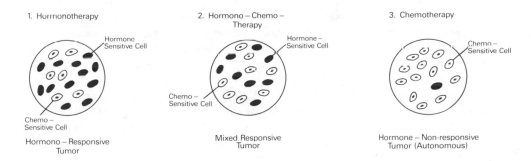

1. Hormonotherapy

Hormone Sensitive Cell

Chemo – Sensitive Cell

Hormono – Responsive Tumor

2. Hormono – Chemo – Therapy

Hormone – Sensitive Cell

Chemo – Sensitive Cell

Mixed Responsive Tumor

3. Chemotherapy

Chemo – Sensitive Cell

Hormone – Non-responsive Tumor (Autonomous)

FIGURE 5.   Distribution of cell populations in hormonotherapy, hormonochemotherapy, and chemotherapy.

effects as surgery, chemotherapy, radiation, or immunotherapy, but with less toxic effects; it is less disfiguring, is without major psychologic complications, and thus, should be considered as an ideal therapeutic method and used more frequently in cancer treatment, especially in advanced metastatic disease. However, keep in mind, that hormones are not completely inoffensive agents, especially used in pharmacologic doses. Some of their side effects are mentioned in Table 2. The development of resistance to hormone therapy is an important factor which often leads to hormone independence with a progressive disease and the occurrence of a more aggressive tumor.

The mechanism of hormone resistance and hormonal escape is complex and varies with the type of tumor. There are several contributing factors: (1) tumor cell heterogeneity; (2) decrease in receptor number; (3) loss of receptor function or occurrence of defective hormone receptors; (4) postreceptor defects; (5) production of autocrine and paracrine growth factors, which might bypass the hormonal regulation, and (6) proper "hormonal milieu". Tumor heterogeneity is an important factor. The hormone-independent or autonomous cells occur prior to any hormonal therapy and are due to a genetic or chromosomal instability which is a fundamental characteristic of cancer cells. Mutations occur in cancer cells in the presence or absence of hormonal treatment, a phenomenon similar to that described in bacteria. Hence, a hormone-independent tumor can originate from a hormone-dependent tumor during hor-monotherapy, due either to selective pre-existing hormone-independent cells or to the oc-currence of a resistant variant during therapy. The hormone-resistance could also result from decreased or absent receptors, or receptor defective, or results from a receptor mutation or postreceptor defect. The production of autocrine growth factors, such as epidermal growth factor (EGF), and TGF-β and insulin-like growth factor-I (IGF-I) allows the cancer cells to bypass steroid tumoral control and become resistant.

Thus, the main goal is to maintain the hormone dependence and responsiveness of cancer patients. A proper "hormonal milieu", during hormonal therapy is also critical for its success or its failure. Recently, it has been shown that more than 90% of hormone-sensitive cells are at the beginning and even at the stage of metastases still hormone sensitive. However, most hormone-insensitive cells develop when tumor cells are exposed to a "low hormonal milieu" provided by the adrenal or gonadal steroids (estrogens, androgens). This shows some analogy with the development of bacterial resistance after inadequate therapy with antibiotics. This transformation of estrogen- or androgen-sensitive cells into hormone-in-sensitive or autonomous clones is analogous to the fact that androgen-sensitive mouse mam-mary tumors that are phenotypically unstable lose their sensitivity to androgens after exposure to an androgen-poor milieu. Also, the mammary carcinoma MT-W9, which is a fully prolactin-dependent tumor, can be transformed to an autonomous tumor by a prolonged exposure of the tumor to lower levels of prolactin. These have major implications for the choice of hormonal therapy and for the decision between early or late hormonal treatment.

One of the most complex and still enigmatic therapeutic problems, is the loss of hormone sensitivity during tumor progression. Namely, why some hormone receptor-positive tumors do not respond to endocrine therapy, while some hormone-negative receptor tumors are still responsive to hormonotherapy. Recent advances in molecular endocrinology suggest some possible mechanisms: (1) loss of hormone receptors; (2) occurrence of abnormal receptors, which can be recognized by epitopes in different parts of the molecule; (3) post-receptor defects in which ligand binding occurred, but did not activate the gene transcription, and, (4) the interference of growth factors, such as stimulators (TGFα and IGFs) and inhibitors (TGFB$_1$). Since growth factors are pluripotent, they can have different effects in hormone-responsive and hormone-unresponsive cells, thus, significantly changing the therapeutic response.[116]

REFERENCES

1. **Huggins, C.,** Control of cancer of man by endocrinologic methods, *Cancer Res.,* 16, 825, 1956.
2. **Huggins, C.,** Two principles in endocrine therapy of cancers: hormone deprival and hormone interference, in *Endocrine Control of Neoplasia,* Sharma, R. K. and Criss, W. E., Eds., Raven Press, New York, 1978, 1.
3. **Huggins, C., Moon, R., and Morii, S.,** Extinction of experimental mammary cancer. I. Estradiol-17β and progesterone, *Proc. Natl. Acad. Sci. U.S.A.,* 48, 379, 1962.
4. **Lipschütz, A. and Vargas, L.,** Prevention of experimental uterine and extrauterine fibroids by testosterone and progesterone, *Endocrinology,* 28, 669, 1941.
5. **Lacassagne, A.,** Hormones and their relation to cancer, *Schweiz. Med. Wochenschr.,* 78, 705, 1948.
6. **Lupulescu, A.,** *Hormonii Steroizi (Steroid Hormones),* Medical Publ. House, Bucharest, 1958, 232, 365.
7. **Beatson, G.,** On the treatment of inoperable cases of carcinoma of the mamma: suggestions for a new method of treatment with illustrative cases, *Lancet,* 2, 104, 1896.
8. **Ingle, J. N.,** Additive hormonal therapy in women with advanced breast cancer, *Cancer,* 53, 766, 1984.
9. **Heilman, F. and Kendall, E.,** The influence of 11-dehydro-17-hydroxycorticosterone (compound E) on the growth of a malignant tumor in the mouse, *Endocrinology,* 34, 416, 1944.
10. **Pearson, O., Eliel, C., Rawson, R., Dobriner, K., and Rhoads, C.,** ACTH and cortisone induced regression of lymphoid tumors in man, *Cancer,* 2, 943, 1949.
11. **Sirbasku, D. A.,** Estrogen induction of growth factors specific for hormone-responsive mammary, pituitary, and kidney tumor cells, *Proc. Natl. Acad. Sci. U.S.A.,* 75, 3786, 1978.
12. **Sporn, M. B. and Todaro, G.,** Autocrine secretion and malignant transformation of cells, *N. Engl. J. Med.,* 303, 878, 1980.
13. **Dickson, R. B., Huff, K. K., Spencer, E. M., and Lippman, M. E.,** Induction of epidermal growth factor-related polypeptides by 17β-estradiol in MCF-7 human breast cancer cells, *Endocrinology,* 118, 138, 1986.
14. **Koga, M. and Sutherland, R. L.,** Epidermal growth factor partially reverses the inhibitory effects of antiestrogens on T47D human breast cancer cell growth, *Biochem. Biophys. Res. Commun.,* 146, 739, 1987.
15. **Maddox, A. M.,** Mechanism of resistance to hormone therapy, *Cancer Bull.,* 41, 52, 1989.
16. **Merkel, D. E. and Osborne, C. K.,** Steroid receptors in relation to response in, *Endocrine Management of Cancer: Biological Bases,* Stoll, B. A., Ed., Karger, London, 1988, 84.
17. **Rose, C. and Mouridsen, H. T.,** Combined cytotoxic and endocrine therapy in breast cancer, in *Progress in Cancer Research and Therapy,* Bresciani, F., King, J. B., Lippman, M. E., Namer, M., and Raynaud, J. P., Eds., Raven Press, New York, 1984, 269.
18. **Gametchu, B.,** Glucocorticoid receptor-like antigen in lymphoma cell membranes: Correlation to cell lysis, *Science,* 236, 456, 1987.
19. **Kennedy, B. J.,** Hormone therapy in cancer, *Geriatrics,* 25, 106, 1970.
20. **Coombes, R. C.,** Endocrine treatment of breast cancer: current concepts and future approaches, in *The New Endocrinology of Cancer,* Waxman, J. and Coombes, R. C., Eds., Edward Arnold, London, 1987, 54.
21. **Lupulescu, A.,** *Hormones and Carcinogenesis,* Praeger Scientific, New York, 1983, 316.
22. **Schinzinger, A. S.,** Über carcinoma mammae, *Beilage Centralbl. Chirurgie,* 16, 55, 1889.
23. **Dodds, E., Goldberg, L., Lawson, W., and Robinson, R.,** Oestrogenic activity of certain synthetic compounds, *Nature (London),* 141, 247, 1938.

24. **Craig, H. I., Harris, J. R., Kinne, D. W., and Hellman, S.,** Cancer of the breast in *Cancer Principles and Practice of Oncology*, DeVita, V. T., Hellman, S., and Rosenberg, S. A., Eds., Lippincott, Philadelphia, 1989, 1197.

25. **Kardinal, C. G.,** Endocrine therapy of breast cancer, in *Cancer of the Breast*, Donegan, W. L. and Spratt, J. S., Eds., W. B. Saunders, Philadelphia, 1988, 501.

26. **Harmsen, H. J. and Porsius, A. J.,** Endocrine therapy of breast cancer, *Eur. J. Cancer. Clin. Oncol.*, 24, 1099, 1988.

27. **Loeb, L.,** Further observations on the endemic occurrence of carcinoma on the inoculability of tumors, *Univ. Penn. Med. Bull.*, 20, 2, 1907.

28. **Farrow, J. H. and Adair, F. E.,** Effect of orchiectomy on skeletal metastasis from cancer of the male breast, *Science*, 95, 654, 1942.

29. **Adami, H. O., Holmberg, L., Malker, B., and Ries, L.,** Long-term survival in 406 males with breast cancer, *Br. J. Cancer*, 52, 99, 1985.

30. **Resnick, M. I.,** Hormonal therapy in prostate carcinoma, *Urology*, 24 (Suppl.), 18, 1984.

31. **Scott, W. W., Menon, M., and Walsh, P. C.,** Hormonal therapy of prostatic cancer, *Cancer*, 45, 1929, 1980.

32. **Freiha, F. S., Bagshaw, M. A., and Torti, F. M.,** Carcinoma of the prostate: pathology, staging and treatment, *Curr. Probl. Cancer*, 12, 335, 1988.

33. **Moore, F. D., Van Devanter, S. B., Boyden, C. M., Lokich, J., and Wilson, R. E.,** Adrenalectomy with chemotherapy in the treatment of advanced breast cancer. Objective and subjective response rates. Duration and quality of life, *Surgery*, 76, 376, 1974.

34. **Yonemoto, R. H., Tan, M. S., Byron, R. L., Riihimaki, D. U., Keating, J., and Jacobs, W.,** Randomized sequential hormonal therapy vs adrenalectomy for metastatic breast carcinoma, *Cancer*, 39, 547, 1977.

35. **Harvey, H. A., Santen, R. J., Osterman, J., Samojlik, E., White, D. S., and Lipton, A.,** A comparative trial of transsphenoidal hypophysectomy and estrogen suppression with aminoglutethimide in advanced breast cancer, *Cancer*, 43, 2207, 1979.

36. **Pollen, J. J.,** Endocrine treatment of prostatic cancer, *Urology*, 21, 555, 1983.

37. **Whitmore, W. F.,** The natural history of prostatic cancer, *Cancer*, 32, 1104, 1973.

38. **Sogani, P. C. and Fair, W. R.,** Treatment of advanced prostatic cancer, *Urol. Clin. North Am.*, 14, 353, 1987.

39. **Andersson, L., Edsmyr, F., Jönsson, G., and Könyves, I.,** Estramustine phosphate therapy in carcinoma of the prostate, *Rec. Res. Cancer Res.*, 60, 73, 1977.

40. **Nesto, R. W., Cady, B., Oberfield, R. A., Pazianos, A. G., and Salzman, F. A.,** Rebound response after estrogen therapy for metastatic breast cancer, *Cancer*, 38, 1834, 1976.

41. **Davidson, N. E. and Lippman, M. E.,** Treatment of metastatic breast cancer, in *Diagnosis and Management of Breast Cancer*, Lippman, M. E., Lichter, A. S., and Danforth, D. N., Eds., W. B. Saunders, Philadelphia, 1988, 375.

42. **Goss, P. E., Ashley, S., Powles, T. J., and Coombes, R. C.,** High-dose oral medroxyprogesterone acetate in heavily pretreated patients with metastatic breast cancer, *Cancer Treat. Rep.*, 70, 777, 1986.

43. **Ettinger, D. S., Allegra, J., Bertino, J. R., Bonomi, P., Browder, H., Byrne, P., Greco, F., Catalano, R., Creech, R., Dana, B., Greenwald, E., Holmes, F., Henderson, I., Keller, J., Kinzbrunner, B., Losada, M., Muss, H., Nimeh, N., Weinreb, J., Wheeler, R., and Wiernik, P. H.,** Megestrol acetate vs tamoxifen in advanced breast cancer: correlation of hormone receptors and response, *Semin. Oncol.*, 13, (Suppl. 4), 9, 1986.

44. **Horton, J., Knuiman, M., Keller, A. M., Gale, K. E., Hahn, R. G., Vogel, H., Rosenbluth, R. J., and Tormey, D. C.,** Combination hormone therapy for metastatic breast cancer: an ECOG study of megestrol and aminoglutethimide, *Cancer*, 60, 2137, 1987.

45. **Teulings, F. A., Van Gilse, H. A., Henkelman, M. S., Portengen, H., and Alexieva-Figusch, J.,** Estrogen, androgen, glucocorticoid, and progesterone receptors in progestin-induced regression of human breast cancer, *Cancer Res.*, 40, 2557, 1980.

46. **Allegra, J. C. and Kiefer, S. M.,** Mechanisms of action of progestational agents, *Semin. Oncol.*, 12 (Suppl. 1), 3, 1985.

47. **Greenwald, E. S.,** Megestrol acetate flare, *Cancer Treat. Rep.*, 67, 405, 1983.

48. **Lacassagne, A. and Raynaud, A.,** Sur le mécanisme d'une action préventive de la testostérone sur le carcinome mammaire de la souris, *C. R. Soc. Biol.* (Paris), 131, 586, 1939.

49. **Kennedy, B. J.,** Hormonal therapies in breast cancer, *Semin. Oncol.*, 1, 119, 1974.

50. **Zava, D. T. and McGuire, W. L.,** Human breast cancer: Androgen action mediated via estrogen receptor, *Science*, 199, 787, 1978.

51. **Rochefort, H.,** Biochemical basis of breast cancer treatment by androgens and progestins, in *Hormones and Cancer*, Gurpide, E., Calandra, R., Levy, C., and Soto, R. J., Eds., Alan R. Liss, New York, 1984, 79.

52. **Lopez, M.,** Cyproterone acetate in the treatment of metastatic cancer of the male breast, *Cancer,* 55, 2334, 1985.

53. **Haskell, C. M.,** Principles of cancer treatment, in *Cancer Treatment,* 2nd ed., Haskell, C. M., Ed., W. B. Saunders, Philadelphia, 1985, 82.

54. **Geimer, N. F. and Donegan, W. L.,** Role and mechanism of corticosteroid therapy in breast cancer, *Rev. Endocr.-Relat. Cancer,* 6, 5, 1980.

55. **Santen, R. J.,** Suppression of estrogens with aminoglutethimide and hydrocortisone (medical adrenalectomy) as treatment of advanced breast carcinoma, a review, *Breast Cancer Res. Treat.,* 1, 183, 1981.

56. **Lawrence, B. V., Lipton, A., Harvey, H. A., Santen, R. J., Wells, S., Cox, C., White, D. S., and Smart, E. K.,** Influence of estrogen receptor status on response of metastatic breast cancer to aminoglutethimide therapy, *Cancer,* 45, 786, 1980.

57. **Harris, A. L., Powles, T. J., Smith, I. E., Ford, A., Morgan, M., White, J., Parsons, C., and McKinna, J.,** Aminoglutethimide for the treatment of advanced postmenopausal breast cancer, *Eur. J. Cancer Clin. Oncol.,* 19, 11, 1983.

58. **Nemoto, T., Rosner, D., Patel, J., and Dao, T. L.,** Aminoglutethimide in patients with metastatic breast cancer, *Cancer,* 63, 1673, 1989.

59. **Vincent, M. D., Clink, H. M., Coombes, R. C., Smith I. E., Kandler, R., and Powles, T. J.,** Aminoglutethimide (with hydrocortisone) induced agranulocytosis in primary breast cancer, *Br. Med. J.,* 291, 105, 1985.

60. **Brodie, A. M., Schwarzel, W. C., Shaikh, A. A., and Brodie, H. J.,** The effect of an aromatase inhibitor 4-hydroxy-4-androstene-3,17-dione, on estrogen-dependent processes in reproduction and breast cancer, *Endocrinology,* 100, 1684, 1977.

61. **Goss, P. E., Powles, T. J., Dowsett, M., Hutchinson, G., Brodie, A. M., Gazet, J. C., and Coombes, R. C.,** Treatment of advanced postmenopausal breast cancer with aromatase inhibitor 4-hydroxyandrostenedione-phase II report, *Cancer Res.,* 46, 4823, 1986.

62. **Dowsett, M., Cunningham, D. C., Stein, R. C., Evans, S., Dehennin, L., Hedley, A., and Coombes, R. C.,** Dose-related endocrine effects and pharmacokinetics of oral and intramuscular 4-hydroxyandrostenedione in postmenopausal breast cancer patients, *Cancer Res.,* 49, 1306, 1989.

63. **Barbieri, R. L. and Ryan, K. J.,** Danazol: endocrine pharmacology and therapeutic applications, *Am. J. Obstet. Gynecol.,* 141, 453, 1981.

64. **Broekmans, A. W., Conard, J., Van Weyenberg, R. G., Horellou, M. H., Kluft, C., and Bertina, R. M.,** Treatment of hereditary protein C deficiency with stanozolol, *Thromb. Haemost.,* 57, 20, 1987.

65. **Coombes, R. C., Perez, D., Gazet, J. C., Ford, H. T., and Powles, T. J.,** Danazol Treatment for advanced breast cancer, *Cancer Chemother. Pharmacol.,* 10, 194, 1983.

66. **Clayton, R. N.,** Gonadotrophin releasing hormone: from physiology to pharmacology, *Clin. Endocrinol.,* 26, 361, 1987.

67. **Schally, A. V., Redding, T. W., and Comaru-Schally, A. M.,** Potential use of analogs of luteinizing hormone-releasing hormones in the treatment of hormone-sensitive neoplasms, *Cancer Treat. Rep.,* 68, 281, 1984.

68. **Waxman, J.,** Gonadotrophin releasing hormone analogues for prostatic cancer: an overview, *Semin. Oncol.,* 15, 366, 1988.

69. **Harvey, H. A., Lipton, A., Max, D. T., Pearlman, H. G., Diaz-Perches, R., and de la Garza, J.,** Medical castration produced by the GnRH analogue leuprolide to treat metastatic breast cancer, *J. Clin. Oncol.,* 3, 1068, 1985.

70. Leuprolide Study Group: Leuprolide versus diethylstilbestrol for metastatic prostate cancer, *N. Engl. J. Med.,* 311, 1281, 1984.

71. **Labrie, F., Dupont, A., Bélanger, A., Lefebvre, F. A., Cusan, L., Raynaud, J. P., Husson, J. M., and Fazekas, A. T.,** New hormonal therapy in prostate cancer: combined use of a pure antiandrogen and an LHRH agonist, *Horm. Res.,* 18, 18, 1983.

72. **Bouffioux, C.,** Total androgen blockade in advanced prostatic cancer, *Eur. Urol.,* 15, 187, 1988.

73. **Santen, R. J., Manni, A., and Harvey, H.,** Gonadotropin releasing hormone (GnRH) analogs for the treatment of breast and prostatic carcinoma, *Breast Cancer Res. Treat.,* 7, 129, 1986.

74. **Conn, P. M.,** The molecular basis of gonadotropin-releasing hormone action, *Endocr. Rev.,* 7, 3, 1986.

75. **Krulich, L., Dhariwal, A. P., and McCann, S. M.,** Stimulatory and inhibitory effects of purified hypothalamic extracts on growth hormone release from rat pituitary *in vitro, Endocrinology,* 83, 783, 1968.

76. **Reichlin, S.,** Somatostatin, *N. Engl. J. Med.,* 309, 1495, 1983.

77. **Fine, A.,** Peptides and Alzheimer's disease, *Nature (London),* 319, 537, 1986.

78. **Schally, A. V. and Redding, T. W.,** Somatostatin analogs as adjuncts to agonists of luteinizing hormone-releasing hormone in the treatment of experimental prostate cancer, *Proc. Natl. Acad. Sci. U.S.A.,* 84, 7275, 1987.

79. **Lamberts, S. W.,** A guide to the clinical use of the somatostatin analogue SMS 201-995 (Sandostatin), *Acta Endocrinol.,* (Kbh), 286 (Suppl.), 54, 1987.

80. **Bloom, S. R. and Polak, J. M.,** Somatostatin, *Br. Med. J.,* 295, 288, 1987.
81. **Parmar, H., Bogden, A., Mollard, M., de Rougé, B., Phillips, R. H., and Lightman, S. L.,** Somatostatin and somatostatin analogues in oncology, *Cancer Treat. Rev.,* 16, 95, 1989.
82. **Mazzaferri, E. L.,** Papillary thyroid carcinoma: factors influencing prognosis and current therapy, *Semin. Oncol.,* 14, 315, 1987.
83. **Danforth, D. N., Tamarkin, L., Mulvihill, J. J., Bagley, C. S., and Lippman, M. E.,** Plasma melatonin and the hormone-dependency of human breast cancer, *J. Clin. Oncol.,* 3, 941, 1985.
84. Consensus Conference, NCI (Natl. Cancer Institute): adjuvant chemotherapy for breast cancer, *JAMA,* 254, 3461, 1985.
85. **Legha, S. S.,** Tamoxifen in the treatment of breast cancer, *Ann. Intern. Med.,* 109, 219, 1988.
86. Controlled trial of tamoxifen as a single adjuvant agent in the management of early breast cancer, Analysis of eight years by Nolvadex adjuvant trial organization, *Br. J. Cancer,* 57, 608, 1988.
87. **Craig Henderson, I., Hayes, D. F., Come, S., Harris, J. R., and Canellos, G.,** New agents and new medical treatments for advanced breast cancer, *Semin. Oncol.,* 14, 34, 1987.
88. **Patterson, J. S., Battersby, L. A., and Edwards, D. G.,** Review of clinical pharmacology: an international experience with tamoxifen in advanced breast cancer, *Rev. Endocr.-Relat. Cancer,* (Suppl.) 9, 563, 1982. 9, 563, 1982.
89. **Taylor, C. M., Blanchard, B., and Zava, D. T.,** Estrogen receptor-mediated and cytotoxic effects of the antiestrogen tamoxifen and 4-hydroxy-tamoxifen, *Cancer Res.,* 44, 1409, 1984.
90. **Hortobagyi, G. N., Hug, V., Buzdar, A. U., Kau, S. W., Holmes, F. A., and Fritsche, H. A.,** Sequential cyclic combined hormonal therapy for metastatic breast cancer, *Cancer,* 64, 1002, 1989.
91. **Donaldson, V. H.,** Danazol, *Am. J. Med.,* 87, 3-49N, 1989.
92. **Schacter, L., Rozencweig, M., Canetta, R., Kelley, S., Nicaise, C., and Smaldone, L.,** Megestrol acetate: clinical experience, *Cancer Treat. Rev.,* 16, 49, 1989.
93. **Vennin, P. H., Peyrat, J. P., Bonneterre, J., Louchez, M. M., Harris, A. G., and Demaille, A.,** Effect of the long-acting somatostatin analogue SMS 201-995 (Sandostatin) in advanced breast cancer, *Anticancer Res.,* 9, 153, 1989.
94. **Hultborn, R., Friberg, S., Hultborn, K. A., Peterson, L. E., and Ragnhult, I.,** Male breast carcinoma, *Acta Oncol.,* 26, 327, 1987.
95. **Huben, R. P. and Murphy, G. P.,** Prostate cancer: an update, *Ca-A Cancer J. Clinicians,* 36, 274, 1986.
96. **Hilaris, B. S., Dattatreyudu, N., and Batata, M.,** Cancer of the prostate: current perspectives, *Cancer Invest.,* 5, 459, 1987.
97. **Paulson, D.,** Diseases of the prostate, *Ciba Clin. Symp.,* 41, 17, 1989.
98. Consensus Conference: The management of clinically localized prostate cancer, *JAMA,* 258, 2727, 1987.
99. **Brendler, C. B.,** The current role of hormonal therapy in the clinical treatment of prostatic cancer, *Semin. Urol.,* 6, 269, 1988.
100. **Debruyne, F. M., Denis, L., Lunglmayer, G., Mahler, C., Newling, D. W., Richards, B., Robinson, M. R., Smith, P. H., Weil, E. H., and Whelan, P.,** Long-term therapy with a depot luteinizing hormone-releasing hormone analogue (Zoladex) in patients with advanced prostatic carcinoma, *J. Urol.,* 140, 775, 1988.
101. **Flamm, J. and Fischer, M.,** Komplette Androgen Blockade (Orchiektomie + Flutamid) versus Androgen Blockade mit zytostase (Orchiektomie + Estramustin) in der Behandlung des Virginellen Fortgeschritten Prostatakarzinoms, *Wien. Klin. Wochenschr.,* 100, 589, 1988.
102. **Nesbit, R. M. and Baum, W. C.,** Endocrine control of prostatic carcinoma: clinical and statistical survey of 1818 cases, *JAMA,* 143, 1317, 1950.
103. **Berek, J. S., Hacker, N. F., and Hatch, K. D.,** Uterine corpus and uterine cancer, *Curr. Probl. Cancer,* 12, 65, 1988.
104. **Kneale, B. G.,** Adjuvant and therapeutic progestins in endometrial cancer, *Clin. Obstet. Gynaecol.,* 13, 789, 1986.
105. **Piver, M. S.,** Progesterone therapy for malignant peritoneal cytology surgical Stage I endometrial adenocarcinoma, *Semin. Oncol.,* 15, 50, 1988.
106. **Slotman, B. J. and Rao, B. R.,** Ovarian cancer (review), *Anticancer Res.,* 8, 417, 1988.
107. **Freedman, R. S., Saul, P. B., Edwards, C. L., Jolles, C. J., Gershenson, D. M., Jones, L. A., Atkinson, E. N., and Dana, W. J.,** Ethinyl estradiol and medroxyprogesterone acetate in patients with epithelial ovarian carcinoma: a Phase II study, *Cancer Treat. Rep.,* 70, 369, 1986.
108. **Greenway, B. A.,** Carcinoma of the exocrine pancreas: a sex hormone responsive tumor? *Br. J. Surg.,* 74, 441, 1987.
109. **Isaacs, J. T.,** Cellular factors in the development of resistance to hormonal therapy, in *Drug and Hormone Resistance in Neoplasia,* Bruchovsky, N. and Goldie, J. H., Eds., CRC Press, Boca Raton, FL, 1982, 139.
110. **Allegra, J. C.,** Methotrexate and 5-fluorouracil following tamoxifen and premarin in advanced breast cancer, *Semin. Oncol.,* 10 (Suppl. 2), 23, 1983.

111. **Weissman, D. E.,** Glucocorticoid treatment for brain metastases and epidural spinal cord compression: a review, *J. Clin. Oncol.,* 6, 543, 1988.
112. **Tchekmedyian, N. S., Tait, N., Moody, M., and Aisner, J.,** High-dose megestrol acetate: A possible treatment for cachexia, *JAMA,* 257, 1195, 1987.
113. **Moricca, G.,** Chemical hypophysectomy for cancer pain, in *Advances in Neurology,* Bonica, J. J., Ed., Raven Press, New York, 1974, 707.
114. **Szántó, J. József, S., Radó, J., Juhos, É., Hindy, I., and Eckhardt, S.,** Pain killing with calcitonin in patients with malignant tumours, *Oncology,* 43, 69, 1986.
115. **Chrubasik, J.,** Analgetische wirkung von somatostatin, *Münch. Med. Wochenschr.,* 131, 199, 1989.
116. **King, R. J.,** Receptors, growth factors and steroid insensitivity of tumours, *J. Endocr.,* 124, 179, 1990.

Chapter 3

HORMONE ANTAGONISTS AND HORMONE AGONISTS

I. GENERAL CONSIDERATIONS AND PROSPECTS OF MEDICAL ENDOCRINE ABLATION

Hormone antagonists are a recent development in endocrine pharmacology and cancer treatment. These agents are likely to provide new and better therapy, replacing in many cases, the ablative endocrine therapy, such as surgical or radiation castration (ovariectomy or oophorectomy and orchiectomy), surgical adrenalectomy, and hypophysectomy.

They provide similar or even identical beneficial therapeutic effects to surgical or radiation ablation, without disfigurement and psychologic effects, and consequently they are replacing the conventional surgical castration and surgical adrenalectomy with medical castration and medical adrenalectomy, which are less life-threatening and preferable to many cancer patients. Several hormone antagonists are under study in clinical trials, which already indicate that their physiologic and pharmacologic effects, in lowering the steroid hormone levels to basal line or near "castrate" levels, are almost identical to that provided by surgical removal of ovary, testis, or adrenal gland.[1-3] Hormone antagonists, such as tamoxifen, aminoglutethimide, and LHRH agonists are significantly superior to cytotoxic chemotherapy in extending the disease-free interval and response rate, but with minimal toxic side effects.

A. HORMONE ANTAGONISTS

Hormone antagonists act on cancer cells by different mechanisms related to species or type of tumor. Two of these mechanisms are better known: (1) by competing with the same hormone receptors, thus inhibiting the effect of hormones on target cells, e.g., antiestrogen tamoxifen, and (2) by inhibiting the steroid hormone synthesis (at different enzyme levels), thus decreasing the endogenous hormone synthesis, such as aromatase inhibitors, aminoglutethimide (AG). The most important and commonly used hormone antagonists in cancer treatment are: (1) antiestrogens, (2) antiandrogens, (3) antiprogestins, (4) antiprolactin, (5) antiglucocorticoids, (6) LHRH antagonists, (7) aromatase inhibitors, (8) somatostatin synthetic analogs, and (9) prostaglandin synthesis inhibitors.

1. Antiestrogens

The antiestrogens, tamoxifen (TAM), trioxyphene, clomiphene, and nafoxidine, are triphenylethylene derivatives which are, depending upon the species and organ under study, antagonists or partial agonists on the circulating estrogens. Tamoxifen is a nonsteroidal antiestrogen synthesized in 1966, and originally used as an antifertility drug.[4] Since 1970, it has been used for treatment of postmenopausal women with metastatic breast cancer. Due to its antitumor activity and lack of toxicity, tamoxifen is widely used in several clinical trials in the U.S., as elsewhere. The physiologic effect of Tamoxifen has a paradoxical species-specific pharmacology. Thus, the drug is a full estrogen in the mouse, a partial estrogen/antiestrogen in the humans and the rat, and an antiestrogen in the chick oviduct.[5] Tamoxifen is a nonsteroidal antiestrogen, structurally related to diethylstilbestrol (DES) (see Figure 1). The drug is easily synthesized and it is available as a monocitrate salt (Nolvadex) in 10 mg tablets. Pharmacokinetic studies using radiolabeled tamoxifen [^{3}H]-tamoxifen in animals and women have shown that the drug has a long plasma half-life. In women, the peak plasma radioactivity level was reached within 4 to 7 hours after a single oral dose, but only 20 to 30% of the radioactive material was tamoxifen, the remainder being its metabolites. After an initial serum half-life, 7 to 14 h, the concentration of total radioactivity with a

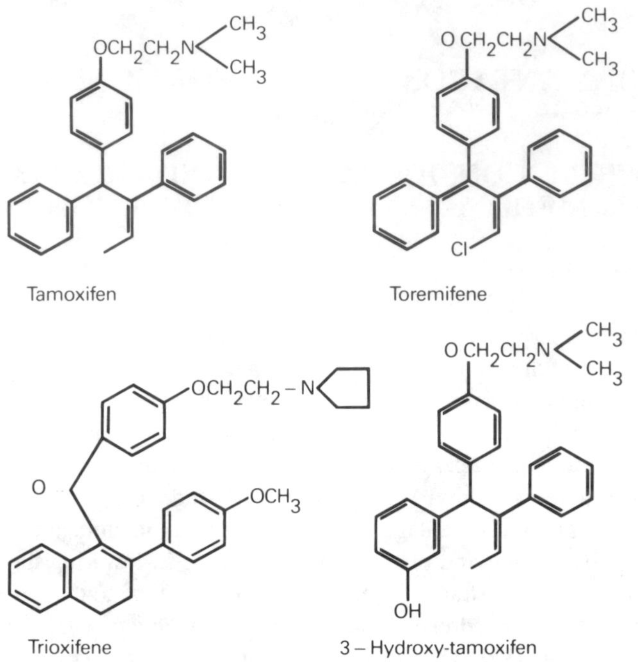

FIGURE 1.   Major antiestrogens and their chemical configuration.

terminal half-life of more than 7 d remained. Studies with [³H]-tamoxifen revealed that this drug undergoes extensive metabolic conversion by hydroxylation and conjugation. It recently has been shown that the major metabolite of tamoxifen in patients is *N*-des-methyl-tamoxifen, and this metabolite has a very similar pharmacology to tamoxifen. However, hydroxylation of tamoxifen forms 4-hydroxytamoxifen, which is the major metabolite in rats and athymic mice and is found only in minor proportion in serum from tamoxifen-treated patients. After oral administration of tamoxifen, a steady-state serum concentration is not achieved until 4 weeks of treatment with the standard dose of 10 mg b.i.d. The approximate biologic half-lives of tamoxifen and *N*-desmethyltamoxifen, are 7 to 14 d, respectively. Consequently, tamoxifen can be detected for 4 weeks in the serum after the treatment was discontinued. Therefore, interpretation of tumor-receptor content may not be reliable until 6 weeks after treatment cessation.

Several antiestrogens, including clomiphene, nafoxidine, and tamoxifen, were tested as potential antitumor agents, but only tamoxifen is available for cancer therapy because it has a low incidence of side effects.[6] A number of other antiestrogens, such as toremifene, trioxifene, 3-hydroxytamoxifen, and MER25, are also undergoing evaluation in early clinical studies (see Figure 1).

New antiestrogens, such as trioxifene, had a similar therapeutic efficacy and toxicity to tamoxifen when used in the management of advanced breast cancer. In several patients who had previously responded to tamoxifen, and then relapsed, partial remissions were achieved with trioxifene. Its affinity for ER is about 10 times higher than that of TAM, and it induces a dose-dependent reduction of LH an FSH levels. The hormonal and antitumor properties of toremifene (chlorotamoxifen) have recently been described. The half-life of distribution of toremifene in the rat is 4 h, and the t $\frac{1}{2}$ for elimination is approximately 24 h. The major route of elimination of its metabolites is via biliary excretion in the feces, and very little is eliminated in the urine. In humans, the distribution and elimination t $\frac{1}{2}$ of toremifene are 4 h and 5 d, respectively. Toremifene is also effective in postmenopausal patients with advanced breast cancer, but it does not offer clear advantages over tamoxifen. However, it is interesting that clinical studies with toremifene are using much higher doses (60 to 100 mg/d) than those recommended for tamoxifen (20 to 40 mg/d). It has been reported that high doses of toremifene (200 mg/d) have induced clinical responses in tumors resistant to tamoxifen. The use of 3-hydroxytamoxifen (droloxifene), has been reported in metastatic breast cancer. By using an intermittent dosage regimen (100 mg every second or third day), a complete response lasting for at least 6 months in 3/10 patients has been reported. Toremifene has also recently been reported to be an active chemosensitizer that reverses the phenomenon of multidrug resistance (MDR).

a. Mechanism of Action

Most studies at present have focused upon the interaction of antiestrogens with the estrogen receptor. (1) Antiestrogens inhibit the binding of [^{3}H]-estradiol to the estrogen receptor. [^{3}H]-tamoxifen can bind directly to the estrogen receptor. (2) Studies with radiolabeled estrogens and antiestrogens demonstrate that the ligands interact with the receptor in different ways. Estrogens and antiestrogens may have a different method of "activating" receptors (3) Differences in the size of nuclear estrogen and antiestrogen receptor complexes have been noted. (4) Differences in the interaction of estrogen and antiestrogen receptor complexes with DNA have been described. This may be related to the observation that antiestrogen-receptor complexes are more easily extracted from nuclei by $0.4\ M$ of KCl than estradiol-estrogen receptor complexes. (5) The concentration of estradiol-estrogen receptor complexes extracted with $0.4\ M$ of KCl decreases over the first 6 h of estrogen exposure, whereas antiestrogen-estrogen receptor complexes do not. (6) Antiestrogens may inhibit the estrogen receptor resynthesis by blocking the recycling of spent receptors or synthesis *de novo*. (7) Antiestrogens may affect the circulating levels of plasma estradiol and lower the release of gonadotropins and prolactin from the pituitary gland. (8) In addition, antiestrogens affect the cell cycle and induce a dose-dependent decrease in the percentage of cells in the S-phase, and a relative increase in the number of cells in either the G_o/G_1-phase or G_1/G_2 phase.[7] The G_1-phase blockade of tamoxifen can be reversed by estrogens ("estrogen rescue") in MCF-7 cells in culture. (9) Antitumor effect is a dose-dependent effect. At low concentrations of tamoxifen, there is a cytostatic effect, by which ER positive cells are blocked by the drug in the early G_1-phase of the cell cycle; whereas, at higher concentrations of tamoxifen (more than 4 μm), it has cytotoxic effects characterized by cell death of both ER + and ER − cells. Antiestrogens inhibit the initiation and growth of dimethyl-benz(α)anthracene (DMBA)-induced rat mammary carcinoma. This tumor is more prolactin dependent. Antiestrogens also inhibit the growth of NMU (*N*-nitrosomethylurea) induced hormone-dependent tumors in female rats which are more estrogen-dependent than DMBA-induced tumors. (10) Tamoxifen is a potent inhibitor of calmodulin. This protein binds calcium ions (Ca^{2+}), and inhibitors of calmodulin, such as trifluoperazine, will produce a block in the G_1-phase of the cell cycle. (11) Tamoxifen exerts mild estrogenic effects at low concentrations. It also enhances the natural killer (NK) cell activity (additive to interferon). It also inhibits the synthesis of estrogen-regulated stimulating growth factors, while stimulating the synthesis of inhibitory growth factors, (TGF-β).[7] Finally, (12) tamoxifen suppresses the expression of some oncogenes (myc, ras, and fos).

b. Clinical Use of Tamoxifen

Before tamoxifen, the approach to primary hormonal treatment in patients with metastatic breast cancer whose tumors contain ER (approximately 60%), was oophorectomy for premenopausal women and DES for postmenopausal women. In patients who responded to primary endocrine treatment, secondary treatment included adrenalectomy or hypophysectomy, and androgens and progestins were used later as tertiary treatment. Over the past 10 years there has been a major shift from this sequence of treatment to use of tamoxifen, either as a primary treatment or as secondary hormonal treatment.

As regards the tamoxifen dose used, it is now concluded that tamoxifen does not have a significant dose-responsive curve. Usually, the antiestrogenic effects of tamoxifen are manifest to the standard dose of 10 mg b.i.d. Response to the standard dose of 10 mg b.i.d. are equivalent to those for 20 mg b.i.d. and doses up to 90 mg/d have no advantage. Thus, the standard dose is now accepted to be 10 mg b.i.d.[8] Although tamoxifen is used in a twice-daily schedule, it is possible to obtain the same biologic effects with a single daily dose (a loading dose), due to the long half-life of tamoxifen and its metabolites. This loading dose allows a steady-state serum drug concentration to be achieved within 1 week of treatment instead of 4 weeks with the standard dose.[8] However, the frequency of responses and overall survival are the same in both schedules.

Tolerance to tamoxifen is excellent. The most frequent side effects have been hot flushes, menstrual dysfunction, and rarely uterine bleeding, all related to estrogen-blockade. Sometimes (approximately 10%) patients have nausea and vomiting. A less frequent side effect is increased bone pain or soft tissue pain and occasionally hypercalcemia, a phenomenon called tumor flare or tamoxifen flare, which is believed to be due to the mild estrogenic effect. Tumor flare usually heralds a hormone responsiveness in the primary tumor as well as in the metastases, especially bone metastases. Tumor flare should be treated with analgesics, and full doses of tamoxifen should be continued. Tumor flare is observed, generally 12 to 21 d after starting most hormonal therapies in the following percentages of patients:

1. LHRH agonists, 3 to 10%
2. Androgens, 3%
3. Antiestrogens (tamoxifen), 2.2%
4. Estrogens, 1%
5. Progestins, 1%
6. Aminoglutethimide, not reported

The treatment for patients with tumor flare includes supportive care (analgesics); sometimes prednisone is added to the treatment for 1 to 2 weeks. Other rare side effects include thrombophlebitis and ocular toxicity. Reversible ocular toxicity (retinal hemorrhage, visual impairment) has recently been described in a patient with metastatic breast cancer which resolved completely after cessation of tamoxifen therapy.[9] However, the carcinogenic potential of antiestrogens in mice warrants extreme caution with regard to the use of the drug in high-risk groups. Recently, new compounds have ben synthesized with reduced estrogenic activity, such as LY117018 and LY139481, hydroxylated compounds which bind to estrogen receptors with the same affinity as estradiol, but have minimum estrogen-like activity. Unfortunately, hydroxylation shortens biologic half-life as well as their antitumor activity, and they are less active than tamoxifen against prolactin-dependent carcinogen induced mammary tumors.[10] Overall, tamoxifen withdrawal because of toxicity is necessary in less than 3% of patients.

Initially, tamoxifen use was restricted to postmenopausal women with metastatic breast cancer. At present, however, tamoxifen has a broader use to include premenopausal women with metastatic disease and also to control micrometastases in women with early breast cancer. In metastatic breast cancer, tamoxifen is currently the treatment of choice for all patients with ER + and PR + tumors without extensive visceral metastases. Because the response to tamoxifen is better than 50% in elderly patients, tamoxifen is preferred, not only for patients with recurrent disease, but also for those with advanced primary tumors that are not suitable for surgical removal.[11] Although the role of tamoxifen in the treatment of metastatic cancer in postmenopausal women is well defined, its use in premenopausal women is still controversial. Tamoxifen, however, does not block the effects of circulating estrogens completely, even in higher doses of 40 mg/d. Consequently, some of these patients may respond to bilateral ovariectomy. The response to bilateral ovariectomy in patients that respond to tamoxifen is significantly higher (50 to 60%) compared with a response rate of 15 to 20% in patients who did not respond to the drug. A recent controlled trial of tamoxifen as a single adjuvant agent in the management of early breast cancer, made by Nolvadex Adjuvant Trial Organization (NATO) using tamoxifen 20 mg/d for 2 years vs. no treatment, revealed a significant advantage for patients receiving tamoxifen. This advantage is independent of menopausal status, stage, grade, and ER status.[12] In a recent study performed in 1846 postmenopausal patients, and using tamoxifen as an adjuvant to primary surgery for early breast cancer, the median followup was 4.5 years; it was found that in tamoxifen patients, second breast cancers occurred less often and endometrial cancer occurred more often than in the controls.[13]

Interestingly, in a randomized trial in 122 premenopausal women with advanced breast cancer, half treated with tamoxifen and half with oophorectomy, it was found that duration of response and overall survival were similar in both groups, although toxicity was greater in those undergoing oophorectomy.[14] Recently, several comparative randomized trials (more than 26) which compared tamoxifen with other endocrine therapies revealed that tamoxifen has become the most commonly used endocrine therapy of advanced breast cancer due to its few side effects and an overall response rate of 35% compared with either ablative, additive, or inhibitive hormone treatments. Thus, tamoxifen may replace the oophorectomy in premenopausal women, and aminoglutethimide or progestins in postmenopausal women.

Presently, there is controversy regarding the time needed for adjuvant treatment with tamoxifen to be effective. It is believed tamoxifen treatment should be continued for at least 2 years and possibly longer (to 5 years) after mastectomy, and beneficial therapeutic effects are higher than in shorter trials. This is concordant with the experimental studies which showed that long-term administration of tamoxifen providing a continuing cytostatic effect in rats and prevented metastases as long as tamoxifen was used.[15]

A randomized, controlled trial of tamoxifen as a single adjuvant agent after mastectomy for early breast cancer (followed up until 6 years) in both premenopausal women with positive axillary nodes and postmenopausal women with positive and negative axillary nodes were randomized to receive either tamoxifen 10 mg b.i.d. for 2 years or to the untreated control group; there has been a highly significant reduction in death rate, with 34% fewer deaths observed in the treatment group than in the control group. This benefit appeared to be independent of menopause, nodal, or ER status.[16,17] Similarly, tamoxifen combined with chemotherapy is not established to be superior to tamoxifen alone. Tamoxifen should be used in a standard dose of 10 mg twice a day for a minimum 4 to 6 weeks before it can be judged ineffective. Frequently, a period of 8 to 12 weeks is desirable for an adequate trial. Thus, tamoxifen should be given as a single agent, and the duration of the entire treatment is approximately 2 years. A longer duration (at least 2 years) is more effective than 1 year.

There is some experimental evidence that antiestrogens can prevent the induction of rat mammary carcinomas by carcinogens. Thus, antiestrogens can be used as chemopreventive agents in patients at risk for breast cancer. Although tamoxifen (Nolvadex) has been available for more than 10 years for the treatment of breast cancer, the complete or partial response rate in 68 published studies involving 4000 patients treated with Nolvadex has remained unchanged from the earliest publication and remarkably constant at 33%. A further 20% of patients show disease stabilization.[16] Thus, only 55% of patients with ER+ are seen to respond. However, tamoxifen is less toxic than other antiestrogens, nafoxidine, and MER-25, which have shown unpredicted phototoxicity and central nervous system problems in man.

Patients with long history of cardiovascular and clotting disorders, should be excluded from chemosuppressive trials. Experimental results indicate that the estrogen-like effects of tamoxifen may maintain the bone density in ovariectomized rats. Studies in women by measuring bone mineral density (BMD), in postmenopausal women treated with tamoxifen (2 years), suggest that tamoxifen does not have "anti-estrogenic" side effects on bone mineral density.[18]

Recently, other new antiestrogens with superior antiestrogenic properties, such as trioxifene mesylate have been used in the treatment of advanced breast cancer. This agent showed significant antitumor activity in the DMBA-induced rat mammary carcinoma, and also a higher binding affinity to ER, compared to estradiol or tamoxifen. It has been used in doses of 5 mg, 10 mg, and 20 mg orally twice daily. This limited clinical trial including only 69 patients suggests that trioxifene mesylate is an active agent and has similar therapeutic efficacy compared with those reported for tamoxifen.[19]

A recent study using a loading dose schedule of 100 mg/m² tamoxifen followed by a maintenance dose of 20 mg twice daily in 53 patients with stage III or IV ovarian cancer who had relapsed following cytotoxic chemotherapy, showed only a minimal activity. However, the presence in ovarian cancer cells of steroid hormone receptors, such as ER, PR, and AR (androgen receptors), should continue to stimulate investigation of other hormonal manipulation in this disease.[20] Also, tamoxifen in combination cytotoxic chemotherapy in patients with stage III and IV epithelial ovarian cancer showed no correlation between therapy and ER and PR.[21] Studies on the MCF-7 breast cancer line in the presence of various concentrations of these antiestrogens, 4-hydroxytamoxifen, tamoxifen, and ICI, show that pretreatment of MCF-7 cells for 2 d with other antiestrogens did not inhibit EGF-induced in-cell proliferation, and suggest that antiestrogen therapeutic failure may be caused by the paracrine mechanism of growth factors from neighboring cells.[22]

Antiestrogens are used also in different types of tumors, which are not hormone dependent; in some of them hormone receptors were found, such as exocrine pancreas cancer, gastric cancer, colorectal cancer, and desmoid tumors. Recently, estrogen receptors and antiestrogen binding sites (AEBSs) were found in desmoid tumors (aggressive fibromatosis). Thus, ERs were determined in cytosol and were found in 33% of desmoid tumors (DT), whereas AEBS were detected in 79% of the cases, in the microsomal fraction. These preliminary studies suggest that the therapeutical use of tamoxifen and the use of high-dose tamoxifen led to complete relief of pain and a decrease in size of desmoid tumor.[23] Also, tamoxifen therapy has been used in melanoma and more recently in eccrine adenocarcinoma. In patients with ER+ following tamoxifen, the lymph node metastasis regressed completely and was associated with full relief of pain from bone metastases for nearly 3 years. Tamoxifen produced excellent palliation and metastatic regression eccrine adenocarcinoma.[24] Tamoxifen binds also to antiestrogen binding sites. However, the antiestrogen and tumor growth-inhibiting actions of TAM correlate only with its binding affinity for ER, but not with that for AEBS, e.g., ER positive and ER negative tumors contain equal concentrations of AEBS.

Studies on the existence of ER subpopulations could also shed light on the mode of action of the antiestrogens. Clomiphene and nafoxidine are full agonists of the Type I subpopulations and are very weak agonists of the Type II ER. Nafoxidine causes a persisting increase in ER without PR synthesis, whereas TAM exhibits a slower and longer lasting increase followed by a slower decrease of ER and PR synthesis. A correlation between AEBS and antiestrogenic activity has not been reported. While more information is needed regarding the basic mechanism of action, toxicology, and pharmacology of tamoxifen, the available data are supportive of a hormonal mode of action by blocking the action of estrogen (binding to the estrogen receptor) and also slowing down of the cell cycle of breast cancer cells by accumulating them in G_0/G_1-phases of the cell cycle. Thus, tamoxifen is not usually cytocidal, but mainly cytostatic, and treatment with tamoxifen should be considered as chemosuppressive therapy.

In humans, tamoxifen exhibits both estrogen agonist and antagonist properties. Hence, as is seen in animal models, tamoxifen is more effective in inhibiting developing tumors than in controlling advanced disease. It appears that tamoxifen therapy in early cancer disease should not be "curative", but only "suppressive" with a delaying effect. Clinical trials of tamoxifen for 1 to 2 years in primary breast cancer demonstrates consistent beneficial effects on disease-free survival.[25] Currently only tamoxifen seems suitable for the treatment of premenopausal women with metastasized hormone-dependent breast cancer. Also, it is the drug of first choice for soft tissue and lung metastases. It has been reported that there are some differences regarding pharmacology of tamoxifen in premenopausal and postmenopausal women. Thus, in premenopausal women the major changes in FSH and LH do not occur, but elevations in serum estrogens, estradiol, and progesterone are common; whereas, in postmenopausal women, the normally elevated levels of FSH and LH decrease to normal, and estrogen and progesterone levels remain unchanged. Women on tamoxifen have been reported to develop endometrial cancers; however, only women with breast cancer are at high risk of this neoplasm.[26] Most of its side effects are mild and reversible. However, high-dose therapy for a long time can produce encephalopathy and retinopathy, and optic neuritis may occur. Hence, antiestrogen therapy with tamoxifen has replaced additive hormone therapy as well as ablative therapy, such as adrenalectomy and hypophysectomy, as the first-line hormonal treatment in postmenopausal women, and it may replace ovariectomy in premenopausal women.

2. Antiandrogens

Recently, both steroidal and nonsteroidal antiandrogens have been developed; however, many of the steroidal antiandrogens have progestational properties. This is not a drawback since many progestins inhibit androgen production through their antigonadotrophic actions without inducing feminization.

The mechanism of action of antiandrogens is complex and yet not well defined.

1. They may act by inhibiting the synthesis of testosterone from cholesterol by blocking the enzymes involved in this process. Thus, aminoglutethimide blocks the enzyme 20,21-desmolase and consequently, the early steps of cholesterol conversion to pregnenolone. Spironolactone, cyproterone acetate, and ketoconazole act further down the chain of synthesis by inhibiting the 17,20-desmolase enzyme, and interfere only with androgen synthesis. Other agents, including cyproterone acetate and medrogestone, all inhibit the 3β-hydroxysteroid dehydrogenase.
2. They may act by competing with natural androgens for their intracellular receptor proteins and thus, preventing translocation of androgen-receptor complexes to the nucleus.
3. They may act by interfering with the regulation of nuclear receptors of dihydrotestosterone by some nonreceptor-mediated process.[27]

Cyproterone acetate (CPA) is the best known steroidal antiandrogen and also the most frequently used. Although CPA has been shown in clinical trials to be no more effective than diethylstilbestrol (DES) in inducing tumor remission, its less toxic side effects warrants its clinical use.[28] The best known nonsteroidal antiandrogens are flutamide and anandron. In clinical trials, neither DES nor flutamide showed significant superiority. "Pure" antiandrogens, such as flutamide, anandron, and cyproterone, act directly at the receptor level, and thus interact in this manner at the hypothalamus. Consequently, an increased release of gonadotropin and enhanced synthesis of testosterone occurs.

Flutamide (SCH-13521) is a synthetic anilide which has been found in a variety of laboratory animals to be a potent antiandrogen without estrogenic, progestational, or antigonadotrophic activities, when administered to intact male rats; it if functionally specific for androgen-dependent accessory sex organs (seminal vesicles and prostate). The exact mechanism by which it exerts its antiandrogenic effect is yet not known. However, evidence suggests that flutamide or its metabolites inhibit the uptake of testosterone (or the binding of testosterone or DHT, to the nuclear receptor) and thus, prevent androgens from exerting their biologic effects on the accessory sex organs.

Administration of flutamide orally in pharmacologic doses in dogs, rats, or baboons induced a marked reduction and atrophy of the prostate gland, without structural changes in the testes. When flutamide is administered to mature animals, a significant decrease in the uptake of radiolabeled testosterone by prostatic cell nuclei is observed. In human, the drug is well absorbed from the GI tract, rapidly metabolized, and excreted in urine. Several metabolites have been identified; the major metabolite is SCH-16423 (hydroxyflutamide) with a plasma half-life of 5 to 6 h. The rapid conversion of flutamide to hydroxyflutamide and the high plasma levels of hydroxyflutamide suggest that this metabolite may be an active form of flutamide. At high doses flutamide produces an elevation of serum LH without a decrease in the level of plasma testosterone. In comparing the effect of flutamide and cyproterone acetate on levels of pituitary and gonadal hormones in healthy male subjects, it was found that there are important physiologic differences. Thus, administration of flutamide is associated with significant increases in serum levels of testosterone, estradiol, and luteinizing hormone (LH), whereas cyproterone acetate administration was associated with a notable reduction of serum testosterone, estradiol, DHT, LH, and FSH. Flutamide does not influence serum prolactin and presumably has no effect on aromatase activity. Several clinical trials of flutamide have been conducted in the U.S. as elsewhere, and reported favorable response rates in range between 66 to 85 to 90% in previously untreated patients with advanced prostate cancer. The drug was administered at a dose of 250 mg t.i.d. and now is approved by the FDA as Eulexin.

Flutamide may: (1) improve bone pain; (2) decrease the elevated serum acid phosphatase level to normal levels; (3) decrease the size, nodularity or induration of the prostate gland as determined by serial digital rectal examination; (4) decrease the number and size of bone metastases in bone scan; (5) improve hydronephrosis secondary to ureteral obstruction; (6) improve the symptoms of bladder outlet obstruction; and (7) improve the general physiologic status, gain in weight of more than 3%, not due to edema. However, flutamide has only minimal effectiveness after conventional endocrine treatment in refractory cancer patients. Thus, flutamide appears to be as effective as orchiectomy or estrogen therapy in untreated patients, but offers no therapeutic benefits to hormonally refractory patients. Recently the association of flutamide with Leuprolin significantly increased by 27% the survival of patients with advanced prostate cancer, as compared to each drug alone. Their clinical use in combination with LHRH agonists (antiandrogens + LHRH agonists) or so-called total or complete androgen blockade, has been previously described (see Chapter 2).

Ketoconazole, a nonestrogenic antifungal agent causes a rapid decrease in adrenal and testicular androgen synthesis. The mechanism of action of ketoconazole is believed to be interference with cytochrome P-450 dependent 14-demethylation. The predominant effect is an inhibition of androstenedione, dehydro-3-epiandrosterone, and testosterone. Further testing of this drug will be necessary to determine its therapeutic value. Megestrol acetate (Megace) is a progestin which acts as an antiandrogen. Megace exerts its therapeutic effect in the following ways: (1) it acts as a competitive bind to the DHT receptor and thus acts as an antiandrogen; (2) it causes reduction in the conversion of testosterone to DHT by blocking the enzyme 5-α-reductase; (3) it reduces the testosterone production by interfering directly with Leydig cell metabolism; and (4) it decreases serum testosterone indirectly by suppression of pituitary LH. Megestrol acetate used in dose of 120 mg/d produced different response rates, reaching 92% in untreated patients with prostate cancer and 30% in patients who had relapsed after castration or DES.

3. Antiprogestins

The growth of hormone-dependent breast cancer may be inhibited by high concentrations of progestins mediated by their own receptors. Unfortunately, they have many undesirable side effects. The new developed antiprogestin drugs are R2323 and RU38486, and they are currently tested in clinical trials. R2323 is an antiprogestin that can inhibit the endometrial response to progesterone and prevent the maintenance of pregnancy in rodents. When injected daily for a prolonged period of time to rats following the administration of DMBA (7,12-dimethylbenz(a)anthracene), it reduces both tumor size and incidence. R2323 exerts its action by a competitive inhibition of the binding of progesterone to its receptors. R2323 is also a potent inhibitor of gonadotropin secretion, and its antitumor activity may be mediated in part through its effects on the hypothalamic-pituitary axis.

Recently, another steroidal compound RU38486 (Mifepristone) has been reported to be a potent antiprogestin and antiglucocorticoid steroid. This compound binds with high affinity to the progesterone (PR) and glucocorticoid receptors (GR), inhibits egg implantation and decidua function, and has been proposed as a contraceptive agent (contragestion).[30] When administered either prophylactically or therapeutically to rats previously treated with DMBA, RU38486 delays mammary tumor development and causes stasis of established lesions. It has also been demonstrated that the antiproliferative actions of RU38486 were only seen in progesterone positive (PR +) cell lines where the extent of the effect was proportional PT concentration. Thus, RU38486 appears as an ideal candidate for clinical evaluation in the treatment of breast and endometrial cancer. RU38486 exerts significant inhibitory effects of DMBA-induced rat mammary tumors (75% vs. controls) at a dose of 10 mg/kg/d. The considerably increased levels of LH, estradiol, and progesterone, in combination with unchanged levels of FSH and corticosterone, suggest that Mifepristone acts mainly by its antiprogestin activity, rather than by its antiglucocorticoid activity. Clinical trials using RU 38486 given alone at a dose of 200 mg/d in oophorectomized or postmenopausal patients was well tolerated and showed a 50% response rate at 4 to 6 weeks and 18% at 3 months, suggesting that it could be useful as second- or third-line hormonal therapy in advanced breast cancer.[31]

4. Antiprolactins

Despite the fact that antiprolactin agents inhibit the growth of carcinogen-induced mammary carcinomas in mice and rats, they have disappointing therapeutic results in patients. Thus, when L-dopa, a drug which lowers prolactin levels, was compared in a randomized clinical trial with the antiestrogen nafoxidine, no tumor remissions were observed in 40 patients treated with L-dopa, whereas 7 of 36 patients treated with the antiestrogen responded.

Bromocriptine, another antiprolactin agent, also failed to induce tumor remissions in breast cancer patients, despite being more effective than L-dopa at reducing circulating prolactin concentrations. In a randomized study, bromocriptine with medroxyprogesterone acetate (MPA) produced a 55% remission rate among 69 patients.[7] However, bromocriptine used perioperative (after mastectomy) in women with axillary nodal metastases reduced significantly the prolactin levels and tumor cells in the S-phase within the primary infiltrating breast carcinoma. Thus, perioperative bromocriptine may provide another approach to adjuvant therapy, for patients with axillary lymph nodes.[32] Another antiprolactin, an ergot derivative, lergotrile mesylate, has also failed to induce tumor remissions in breast cancer patients, although serum prolactin levels were very much reduced. However, bromocriptine mesylate, (Parlodel) is used with some therapeutic benefits in patients with prolactin-secreting pituitary tumors and galactorrhea, cyclical mastalgia or infertility, in doses of 2.5 mg b.i.d. with meals for 10 to 14 d. Side effects have been noted, such as mild postural hypotension, nausea, diarrhea, headache, and dizziness. Hypertension and myocardial infarction have also been reported in a small number of patients. Thus, blood pressure should be carefully monitored and the treatment discontinued if blood pressure increases. Bromocryptine decreases the prolactin levels in patients with hyperprolactinemia; it can reduce the serum growth hormone (GH) by 50% or more in approximately one half of treated patients. With its use reduction in tumor size has been demonstrated in both male and female patients with pituitary macroadenomas. Bromocryptine may be used also to reduce the tumor mass prior to hypophysectomy.

5. Antiglucocorticoids

Some antiprogestins, such as steroidal compound RU38486, exhibit an antiglucocorticoid activity due to their affinity and binding to glucocorticoid receptors (GR). Also, inhibitors of steroid synthesis, such as aminoglutethimide (AG), inhibit the C-21 (glucocorticoids) synthesis. At present, there have been no specific drugs synthesized which exhibit a significant antiglucocorticoid activity.

6. LHRH Antagonists and Agonists

Naturally occurring LHRH is a decapeptide produced by the hypothalamus which stimulates luteinizing hormone (LH) and follicle stimulating hormone (FSH) release from the anterior pituitary. These hormones are central to normal reproductive function and control of spermatogenesis and testicular function in the male, and follicular maturation and ovarian hormone synthesis in the female. The administration of potent LHRH agonists, although initially stimulating LH and FSH release, quickly results in pituitary desensitization to LHRH and a paradoxical fall in the circulating of the gonadotropins.[33] Several studies have shown that these effects can be achieved within 4 to 7 d of continuous LHRH agonist treatment, are sufficient to promote regression of hormone dependent mammary tumors and Dunning prostate tumors in rodents, similar to "castration-like"; and form the basis for therapeutic use of LHRH agonists in breast and prostate cancer patients. The reduction of LHRH release is caused by a Ca^{2+}-independent densensitization, due to a decrease in LHRH receptors. Since the isolation and structural elucidation of LHRH more than 2000 analogs have been synthesized. While repeated administration of LHRH agonists is required to lower the levels of LH, FSH, and sex steroids, similar effects can be obtained with single administration of LHRH antagonists. Competitive antagonists of LHRH were developed by multiple modifications of the parent molecule, Glu-His-Trp-Ser-Tyr-Gly-Leu-Arg-Pro-Gly-NH$_2$. Agonist activity is reduced by substitution of aromatic D amino acids at positions 2 and 3, and receptor affinity is retained when there is replacement at residues 1 and 6. LHRH antagonists are frequently characterized by the nature of the residue in position 6.

Analogs with hydrophobic D residues, such as D-Trp are known as hydrophobic antagonists, and those with hydrophilic antagonists, such as D-Arg, are known as hydrophilic antagonists. Hydrophobic D residues do not exhibit edematogenic effects.[34] The use of antagonists will avoid the transient stimulation that occurs initially in response to LHRH agonists and prevents the clinical "flare-up" of the disease. Thus, the use of LHRH antagonists could be useful for the treatment of hormone-dependent tumors, contraception, and prevention of gonadal damage caused by radiation and chemotherapy. Replacement of the sixth amino acid variety of D amino acids and deletion of the tenth amino amide group in LHRH formula results in a molecule with increased affinity for hypothalamic receptors. Thus, a variety of LHRH analogs have been synthesized that are capable of releasing 15 to 120 times more LH than is the native hormone.[35] They exert paradoxical effects: acute administration of LHRH analogs results in increased levels of testosterone, the so-called "flare" period, whereas chronic administration reduces serum testosterone to castrate levels. The mechanism by which this occurs seems to involve: (1) alterations in the central feedback control of LH release, (2) desensitization of the gonads to LH by reduction in LH receptor sites, and (3) direct inhibition of sex steroid synthesis.

Recent studies showed that the pulsatile secretion of gonadotropin-releasing hormone (GnRH) from mediobasal hypothalamus can be suppressed by an α-adrenergic antagonist phentolamine in ovariectomized monkey (*Rhesus macaques*), and suggests that adrenergic neuronal activities are critical for the pulsatile release of hypothalamic GnRH in gonadectomized animals.[36] Also, dexamethasone suppresses hypothalamic GnRH secretion, thereby preventing the postcastration rises in GnRH receptors (GnRH-R) and gonadotropins in male rats.

Previous studies showed that chronic administration of highly potent GnRH analogs, leuprolide (Lupron), results in the inhibition of gonadotropin release, and the ovarian and testicular function are suppressed similar to castrate levels. Administration of leuprolide (Lupron) to premenopausal women with metastatic breast cancer showed that 44% had a partial response with a median duration of 39 weeks and 20% remained stable. Leuprolide induced amenorrhea in all patients who received treatment for 10 weeks or longer. Toxicity was mild and included hot flashes, nausea, vomiting, and headache. It was concluded that LHRH analogs produced a safe and effective medical castration in premenopausal patients with metastatic breast cancer.[37] On continued treatment, estradiol and progesterone concentrations fall to the levels observed in ovariectomized or postmenopausal women, and tumor remissions are recorded in approximately one third of women. Tumor regression was observed largely in patients with ER + tumors and rarely, if ever, in ER − tumors. Thus, new "superagonist" analogs of GnRH may well produce a more complete "medical oophorectomy" than antiestrogens in premenopausal breast cancer patients.[38]

Short-term objective tumor remissions have also been reported in 12 out of 31 postmenopausal patients. Similarly, partial objective clinical responses have been recorded in postmenopausal women with asymptomatic metastatic breast cancer treated with the LHRH agonist ICI 118630. In this study, the LHRH agonist was without effect on the low plasma concentrations of estradiol, progesterone, testosterone, and androstenedione. These data suggest extra gonadal actions of LHRH agonists in postmenopausal patients.[28]

Recently, LHRH receptors were found on human breast tumors. Although the predominant clinical application will be in premenopausal patients with ER + tumors, their potential use in postmenopausal women as well as their possible use in the treatment of breast benign disease, points to LHRH agonists as playing a central part in the control of the development and growth of breast cancer. Sustained-release formulations of these agents, such as Zoladex, a long-acting analog, have proven to be active in prostate and breast cancer, leuprolide is also used in the treatment of prostate and breast cancer.[39,40] Decapeptyl (D-Trp-6LHRH) has been producing good responses in patients with prostate cancer. Nasally administered Buserelin 2400 μg/d in 3 divided doses as inhalation for 7 d produced a complete remission of lung metastases in male breast cancer due to its inhibition of androgen synthesis.[41] Also, leuprolide acetate (Lupron) produced a partial response (17%) in patients with refractory epithelial ovarian cancer. The most widely used LHRH analogs are: buserelin, decapeptyl, leuprolide, and zoladex.

Recent studies have also demonstrated the clinical usefulness of LHRH agonists in the treatment of advanced prostate cancer. In patients with advanced prostate cancer treated with LHRH agonists, circulating levels of testosterone in serum are significantly reduced to castrate values after approximately three weeks. Hormonal changes are accompanied by clinical improvement and a reduction in serum acid phosphatase levels. Response was also assessed by fine needle aspiration biopsy of the prostate which showed cytologic evidence of tumor regression. The side effects associated with LHRH agonist therapy are minimal, and tumor flare has been reported to occur in a small percentage of patients (3 to 10%).

Combinations of endocrine therapies improve the outcome of treatment. Thus, the addition of buserelin to the antiestrogen tamoxifen in the treatment of breast cancer in premenopausal women reduces ovarian function and inhibits the residual estrogen action. Greater success has been reported by Labrie and associates using LHRH agonist buserelin in combination with the pure antiandrogen RU 23908 (anandron). The rationale for this approach is as follows: 95% of circulating androgens are testicular in origin and 5% are adrenal. In a cancer which is androgen dependent, the elimination of all androgen sources are important. Using this combination, so-called "total or complete androgen blockade", objective responses were observed in over 95% of patients, as compared to the standard methods which gave 60 to 70% positive response.[42] However, not all investigators obtained the same beneficial therapeutic results. Zoladex and buserelin are both available as implants and decapeptyl as a microencapsulated injection. Long-acting depot treatments will achieve gonadal regulation for a period in excess of 3 months, and a patient could attend his physician every 3 months for an injectable implant. Recently, leuprolide at doses of 1 mg/d s.c. for at least 4 months was used for treatment of patients with benign prostatic hypertrophy (BPH); it was found by transrectal ultrasonography that an average shrinkage or prostate by 40% occurred after 4 months and 46% after 6 months of treatment. The serum testosterone, and dihydrotestosterone, concentrations fell to very low levels within 4 to 6 weeks after treatment. Thus, the leuprolide treatment results in shrinkage of prostatic size and concomitant improvement in the obstructive symptoms of prostatism. The prostatic shrinkage reverses when treatment is discontinued or combined with androgens.[43]

a. LHRH Antagonists

Antagonistic analogs of LHRH were first produced by substitution of L-histidine and L-tryptophan at positions 2 and 3 of LHRH by D-amino acids. These modifications plus alterations at position 6 have produced antagonists, which in animals can suppress circulating gonadotrophin levels over relatively short periods of time. The earliest clinical study of an LHRH antagonist was performed in healthy men and resulted in a slight suppression of the pituitary gonadotropin reserve. Administration of the same dose of the LHRH antagonist (90 mg) to healthy women in the preovulatory phase of the menstrual cycle disrupted ovulation. More potent inhibitory analogs of LHRH have been synthesized by substitutions made in 5 positions, 1, 2, 3, 6, and 10. These penta-substituted inhibitory analogs inhibit ovulation in monkeys at doses of 1 mg/d and 200 μg/d. Recently, more potent LHRH antagonists have been synthesized by substitution at positions 4 and 5 throughout decapeptide. These molecules are highly active and have been shown to inhibit ovulation in rats at doses as low as 2.5 μg/rat. Significant improvements in LHRH antagonists were made; and acetyled hydroPro[1], *p*-fluoro-D-Phe[2], D-Trp[3,6], LHRH has been found to be 300 to 1000 times more potent than D-Phe[2], D-Ala[6], LHRH at inhibiting ovulation in rats. Most LHRH antagonists exhibit antitumor activity, and the suppressive mechanisms appear to be largely passive.

Antagonists always act in higher doses to produce similar results, than doses required for agonists. Although specific gonadal receptors for LHRH-like material bind both agonists and antagonists, it has been noted that only the agonists display a biologic function, which is inhibitory in nature. Antitumor effects of LHRH antagonists have been identified in several experimental models. Similarly, LHRH antagonists induce a decrease in the growth rate of Dunning-R3327H prostate adenocarcinoma as well as an increase in their tumor cell doubling time. LHRH antagonists produced tumor remissions in experimental mammary tumors, and the reduction in tumor size was associated with a fall in the level of LH, estrogen, and progesterone. Thus, LHRH antagonists possess significant antitumor activity, and may ultimately make them the LHRH analogs of choice in the therapy of these hormone-dependent cancers.

b. Antigonadotrophins not Based on LHRH

Danazol (17α-pregna-2,4-dien-20-yno[2,3-d]isoxazol-17-ol) has an inhibitory effect on both the synthesis and release of LH and FSH and reduces the peripheral androgen concentrations in women and men. It is also a weak synthetic progestin. It is widely and successfully used in the treatment of endometriosis and benign breast disease. Its mode of action is partly due to inhibition of secretion of gonadotropins (LH, FSH), but it can also bind to the progesterone and androgen receptors. Thus, it has been reported to reduce serum of LH, FSH, prolactin, estradiol, and progesterone concentrations.[44] Danazol decreases sex hormone-binding globulin (SHBG) and may displace testosterone from SHBG, thus causing an increase in free testosterone. It acts centrally on the hypothalamus and pituitary, exhibiting antigonadotrophic activity with actions on pituitary synthesis and storage of gonadotrophins as well as direct pituitary inhibition of hormone release.[44] Studies in tissue culture suggest that danazol also acts peripherally on target organs, binding with steroid receptors (ER, PR, and AR) and inhibiting multiple enzymes of gonadal steroidogenesis.[45]

In summary, the endocrine pharmacology of danazol reveals that: (1) danazol prevents the midcycle surge of LH and FSH; (2) danazol does not significantly suppress basal LH or FSH in gonadally intact human beings; (3) in castrated animals, danazol can prevent the compensatory increase in LH and FSH; (4) danazol binds to androgen, progesterone, and glucocorticoid receptors; (5) danazol-androgen receptor complex can translocate into the nucleus and initiate androgen-specific RNA synthesis; (6) the danazol progesterone receptor complex translocates poorly and can initiate minimal, if any, RNA synthesis; (7) danazol does not bind to intracellular estrogen receptors; (8) danazol inhibits cholesterol cleavage enzyme, 3β-hydroxysteroid dehydrogenase, 17α-hydroxylase, and 21-hydroxylase; (9) danazol does not inhibit aromatase; and (10) metabolites of danazol are hormonally active.[46] Due to its antiprogestational and androgenic activities, danazol may directly interfere with the growth of breast cancers, especially in postmenopausal women, since the receptors for progesterone (PR) and androgens (AR) are found in approximately 50% of tumors. Danazol has also been proposed for use in those patients with prostatic carcinoma who refuse orchiectomy or have a poor cardiovascular condition. Danazol was administered to 19 patients with advanced prostate cancer from 3 days to 18 weeks with no objective tumor remission, but 3 patients (15.8%) had objective stable disease with complete pain control for 15 to 18 weeks. Thus, danazol has only a limited value in the treatment of advanced prostate cancer. Results from a clinical trial in benign breast disease indicate that danazol started with a standard dose of 100 mg b.i.d. for 6 months; a satisfactory clinical response was achieved in 26 of the 31 patients, but was maintained in only 11.[45] Danazol has been successful in the treatment of endometriosis as well as in metastatic endometriosis, such as pulmonary endometriosis, bowel obstruction, and ureteral obstruction caused by endometriosis. Sometimes danazol caused a reduction in size of uterine cancer (endometriomas), but it rarely causes complete regression. Since danazol is metabolized largely via hepatic mechanism, it can produce mild to moderate hepatic damages. Danazol also affects thyroid function tests, such as marked decrease of thyroid-binding globulin (TBG); consequently, there is a decrease in thyroxine (T_4), but free T_4 and TSH will remain unchanged.[46]

7. Aromatase Inhibitors

Aromatase is an enzyme complex involving a NADPH-cytochrome c-reductase and a cytochrome P450, which mediates the conversion of androgens to estrogens. The reaction involves aromatization of ring A of androstenedione with the loss of the C-19 methyl group to yield estrogens and formic acid. As aromatization of ring A of the steroid molecule is unique to estrogen biosynthesis, a selective of the enzyme is more feasible than for other enzymes. Aromatase is an ubiquitous enzyme and can be found in other tissues; inhibition of aromatase in all estrogen-synthesizing tissues can be a safer method in treating cancer patients than surgical ablation. Following the menopause, aromatization increases in extragonadal sites, such as fat and muscle, and becomes the main sources of estrogens. Approximately 75% of postmenopausal and 60% of premenopausal patients have hormone-dependent breast cancers. The response of the latter group to antiestrogen therapy is less clear. In men, peripheral aromatization also increases with age. Estrogen levels appear to be increased in tissue from patients with benign prostatic hypertrophy (BPH), and possibly estrogens together with androgens mediate the genesis of BPH. The administration of aromatase inhibitors to BPH as well as to prostate carcinoma has been suggested. The commonly used aromatase inhibitors in cancer treatment are: (1) aminoglutethimide (AG), (2) 4-hydroxyandrostene-3,17-dione (4-OHA), (3) Δ^1-testololactone, and (4) trilostane.

a. Aminoglutethimide (AG)

AG is a potent steroid inhibitor as well as aromatase inhibitor, which exerts its mechanism of action by: (1) inhibition of desmolase, (2) possible activation of 3β-OH-steroid dehydrogenase, (3) possible inhibition of C_{21}-hydroxylase, (4) inhibition of 18-hydroxylase, (5) inhibition of aromatase, (6) inhibition of organic binding of iodine in the thyroid gland, and (7) inhibition of prostaglandin synthetase. In postmenopausal women with metastatic breast cancer who were treated with AG, plasma estrone levels declined 72% and the urinary excretion of estrone fell 85% over a 12-week period. Thus, AG has become of major importance with the treatment of women with advanced hormonal-responsive breast cancer, and AG has essentially replaced the surgical adrenalectomy and hypophysectomy in the treatment of advanced breast cancer.[47] AG is well absorbed by the oral route. About 25% of the drug is bound to blood cells or protein, and it is cleared from plasma with a half-life $(t^1/_2)$ of about 12 h. Renal clearance of unchanged drug is 35 to 43% of an administered dose within 48 h. Usually, the inhibition of steroid synthesis in the adrenal gland causes a reflex release of ACTH from the pituitary. To avoid this reflex, AG commonly used as 250 mg q.i.d. (four times/day) is combined with hydrocortisone 20 mg b.i.d. (twice/day) or cortisone acetate (25 mg b.i.d.). It is better to start with 250 mg twice daily for 14 d, increasing to 4 times a day thereafter; plus 100 mg of hydrocortisone (20 mg in the morning, 20 mg at 5 p.m., and 60 mg at bedtime) for 14 d, and then 40 mg/d thereafter. Cytadren is the commercially available drug.

This standard aminoglutethimide/hydrocortisone regimen has been compared to surgical ablative methods of reducing estrogen production, and it is effective as surgical adrenalectomy or surgical hypophysectomy.[48] Inhibition of estrogen biosynthesis with aminoglutethimide has also been compared to antiestrogen therapy, and both modalities of therapy had a near identical antitumor effect. However, patients with bone metastases responded significantly better to aminoglutethimide than to tamoxifen. Although aminoglutethimide and tamoxifen had similar antitumor effects, patients treated with combined therapy (AG + TAM) did not have a superior antitumor effect when compared to tamoxifen alone (37% vs. 30%).[49] However, when AG + TAM was combined with danazol (triple therapy), the objective response rate was seen to be more effective than the sequential administration. Thus, aminoglutethimide can provide similar therapeutic effects to surgical adrenalectomy, and for this reason it is called "chemical adrenalectomy". Also, studies in intact rats with the transplantable Dunning prostatic carcinoma indicate that AG will cause tumor regression comparable to that which occurs following adrenalectomy using various endocrine manipulations (hypophysectomy, orchiectomy, adrenalectomy, estrogen therapy, aminoglutethimide) alone and in combination in this model.

It was found that hypophysectomy and the combination of orchiectomy-DES were the most effective in suppressing tumor growth. The second most effective was adrenalectomy-orchiectomy. Significant inhibition of tumor growth also was seen with aminoglutethimide alone and adrenalectomy alone. However, clinical trials with AG in patients with prostate cancer have shown objective response rates only in approximately 20%. Toxicity of aminoglutethimide is of concern and showed acute side effects occurring in the first 6 weeks, which included lethargy in 48%, macular rash (33%), orthostatic hypotension with dizziness

(20%), ataxia (10%), drug fever (2.5%), and hypothyroidism (5%). Severe hematologic toxicity with leucopenia, thrombocytopenia, or even pancytopenia, may occur in 4%. This major problem of toxicity can now be overcome using a more potent and specific inhibitor of aromatase, 4-OHA.

b. 4-OHA

4-OHA (4-hydroxyandrostene-3,17-dione) is a more potent inhibitor of aromatase *in vitro* than aminoglutethimide, but is less toxic. 4-OHA reduces ovarian estrogen production and causes regression of carcinogen (DMBA)-induced mammary carcinoma in rats. In the primates, 4-OHA has been shown to inhibit peripheral aromatization as well as to reduce estrogen level during the cycle. The most recent studies with aromatase inhibitors suggest that 4-OHA is effective in postmenopausal patients with advanced disease who have relapsed from tamoxifen. From a total of 128 postmenopausal breast cancer patients with advanced metastatic disease who received 4-OHA i.m. weekly, 34% had partial or complete response, while in 16% of the patients, the disease was stabilized. 4-OHA was well tolerated by the patients and did not produce systemic side effects. Patients with ER + tumors responded better than those with ER − tumors. Standard doses were 250 mg/d or 500 mg i.m. every 2 weeks. Furthermore, some patients who did not respond to tamoxifen, responded to 4-OHA treatment. In conclusion, 4-OHA or the suicide inhibitor, is a more potent and selective aromatase inhibitor, and produces tumor regression in postmenopausal women with advanced breast cancer. A dosage of 500 mg given once weekly by i.m. injection produced an overall response rate of 27% similar to other major forms of endocrine treatment. Other suicide inhibitors, such as PEP, are now undergoing animal toxicity and should be available for clinical trial.[50] Also, responses to treatment with 4-OHA have been observed in a number of patients with prostatic cancer. Of 11 patients receiving 4-OHA, 3 had complete subjective response (CR) while 3 other patients had partial subjective responses. However, 4-OHA is the first agent to be used that selectively inhibits aromatase, and has fewer side effects. Also, it does not inhibit cortisol synthesis, and therefore substitution therapy is not required.

c. Testololactone (Δ¹-Testololactone)

Testololactone, a weak androgen, introduced in the early 1960s for treatment of patients with breast carcinoma, is now known to act as an aromatase inhibitor. In MCF-7 breast carcinoma cells grown in culture, testololactone inhibits aromatization with a dose-response characteristic similar to aminoglutethimide. When testololactone is given to normal post-menopausal women, it produces a marked inhibition of the conversion of radioactive androstenedione to estrone. These isotopic kinetic studies were confirmed by the presence of low plasma levels of estrone during testololactone administration. Clinical studies with testololactone in patients with breast carcinoma showed that it is less effective than major surgical ablative treatments, but clearly produced objective tumor regression in patients with hormone-dependent breast carcinoma. This drug is well tolerated and has no major side-effects. It causes a 90% inhibition of aromatization *in vivo*, but only 10 to 14% clinical response rate in postmenopausal breast cancer patients.[50]

d. Trilostane

Trilostane is a synthetic compound which inhibits the 3β-hydroxy-steroid-dehydrogenase-3 oxosteroid isomerase system, and subsequently, the conversion of pregnenolone to progesterone, and of DHEA to androstenedione. However, in clinical trials for patients with advanced breast cancer in doses ranging from 240 to 900 mg/d, trilostane produced only a weak therapeutic effect. Many patients (25%) had lethargy and nausea. Since trilostane alone causes an increase in Δ5-adrenal steroids, but a decrease in hydrocortisone synthesis, combined therapy of trilostane with hydrocortisone demonstrated a significant antitumor activity

(19 to 32% overall response rate) against metastatic breast cancer in postmenopausal women. Major toxic effects included nausea/vomiting, flushing, and abdominal cramping.[51] Remarkably, the three aromatase inhibitors, aminoglutethimide, 4-OHA, and Δ^1-testololactone, behave additively on the microsomal system.

Recently, a new potent nonsteroidal aromatase inhibitor (CGS16949A) has been used to treat postmenopausal women with advanced metastatic breast cancer at a dose of 1 mg b.i.d. orally in ER+ and ER unknown. Following 4 months of treatment in 28 patients, it has been assessed that 71% responded (18% complete responses and 53% PR or stabilized disease). Thus, CGS16949A is a clinically effective aromatase inhibitor; its half-life in circulation is 10.5 h. Also, treatment of premenopausal women with 4-OHA alone showed not results, whereas the combination of 4-OHA and LHRH analogs (Zoladex) produced a profound estrogen suppression; this combination is a more effective treatment than 4-OHA or Zoladex alone in premenopausal women with breast cancer. The aromatization reaction and its inhibitory mechanism reveal the importance of extra-ovarian estrogens (peripheral estrogens) in the etiopathogenesis of breast cancer.

8. Somatostatin and Its Synthetic Antagonists

Somatostatin and its synthetic analogs are called "endocrine cyanide" because they inhibit several peptide hormones; its long-acting analogs exhibit a significant antitumor activity in several endocrine and nonendocrine dependent cancers. It has been found that somatostatin and its analogs inhibit the secretion of growth hormone (GH), some growth factors, and most gastrointestinal hormones, some of which are involved in the growth regulation of pancreatic tumor cells. Due to its multiple effects and long plasma half-life (2 h instead of 3 min for the natural hormone), the somatostatin analog SMS201-995 has been used to ameliorate the symptoms of many endocrine tumors, such as acromegaly, islet cell carcinoma, carcinoid syndrome, glucagonomas, lipomas, APUDomas, VIPomas, hypercalcitoninemia, inappropriate TSH-hypersecretion, and an islet cell tumor-secreting, growth hormone-releasing factor.[52,53] This SMS201-995 is an octreotide which contains only 8 amino acids as compared to somatostatin which contains 14 amino acids. The schematic representation of the amino acid sequence of native somatostatin or SRIF (somatotropin release-inhibiting factor) and Sandostatin (SMS201-995) is shown in Figure 2.

In monkeys, SMS201-995, in comparison with natural SRIF, was shown to be 45 times more active in its GH release-inhibitory effects, 11 times more active in its glucagon release-inhibitory effects, and only 1 to 3 times more active in its insulin release-inhibitory effects. Sandostatin was shown to be highly resistant to enzymatic degradation both *in vitro* and *in vivo*. Pharmacokinetic studies in man involved s.c. injections of 50 and 100 μg SMS201-995 in normal volunteers and showed that clearance was slow, with an elimination half-life ($t^1/_2$) of 113 min for both doses. It can be concluded that Sandostatin has four advantages over the native somatostatin: (1) it inhibits GH preferentially above insulin; (2) it has a long half-life in the circulation, causing a prolonged inhibitory effect in target organs of SRIF; (3) it is active after s.c. and at higher doses, even after oral administration; and (4) no rebound hypersecretion of hormones was observed.

Thus, Sandostatin inhibits the release of a variety of peptide hormones including GH, TSH, insulin and glucagon, gastrin, secretin, cholecystokinin, and vasoactive intestinal peptide (VIP). Its main therapeutic effects are in pituitary tumors, notably in acromegaly, being 45 times more active in the inhibition of GH than somatostatin. The clinical introduction of the long-acting SMS201-995 has added a new dimension to the medical therapy of acromegaly, especially in patients with large pituitary tumors (macroadenomas) which cannot be cured by surgery and/or radiotherapy. In all patients, a marked clinical improvement with few side effects is observed during the first weeks of therapy with the drug in a dose of 100 μg three times daily. However, the effects of SMS201-995 in acromegaly are reversible,

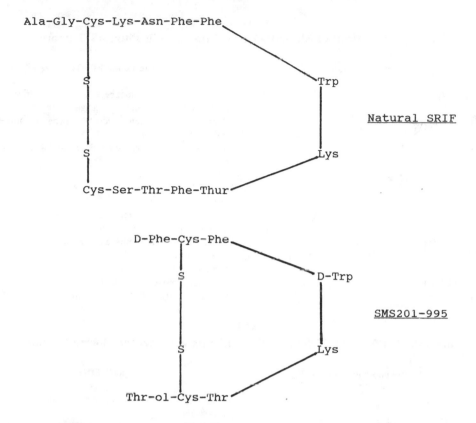

FIGURE 2. Schematic representation of the amino acid sequence of native SRIF and the analog SMS201-995 sandostatin.

after treatment with Sandostatin was stopped. Some clinical investigators suggest that SMS201-995 should be reserved for those 25 to 30% of acromegalic patients who do not benefit from transsphenoidal surgery or radiotherapy. Thus, inhibition of hormone release and tumor shrinkage have been reported during treatment with SMS201-995 in patients with TSH- and ACTH- (Nelson syndrome) secreting pituitary tumors (see Table 1).

Recently, somatostatin and high affinity receptors for it, were found in several human breast cancer cell lines, and these are inhibited by Sandostatin *in vitro*. Some human breast cancer cell lines, such as ZR-75-1 and MCF-7 can synthesize somatostatin. Sandostatin can inhibit the somatostatin synthesis and cell proliferation, but only after 3 d of continuous exposure.[54] These results suggest that higher doses of sandostatin may be effective in some types of breast cancer.[55] Somatostatin has direct inhibitory effects on insulin, glucagon, GH, TSH, and gastrin. Upon entering the lumen of the gut, it modifies the secretion of acid and gastrin, and for this action has been termed a "lumone". It inhibits also VIP (vasoactive intestinal polypeptide), pepsin, motilin, gastric acid secretion, and decreased absorption of water, glucose and calcium. It exerts antiproliferative effects with inhibitory action ties on numerous cellular processes being an important anticancer agent both in curative and palliative treatment. Its half-life is 113 min.

A new octapeptide called somatuline (BIM-23014) has little effect on insulin and glucagon secretion, has a prolonged duration of action, and has a molecular weight of 1096.34. Somatuline produces only 39% inhibition of gastric secretion. At doses of 500 μg s.c./d the GH secretion is immediately suppressed for almost 6 h. Mild diarrhea, abdominal pains, and cramps have been reported in volunteers given doses up to 2 to 4 mg/24 h. Somatostatin receptors have been demonstrated in the central nervous system and peripheral organs in

TABLE 1
Therapeutic Effects of SMS201-995 in Patients with Pituitary Tumors

Pituitary Tumors	Theraputic Effects
Acromegaly	Inhibition of GH secretion; beneficial clinical effects in most patients with tumor shrinkage in 50% of cases
TSH-secreting tumors	Inhibition of TSH secretion, control of hyperthyroidism, and shrinkage of tumors
Inappropriate TSH hypersecretion	Inhibition of TSH secretion and control of hyperthyroidism
Cushing's syndrome	
Cushing's disease	No effect
Adrenal tumors	No effect
Nelson's syndrome (postadrenalectomy)	Inhibition of ACTH secretion and preliminary evidence of control of tumor growth in few cases
Ectopic ACTH secretion	Inhibition of ACTH secretion and control of tumor growth in few cases
Prolactinomas	No effect
Mixed PRL/GH tumors	Partial suppressive effects on GH and PRL secretion
Gonadotropinomas	No data; although SRIF receptors often present

TABLE 2
Therapeutic Effects of SMS201-995 in Patients with Neuroendocrine Tumors

Neuroendocrine Tumors	Theraputic Effects
Glucagonomas	Partial response; palliative effects; reduction in glucagon secretion
Islet cell carcinomas (insulinomas)	Tumor regression in some cases; reduction in insulin secretion
VIPomas	Partial tumor regression; beneficial effect on the gut
Carcinoid syndrome	Significant amelioration of clinical symptoms
APUDomas[a]	Partial tumor regression and palliative effects
Chondrosarcoma	Possible inhibitory effect
Gastrinomas (Zollinger-Ellison syndrome)	Palliative effects
Islet cell tumor-secreting GHRF (growth hormone-releasing factor)	Tumor regression and beneficial clinical effects
Small cell lung cancer	Inhibitory effects *in vitro* and *in vivo*
Breast cancer	Inhibitory effect in experimental mammary carcinoma and human breast cancer cell lines
Prostate cancer	Inhibition in experimental prostate cancer

[a]   APUD (Amine precursor uptake, decarboxylase).

human meningioma, pituitary tumors, breast and carcinoid tumors, and prostate tumors in rats. Somatostatin can act as a paracrine secretory factor (local regulator) or as an autocrine secretory factor (self-regulator). Thus, somatostatin and its synthetic analogs represent a major new pharmacologic approach to the medical treatment of malignant disease.[56] Antitumor effects of Sandostatin can be observed beyond the pituitary tumors, notably in neuroendocrine tumors, and it was used to ameliorate the symptoms of a wide variety of tumors (see Table 2).

Although not a cure for endocrine or neuroendocrine tumors, the SMS201-995 has provided partial response and tumor regression to an increasing number of patients with pituitary tumors and relief from the aggravating effects of hormone hypersecretion by these tumors.[57] Recently, a significant improvement in patients with psoriasis following treatment with SMS201-995 was reported.[58] It is likely that it acts differently than suppression of serum GH, but inhibits substance P and EGF which have been postulated to play a role in the pathogenesis of psoriasis. The synthetic analogs are well tolerated. Most of the reported adverse effects are minor (nausea, pain at injection site, and malabsorption with steatorrhea). Interestingly, tachyphylaxis (a rapid and progressive decrease in physiologic response) was observed after repeated s.c. administration of 2 to 10 μg SMS201-995 b.i.d. to normal rats, which can be due to desensitization through pituitary of the GH-inhibitory effects. Tachyphylaxis is mainly observed on insulin, but not on glucagon secretion.[59] No tachyphylaxis or desensitization has been observed so far in acromegalic patients treated for more than 3 years with 200 to 300 μg SMS201-995/d. Thus, Sandostatin is an exceedingly useful therapeutic tool in the long-term management of neuro-endocrine and pituitary tumors.

In summary, Sandostatin appears to cause inhibitory tumor effects on prostate and mammary cancer, tumors of bone and cartilage, and pancreatic cancer. Specific binding sites for an iodinated derivative of Sandostatin (^{125}1-SMS204-090) appears to be present in MCF-7 cells and pancreatic tumors. In the majority of patients with gastrointestinal tumors chronic Sandostatin treatment decreased plasma IGF-I levels. Sandostatin may act on the tumor cells in different ways: (1) by decreasing secretion of pituitary hormones (GH, PRL) and (2) by acting as a paracrine/autocrine regulator of tumor cell proliferation by inhibiting the secretion of growth factors such as EGF and IGF-I. Thus, the long-acting somatostatin analog (SMS201-995) offers a very useful new therapeutic tool in the treatment of patients with endocrine tumors and neuroendocrine tumors. It appears safe and is well tolerated with minimal side effects.[60]

9. Prostaglandin Inhibitors

Prostaglandins (PGs) are implicated in the development and metastatic process of some cancers (breast, skin, head and neck). It was found that indomethacin, a prostaglandin synthetase inhibitor, reduced the growth of tumors induced in mice by Moloney sarcoma virus. A new prostaglandin synthesis inhibitor, called flurbiprofen, induces a significant inhibition of tumor growth and increases survival rates of mice with tumors. Similar effects were reported, especially a tendency to increase survival time and tumor response to radiation or chemotherapy. High $PGF_{2\alpha}$ levels were positively correlated with histologic differentiation, positive estrogen receptors (ER+), lymph node positive, and low mitotic index (LMI). $PGF_{2\alpha}$ levels are high in tumors with good prognosis. However, investigations regarding significance of prostaglandins in breast cancer are conflicting. Recently, measurements of prostaglandins E_2 and $F_2\alpha$ (PGE_2 and $PGF_{2\alpha}$) by gas liquid chromatography mass spectrometry in extracts of primary tumors from patients with early breast cancer, showed no significant relationship between levels of PG and ER, tumor size, lymph node involvement, and disease-free interval following primary treatment.[61]

It was recently found the Leukotriene B_4 (LTB_4) formed through lipoxygenation of arachidonic acid does play a role in the pathogenesis of squamous cell carcinomas experimentally induced in Syrian hamsters as well as in the head and neck human squamous cell carcinomas (HSCC). Leukotriene-B_4 can play a role as mediator of inflammation and immunoregulation and thus can protect cancerous tissue against radiation therapy.

B. MEDICAL CASTRATION (OVARIECTOMY, ORCHIECTOMY)
1. Castration in Women

(Ovariectomy, Oophorectomy) or in men (orchiectomy) is an important ablative endocrine therapy and consists of complete removal of sex steroid producing organs, such as ovaries in women and testes in men. Castration can be performed either by surgery (surgical castration) or by ovarian radiation (radiation castration). Surgical castration was always preferred to radiation castration because it completely removes the estrogens or testosterone source and brings the hormone levels to basal line. The radiation castration does not totally destroy the steroid-forming tissue and in some cases, menses can persist or recur following radiation. Until a few years ago, castration had been the treatment of choice for premenopausal women with metastatic or inoperable breast cancer.

Surgical castration was first performed for the palliation of metastatic breast cancer by Beatson[1] in 1896. He stated, "We are to look at an altered condition of the ovary and testicle as the real exciting cause of cancer, and there are grounds for the belief that the etiology of cancer lies in an ovarian or testicular stimulus." Later, in 1916, Lathrop and Loeb[62] found that the hormonal milieu of multiple pregnancies predisposed to carcinoma formation and that an early ovariectomy prevented the occurrence of mammary carcinoma in large numbers of mice.[62] Thus, castration exerts significant antitumor effects in animal tumors as well as in human cancer. However, castration, either surgical or radiation, has psychologic adverse effect and sometimes disfiguring consequences and is difficult to be accepted by patients. Because ovariectomy and orchiectomy are irreversible, several workers are investigating medical means for suppressing ovarian estrogen and testicular androgen production. This new procedure using medical means, such as hormone agonists or antagonists, is called "medical castration". It is nontoxic, effective, and easy to administer; is associated with few side effects; and will be a replacement for surgical oophorectomy.

a. Medical Oophorectomy

Medical oophorectomy can be achieved with the use of: (1) antiestrogens (tamoxifen), or (2) LHRH analogs (leuprolide). The first, medical oophorectomy, following antiestrogen (tamoxifen) administration of 10 mg twice a day to premenopausal women, showed a 24% objective response as compared with 21% having an oophorectomy. The median duration of response for tamoxifen (20 months) was longer than that for surgical oophorectomy (7 months). Thus, this randomized, comparative study between tamoxifen and surgical oophorectomy in premenopausal patients with advanced breast cancer has shown a similar objective response rate (tamoxifen 24%, oophorectomy 21%) for the two treatment groups. The report of another randomized trial of surgical oophorectomy vs. tamoxifen in 53 premenopausal women with metastatic disease has shown similar results.[49] Approximately 80% of patients in both treatment groups were ER+; objective response rates were 37% for oophorectomy and 27% for tamoxifen. Tamoxifen was well tolerated with a small number of patients having hot flushes compared with the oophorectomy group. Accordingly, tamoxifen is a suitable alternative to surgical oophorectomy. The second, medical castration, is produced by the LHRH agonists and antagonists. Leuprolide is a potent analog of human gonadotropin-releasing hormone (LHRH). Chronic administration of leuprolide results in the inhibition of gonadotropin release with the suppression of ovarian and testicular function. Leuprolide (Lupron), administered in a dose of 1 mg/d in premenopausal women with metastatic breast cancer, showed a 44% partial response with a median duration of 39 weeks and 20% remained stable. Leuprolide induced amenorrhea in all patients who received treatment for 10 weeks or longer. Toxicity was mild and included hot flushes, nausea, vomiting, and headache. Therefore, chronic administration apparently results in down regulation of the LHRH receptor, inhibition of gonadotropin release, and resultant suppression of ovarian hormone production, e.g., "medical castration". It is concluded that Lupron provides a safe and effective chemical castration in premenopausal women with metastatic breast cancer.[37]

It has been shown that LHRH antagonists are more potent than LHRH agonist, in reducing gonadal activity and suppressing estrus cycle in the female rat and in decreasing the weight of the testes and accessory sex organs in the male rat. Some of these are highly potent antagonists; they produced 100% inhibition of ovulation in cycling rats and suppressed the LH levels in ovariectomized female rats for 47 h, when administered at doses of 25 μg.[34] Thus, antiestrogens (tamoxifen) have largely replaced surgical ablative therapy for postmenopausal women with breast cancer because of efficacy, safety, and lack of side effects. However, the antiestrogens are not ideal for producing a "medical oophorectomy" in premenopausal women. Namely, the current available antiestrogens do not completely block estrogen effects in women with functioning ovaries, and menses often continue. Superagonist analogs of LHRH produce a greater inhibition of gonadotropin release and may well produce a more complete medical oophorectomy than antiestrogens in premenopausal breast cancer patients.

A recent study conducted on 134 pre- and perimenopausal patients with metastatic breast cancer treated with goserelin (Zoladex) depot, injected subcutaneously every 4 weeks, showed that serum concentrations of estradiol, LH, and FSH were significantly suppressed by Zoladex, into the range of castrated or postmenopausal women within 2 to 3 weeks of therapy. The overall objective response was: 10% complete remission (CR) and 35% partial remission (PR). Thus, there was a 45% objective response. Median time to response was 4 months, and duration of response was 8 months. Objective responses were seen for different sites of metastases: loco-regional (62%), bone (46.7%), visceral (45%), and multiple (35.1%). Tumor remission was more common (49.3%) in patients with ER+ tumors or with ER-unknown (44%). Thus, Zoladex produced a "medical castration" better than tamoxifen, which increased estradiol levels and ovarian cysts.[63] The effectiveness of LHRH analogs to suppress ovarian estrogens without significant toxicity, has led to the suggestion that these agents might be ideal for producing a medical ovariectomy. However, there are conceptual differences between the efficacy of antiestrogens and LHRH analogs in producing a medical ovariectomy.

Medical Ovariectomy

Antiestrogens	LHRH Analogs
Incomplete ovarian suppression	Complete ovarian suppression
Menses continue	Menses cease
Reflex rise of estradiol	Estradiol suppressed
Secondary response to surgical ovariectomy	
Lack of complete specificity	Complete specificity
Stimulation of liver proteins, such as TBG through weak estrogen agonist effects	
Possible interaction with cytotoxic chemotherapy	
Nontoxic	Nontoxic

2. Medical Orchiectomy

Surgical castration (bilateral orchiectomy) has been employed to eliminate the principal source of endogenous androgen production, and will effectively lower androgen levels and produce a clinical response in patients with hormone dependent tumors. However, this procedure is often unacceptable to patients because it is irreversible and has psychologic implications. For these reasons, medical alternatives to castration have been used or developed. It has been found that pharmacologic manipulation of the hypothalamic-pituitary-testicular axis, inhibition of testosterone synthesis, or androgen-receptor blockade at the peripheral or cellular level can be equally effective therapy.

LHRH-receptor blockade—Synthetic agonists and antagonists of LHRH, such as leuprolide acetate, can produce pharmacologic orchiectomy. Natural LHRH is released in a pulsatile pattern from the hypothalamus and acts through the pituitary to stimulate testosterone production, whereas synthetic agonists are thought to occupy pituitary LHRH receptors continuously, desensitizing them and thus inhibiting the production of testosterone. Interestingly, acute administration of LHRH agonists, such as leuprolide acetate (Lupron), are stimulating in the early days (1 to 4 d) of treatment, but chronic administration (more than 7 d) produces a significant decrease of LH, and consequently a decreased testosterone

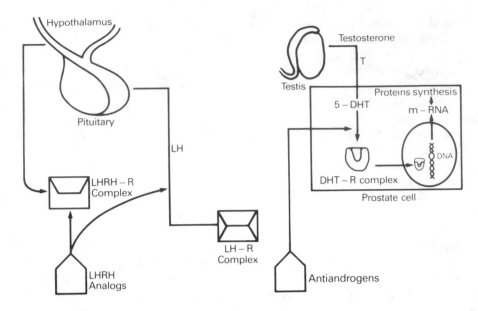

FIGURE 3.   Mechanism of action of LHRH analogs and antiandrogens on cancer cells.

production. Thus, chronic administration of leuprolide (Lupron), has been shown to suppress testicular androgen production in animals to castrate levels. Also, chronic administration of leuprolide to castrate and noncastrate males with prostate cancer (in doses varying 1 to 10 mg) suppressed the pituitary production of LH and FSH and, consequently testicular production of testosterone (T) to baseline or anorchid levels. The development of new long-acting depot treatments, such as Zoladex, decapeptyl, or buserelin depot, given once a month and found effective for up to 3 months, will be offered to the patient with advanced prostate cancer. These treatments can easily replace orchiectomy with its psychologic implications or estrogen treatment with the possibility of toxic effects of the preparations available now; biodegradable Zoladex appears most promising for patient acceptance and ease of administration. Work is underway on developing long-acting preparations that will last for a period in excess of 3 months for an injectable implant and will result in the most acceptable alternative to orchiectomy. Substitution at the second and third amino acid positions of the native molecule of LHRH will result in compounds that still bind tightly to the LHRH receptor. These preparations will inhibit LH without an initial period of increase as observed with the LHRH agonists. These new LHRH antagonists act more rapidly and will be the drug of the future in achieving medical orchiectomy. Hence, depot formulation is a valuable and applicable alternative to other forms of hormonal treatment such as orchiectomy or DES. Recent studies with Nafarelin (LHRH agonist) in combination with a long-acting LHRH antagonist (RS-68439) will be useful, especially in patients with bilateral hydronephrosis, extensive metastatic disease to the lungs or spine, and in those with high cardiovascular risks of estrogen therapy. The LHRH antagonists will produce a rapid medical orchiectomy and make them the therapy of choice.[64] Androgen-receptor blockades, such as DES, block the hypothalamic sex steroid receptors, thus decreasing LH release and producing castration levels of serum testosterone in most men.

Cytoplasmic androgen-receptor blockade—This is achieved by two antiandrogens, flutamide and cyproterone acetate. These drugs block the cytoplasmic receptor for dihydrotestosterone (DHT); DHT-receptor complex cannot be translocated to the nucleus, and elicit m-RNA, new protein synthesis, and cell division (see Figure 3). Therefore, medical orchiectomy can be achieved by using antiandrogens or LHRH agonists and antagonists and is more acceptable to the patients than surgical castration. Preservation of libido and sexual potency appears to be one of the specifically favorable aspects of antiandrogens, namely, flutamide treatment. Interestingly, androgen deprivation (orchiectomy or blockade) destroys only the androgen-dependent or androgen-sensitive cells, but does not retard growth or destroy androgen-independent cell lines, which can proliferate and later transform the whole tumor into a homogeneous androgen-independent autonomous tumor. This is the rationale for sequential hormonal therapy and sequential hormonal and chemotherapy for advanced prostatic cancer (D_2). Initial treatment with DES or orchiectomy showed a significantly higher response rate (81%) to DES than for orchiectomy (62%). Sequential hormonal and chemotherapy using medroxyprogesterone acetate (MPA) and oral chlorambucil or combination chemotherapy, showed a disease stabilization in almost 46% in both treated groups, which indicate that the least toxic form of treatment with MPA should be used.[65]

C. MEDICAL ADRENALECTOMY

The first surgical bilateral adrenalectomy in prostate cancer was performed by Huggins and Scott[66] with appreciable success despite the lack of substitution therapy. Subsequently, bilateral adrenalectomy was used in advanced prostatic cancer, and it has been found to be associated with palliation in 20 to 70% of patients with advanced prostatic carcinoma who were refractory to castration or estrogen therapy. Adrenalectomy also became popular in the 1950s as a treatment of metastatic breast cancer in postmenopausal women or in premenopausal women who had previously responded to oophorectomy. It was found that 30 to 40% of previously castrated women respond to surgical adrenalectomy. Thus, this operation has been recently replaced by the adrenal blocking agent aminoglutethimide (AG), which is a simpler, less expensive and safer way to suppress adrenal steroid synthesis. It appears to be equivalent to surgical adrenalectomy without imposing the risks of major surgery and irreversible adrenal suppression on the patient.

1. Aminoglutethimide

Aminoglutethimide was first used as an anticonvulsant. Inasmuch as it produced side effects including goiter, ovarian dysfunction, and adrenal insufficiency, it was withdrawn and reintroduced as an adrenal blocking agent. Because it is a compound capable of inhibiting adrenal steroid synthesis, this led to its use for treatment of hormone-dependent tumors such as breast cancer, prostate cancer, and endometrial cancer. Because aminoglutethimide is a potent inhibitor of adrenal steroidogenesis, this drug offers the potential for achieving and ideal "medical or chemical adrenalectomy". The mechanism of action of aminoglutethimide has been previously summarized; it suppresses adrenal steroid synthesis by inhibiting the first step in the metabolic pathway, the conversion of cholesterol to pregnenolone, which involves the enzyme 20,22-desmolase. However, the inhibition is less than complete for 18-hydroxylation and 11-hydroxylation, which are involved in the synthesis of Δ^4-type steroids such as testosterone, dihydrotestosterone, and androstenedione. Aminoglutethimide inhibits almost completely the conversion of Δ^4-androstenedione to estrone and testosterone to estradiol in extra-adrenal tissues (aromatization reaction), which is the principal source of estrogens in postmenopausal or castrated women. Studies in animal models revealed that aminoglutethimide blocks the synthesis of adrenal androgens and suppresses the growth of prostate cancer and breast cancer in a manner comparable to adrenalectomy. In intact rats with transplantable Dunning prostate carcinoma, the aminoglutethimide induces tumor regression comparable in extent to that which occurs following adrenalectomy.

Randomized clinical trials of surgical vs. medical adrenalectomy, using aminoglutethimide plus cortisol in a dose of 250 mg orally q.i.d. together with 40 mg hydrocortisone in divided doses (10 mg in a.m., 10 mg at 5 p.m., and 20 mg at bedtime), showed similar results in response rate, response duration, and response of metastatic sites. Thus, it was concluded that medical adrenalectomy with aminoglutethimide plus hydrocortisone can be logically chosen in place of surgical adrenalectomy. In unselected cases with advanced breast cancer, the response rate is about 35% rising to 50% in ER+ patients, with a median duration of response in the 11 to 17 to month range. In the patients treated with aminoglutethimide and cortisol, the urinary cortisol, plasma estrone and estradiol fell significantly. A comparative study between medical adrenalectomy and surgical adrenalectomy showed in both instances that medical adrenalectomy was equal or superior. No permanent adrenal insufficiency or acute crisis was noted. The side effects are seen at the onset of therapy and include lethargy dizziness, blurred vision, and pruritic maculopapular rash, which disappear after approximately 10 d of treatment. Similar effects of medical adrenalectomy were seen in patients with advanced prostatic carcinoma who were treated with 1000 mg of aminoglutethimide and 40 mg of cortisol daily. Their response rate was similar to those treated by surgical adrenalectomy; aminoglutethimide unequivocally suppresses adrenal androgen production, and plasma DHEA, androstenedione, testosterone, and DHT have been shown to be significantly suppressed in multiple trials.

II. COMMENTS AND CONCLUSIONS

The development of new hormone antagonists, which are potent inhibitors of adrenal and gonadal steroidogenesis, are rendering the conventional surgical procedures, such as surgical castration, surgical adrenalectomy, and surgical hypophysectomy, obsolete and they are only seldom used. Important advances in endocrine pharmacology, such as discovery of antiestrogens (tamoxifen), antiandrogens (cyproterone, flutamide), adrenal steroid inhibitors (aminoglutethimide, 4-OHA), LHRH agonists and antagonists, offer to clinical oncologists new tools in cancer treatment with fewer side effects and also with more patient acceptance, as compared to surgical procedures. Experimental studies and clinical trials revealed that the new hormone agonists and antagonists can significantly reduce the hormone plasma levels (estrone, estradiol, testosterone, cortisol, LH, FSH) to castrate (anorchid levels).Thus, medical castration, medical adrenalectomy, and medical hypophysectomy are replacing the old surgical or radiation endocrine ablative therapies, and are providing the same pharmacologic and therapeutic effects on tumor response rate and overall survival rate in cancer patients. Hence, they suppress tumor growth and development in a manner similar to surgical ablative endocrine therapy. Antiestrogen therapy with tamoxifen and LHRH agonists or antagonists has replaced surgical castration, adrenalectomy, and hypophysectomy as the first-choice hormonal treatment in postmenopausal women, and probably will replace oophorectomy in premenopausal women. At the same time, improved techniques of medical adrenalectomy by using aminoglutethimide have permitted its wider application and favorable replacement of the surgical adrenalectomy and hypophysectomy. Inasmuch as medical castration, medical adrenalectomy, and medical hypophysectomy are simpler, safer, and more effective and lack side effects and psychological implications, they largely have replaced the conventional surgical therapy for many patients with breast and prostate cancer. Thus, medical castration and medical adrenalectomy provide the same beneficial therapy, are reversible, less toxic, and less disfiguring, are more acceptable to patients, and recently have become the first-line treatment in hormone-responsive cancer. Hormone agonists and antagonists, such as antiestrogens, antiandrogens, antiprogestins, antiprolactins, LHRH antagonists, adrenal steroid inhibitors, and somatostatin synthetic analogs, replacing additive hormone therapy, are used in a wide variety of tumors, such as endometrial carcinoma, ovarian cancer, kidney tumors, pituitary tumors, insulinomas, glucagonomas, VIPomas, carcinoid syndrome, and gastrinomas. In most comparative randomized trials, they produced a clinical antitumor effect equal to or even greater than surgical or radiation procedures. Also in animal models, notably in hormone-dependent tumors, such as chemically induced

DMBA or NMU-mammary carcinoma in rodents or Dunning prostatic adenocarcinoma in rats, they inhibit the tumor growth and development in a similar manner to surgical ovariectomy, adrenalectomy, or hypophysectomy.

Although their mechanism of action is not yet fully understood, it seems that most hormone antagonists or agonists act at the cellular level:

1. They compete with endogenous hormones (estrogens, androgen) for the cytoplasmic receptors (ER, PR, AR) in hormone-dependent cells forming a hormone-receptor complex (H-R complex). After its translocation to the cell nucleus, the hormone antagonists interfere with the nuclear events so that the cancer cells become insensitive to further stimulation by circulating steroid hormones.
2. They inhibit steroid hormone synthesis via hypothalamic-pituitary-ovarian axis or hypothalamic-pituitary adrenal axis, or by blocking one or more enzymes involved in hormone biosynthesis, and subsequently causing a drastic reduction of circulating plasma hormone levels.
3. They can inhibit steroid hormone conversion in nonendocrine tissue (adipose tissue, muscle, skin) by aromatic reaction.
4. They exert antitumor activity, being cytostatic; they are tumoristatic, not tumoricidal. This can happen by diverting the cancer cells from the G_1-phase of the cell cycle to a dormant stage (Go-phase), where they can remain dormant for several months or years, thus, blocking them from entering the S-phase and increasing the rapidly dividing cells or "growth fraction". However, some investigators believe that hormone antagonists (antiestrogens) can also be tumoricidal, cytotoxic, and kill the cancer cells in high doses.
5. They inhibit *de nuovo* synthesis of cytoplasmic receptors or block the recycling of spent hormone receptors; both mechanisms are poorly understood.

Thus, in the last decade by changing chemical configuration or amino acid sequences in dominant or key positions, it has become possible to obtain new hormone antagonists which exceed by a 100 times (10 to 300) the antitumor activity of their hormone counterparts. Being less toxic, they will become the ideal therapeutic drugs in both ablative and additive hormone therapies. They are promising tools and will open a chapter in cancer therapy. Unlike cytotoxic agents, which have a low therapeutic index and need to be given at toxic level, hormone antagonists may produce antitumor effects in the absence of significant systemic toxicity. For instance, tamoxifen has an incidence of minor side effects of about 10%, and continuous administration is well tolerated for periods of up to 5 years.[12] The development of new endocrine drugs requires a different approach from that used for cytotoxicity. Thus, hormone-dependent animal tumor models, such as NMU or DMBA-induced rat mammary tumors, are available for testing new endocrine agents. Since endocrine treatment is frequently chronic, and some controversy exists regarding tamoxifen and its potential for producing liver tumors in rats and in endometrial tumors in women, all these new hormones and their antagonists should be tested for safety.[67] Despite the fact that somatostatin analog SMS 201-995 (octreotide) is a very promising drug for the treatment of acromegaly and some neuroendocrine tumors, the requirement for multiple subcutaneous injections and the risk of cholelithiasis, make it a little difficult for patients. It is to be hoped that longer acting somatostatin analogs will be developed and cholelithiasis will be safely prevented.[68] Recent advancements were made in developing new prostaglandin analogs such as gemeprost and sulprostone, which in association with mifepristone (RU 486) are very successful and safe (95%) in termination of early pregnancy (49 days or less).[69] Therefore, hormone agonists, synthetic hormones, and hormone antagonists will become one of the most promising areas of cancer therapy today.

REFERENCES

1. **Beatson, G. T.,** On the treatment of inoperable cases of carcinoma of the mamma: suggestions for a new method of treatment, with illustrative cases, *Lancet,* 2, 104, 165, 1896.
2. **Huggins, C. and Hodges, C. V.,** Studies on prostatic cancer. I. The effect of castration, of estrogen and of androgen injection on serum phosphatases in metastatic carcinoma of the prostate, *Cancer Res.,* 1, 293, 1941.
3. **Lupulescu, A.,** *Steroid Hormones,* (Hormonii Steroizi), Med. Publ. House, Bucharest, 1958, 365.
4. **Harper, M. J. and Walpole, A. L.,** A new derivative of triphenylethylene: effect on implantation and mode of action in rats, *J. Reprod. Fertil.,* 13, 101, 1967.
5. **Jordan, C. V. and Robinson, S. P.,** Species-specific pharmacology of antiestrogens: role of metabolism *Fed. Proc.,* 46, 1870, 1987.
6. **Lippman, M. E., Dickson, R. E., Gelmann, E. P., Knabbe, C., Kasid, A., Bates, S., and Swain, S.,** Mechanisms of estrogenic and antiestrogenic regulation of growth of human breast carcinoma, in *Hormonal Manipulation of Cancer: Peptides, Growth Factors and New (Anti) Steroidal Agents,* Klijn, J. G., Paridaens, R., and Foekens, J. A., Eds., Raven Press, New York, 1987, 381.
7. **Harmsen, H. J. and Porsius, A. J.,** Endocrine therapy of breast cancer, *Eur. J. Cancer Clin. Oncol.,* 24, 1099, 1988.
8. **Wilkinson, P. M., Ribiero, G. G., Adam, H. K., Kemp, J. V., and Patterson, J. A.,** Tamoxifen (Nolvadex) therapy — rationale for loading dose followed by maintenance dose for patients with metastatic breast cancer, *Cancer Chemother. Pharmacol.,* 10, 33, 1982.
9. **Ashford, A. R., Donev, I., Tiwari, R. P., and Garrett, T. J.,** Reversible ocular toxicity related to tamoxifen therapy, *Cancer,* 61, 33, 1988.
10. **Wakeling, A. E., Valcaccia, B., Newboult, E., and Green, L. R.,** Non-steroidal antioestrogen — receptor binding and biological response in rat uterus, rat mammary carcinoma and human breast cancer cells, *J. Steroid Biochem.,* 20, 111, 1984.
11. **Bradbeer, J. W. and Kyngdon, J.,** Primary treatment of breast cancer in elderly women with tamoxifen, *Clin. Oncol.,* 9, 31, 1983.
12. Nolvadex Adjuvant Trial Organization, Controlled trial of tamoxifen as a single adjuvant agent in the management of early breast cancer, *Br. J. Cancer,* 57, 608, 1988.
13. **Fornander, T., Rutqvist, L. E., Cedermark, B., Mattsson, A., Skoog, L., Theve, T., Askergren, J., Glas, U., Silfversward, C., Somell, A., Wilking, N., and Hjalmar, M-L.,** Adjuvant tamoxifen in early breast cancer: occurrence of new primary cancers, *Lancet,* 1, 117, 1989.
14. **Rose, C. and Mouridsen, H. T.,** Endocrine therapy of advanced breast cancer, *Acta Oncol.,* 27, 721, 1988.
15. **Legha, S. S.,** Tamoxifen in the treatment of breast cancer, *Ann. Intern. Med.,* 109, 219, 1988.
16. **Patterson, J. S.,** 10 years of tamoxifen in breast cancer, in *Hormonal Manipulation of Cancer Peptides, Growth Factors, and New (Anti) Steroidal Agents,* Klijn, J. G., Paridaens, R., and Foekens, J. A., Eds., Raven Press, New York, 1987, 1.
17. **Wilson, A. J., Baum, M., Brinkley, D. M., Dossett, J. A., McPherson, K., Patterson, J. S., Rubens, R. D., Smiddy, F. G., Stoll, B. A., Richards, D., and Ellis, S. H.,** Six-year results of a controlled trial of tamoxifen as single adjuvant agent in management of early breast cancer, *World J. Surg.,* 9, 756, 1985.
18. **Love, R. R., Mazess, R. B., Tormey, D. C., Barden, H. S., Newcomb, P. A., and Jordan, V. C.,** Bone mineral density in women with breast cancer treated with adjuvant tamoxifen for at least two years, *Breast Cancer Res. Treat.,* 12, 297, 1988.
19. **Lee, R. W., Buzdar, A. U., Blumenschein, G. R., and Hortobagyi, G. N.,** Trioxifene mesylate in the treatment of advanced breast cancer, *Cancer,* 57, 40, 1986.
20. **Osborne, R. J., Malik, S. T., Slevin, M. L., Harvey, V. J., Spona, J., Salzer, H., and Williams, C. J.,** Tamoxifen in refractory ovarian cancer: the use of a loading dose schedule, *Br. J. Cancer,* 57, 115, 1988.
21. **Schwartz, P. E., Chambers, J. T., Kohorn, E. I., Chambers, S. K., Weitzman, H., Voynick, I. M., MacLusky, N., and Naftolin, F.,** Tamoxifen in combination with cytotoxic chemotherapy in advanced epithelial ovarian cancer, *Cancer,* 63, 1074, 1989.
22. **Cormier, E-M. and Jordan, V. C.,** Contrasting ability of antiestrogens to inhibit MCF-7 growth stimulated by estradiol or epidermal growth factor, *Eur. J. Cancer Clin. Oncol.,* 25, 57, 1989.
23. **Lim, C. L., Walker, M. J., Mehta, R. R., and Das Gupta, T. K.,** Estrogen and antiestrogen binding sites in desmoid tumors, *Eur. J. Cancer Clin. Oncol.,* 22, 583, 1986.
24. **Sridhar, K. S., Benedetto, P., Otrakji, C. L., and Charyulu, K. K.,** Response of eccrine adenocarcinoma to tamoxifen, *Cancer,* 64, 366, 1989.
25. **Love, R. R.,** Tamoxifen therapy in primary breast cancer: biology efficacy, and side effects, *J. Clin. Oncol.,* 7, 803, 1989.

26. **Hardell, L.,** Tamoxifen as risk factor for carcinoma of corpus uteri, *Lancet,* 2, 563, 1988.
27. **Callaway, T. W., Bruchowski, N., Rennie, P. S., and Comeau, T.,** Mechanisms of action of androgens and antiandrogens: effects of antiandrogens on translocation of cytoplasmic androgen receptor and nuclear abundance of dihydrotestosterone, *Prostate,* 3, 599, 1982.
28. **Bulbrook, R. D.,** Endocrine aspects of breast and prostatic cancer: an overview, *Cancer Surv.,* 5, 435, 1986.
29. **Sogani, P. C., and Whitmore, W. F.,** Flutamide and other antiandrogens in the treatment of advanced prostatic carcinoma, in *Endocrine Therapies in Breast and Prostate Cancer,* Osborne, C. K., Ed., Kluwer Acad. Publ., Boston, 1988, 131.
30. **Baulieu, E. E.,** RU-486 as an antiprogesterone steroid, *JAMA,* 262, 1808, 1989.
31. **Maudelonde, T., Romieu, G., Ulmann, A., Pujol, H., Grenier, J. Khalaf, S., Cavalie, G., and Rochefort, H.,** First clinical trial on the use of the antiprogestin RU486 in advanced breast cancer, in *Hormonal Manipulation of Cancer: Peptides, Growth Factors and New (Anti) Steroidal Agents,* Klijn, J. G., Paridaens, R., and Foekens, J. A., Eds., Raven Press, New York, 1987, 55.
32. **Fentiman, I. S., Chaudary, M. A., Wang, D. Y., Brame, K., Camplejohn, R. S., and Millis, R. R.,** Perioperative bromocriptine adjuvant treatment for operable breast cancer, *Lancet,* 1, 609, 1988.
33. **Waxman, J.,** Gonadotrophin releasing hormone analogues for prostatic cancer: an overview, *Semin. Oncol.,* 15, 366, 1988.
34. **Bajusz, S., Kovacs, M., Gazdag, M., Bokser, L., Karashima, T., Csernus, V. J., Janaky, T., Guoth, J., and Schally, A. V.,** Highly potent antagonists of luteinizing hormone-releasing hormone free of edematogenic effects, *Proc. Natl. Acad. Sci. U.S.A.,* 85, 1637, 1988.
35. **Brendler, C. B.,** The current role of hormonal therapy in the clinical treatment of prostate cancer, *Semin. Urol.,* 6, 269, 1988.
36. **Pau, H. F., Hess, D. L., Kaynard, A. H., Wei-Zhi, J., Gliessman, P. M., and Spies, H. G.,** Suppression of mediobasal hypothalamic gonadotropin-releasing hormone and plasma luteinizing hormone pulsatile patterns by phentolamine in ovariectomized rhesus macaques, *Endocrinology,* 124, 891, 1989.
37. **Harvey, H. A., Lipton, A., Max, D. T., Pearlman, H. G., Diaz-Perches, R., and de la Garza, J.,** Medical castration produced by the GnRH analogue leuprolide to treat metastatic breast cancer, *J. Clin. Oncol.,* 3, 1068, 1985.
38. **Santen, R. J., Manni, A., and Harvey, H.,** Gonadotropin releasing hormone (GnRH) analogs for the treatment of breast and prostatic carcinoma, *Breast Cancer Res. Treat.,* 7, 129, 1986.
39. **Palmer, W. N.,** Hormone analogs and synthetic hormones in cancer therapy, *Cancer Bull.,* 39, 245, 1987.
40. **Glode, L. M. and Smith, J. A.,** Long-term suppression of luteinizing hormone follicle-stimulating hormone and testosterone by daily administration of leuprolide, *J. Urol.,* 137, 57, 1987.
41. **Vorobiof, D. A. and Falkson, G.,** Nasally administered buserelin inducing complete remission of lung metastases in male breast cancer, *Cancer,* 59, 688, 1987.
42. **Labrie, F., Dupont, A., Cusan, L., Bélanger, A., Giguère, M., Labrie, C., Lacourcière, Y., Monfette, G., and Emond, J.,** Combination therapy with flutamide and (D-Trp^6,Des,Gly-NH$_2$^{10}) LHRH ethylamide in Stage C and D prostate cancer: today's therapy of choice — rationale and 5-year clinical experience, *Prog. Clin. Biol. Res.,* 262, 11, 1988.
43. **Gabrilove, J. L., Levine, A. C., Kirschenbaum, A., and Droller, M.,** Effect of long-acting gonadotropin-releasing hormone analog (leuprolide) therapy on prostatic size and symptoms in 15 men with benign prostatic hypertrophy, *J. Clin. Endocrinol. Metab.,* 69, 629, 1989.
44. **Cole, M., Raghavan, D., Caterson, I., Teriana, N., Pearson, B., Boulas, J., and Rosen, M.,** Danazol treatment of advanced prostate cancer: clinical and hormonal effects, *Prostate,* 9, 15, 1986.
45. **Panahy, C., Puddefoot, J. R., Anderson, E., Vinson, G. P., Berry, C. L., Turner, M. J., Brown, C. L., and Goode, A. W.,** Effect of danazol on incidence of progesterone and oestrogen receptors in benign breast disease, *Br. Med. J.,* 295, 464, 1987.
46. **Donaldson, V. H.,** Danazol, *Am. J. Med.,* 87, 3-49N, 1989.
47. **Santen, R. J., Worgul, T., Samojlik, E., Interrante, A., Boucher, A. E., Lipton, A., Harvey, H., White, D. S., Smart, E., Cox, C., and Wells, S. A.,** A randomized trial comparing surgical adrenalectomy with aminoglutethimide plus hydrocortisone in women with advanced breast cancer, *N. Engl. J. Med.,* 305, 545, 1981.
48. **Brodie, A. M., Dowsett, M., and Coombes, R. C.,** Aromatase inhibitors as new endocrine therapy for breast cancer, in *Endocrine Therapies in Breast and Prostate Cancer,* Osborne, C. K., Ed., Kluwer Acad. Publ., Boston, 1988, 51.
49. **Ingle, J. N., Green, S. J., Ahmann, D. L., Edmonson, J. H., Nichols, W. C., Frytak, S., and Rubin, J.,** Progress report on two clinical trials in women with advanced breast cancer. Trial I: Tamoxifen versus tamoxifen plus aminoglutethimide; Trial II: Aminoglutethimide in patients with prior tamoxifen exposure, *Cancer Res.,* 42(Suppl. 8), 3461, 1982.
50. **Lønning, P. E., Dowsett, M., and Powles, T. J.,** Treatment of breast cancer with aromatase inhibitors — current status and future prospects, *Br. J. Cancer,* 60, 5, 1989.

51. **Chu, P. S., Buzdar, A. U., and Hortobagyi, G. N.,** Trilostane with hydrocortisone in treatment of metastatic breast cancer, *Breast Cancer Res. Treat.,* 13, 117, 1989.
52. **Jackson, I. M., Barnard, L. B., and Lamberton, P.,** Role of long-acting somatostatin analogue (SMS201-995) in the treatment of acromegaly, *Am. J. Med.,* 81, 94, 1986.
53. **Souquet, J. C., Sassolas, G., Forichon, J., Champetier, P., Partensky, C., and Chayvialle, J. A.,** Clinical and hormonal effects of a long-acting somatostatin analogue in pancreatic endocrine tumors and in carcinoid syndrome, *Cancer,* 59, 1654, 1987.
54. **Nelson, J., Cremin, M., and Murphy, R. F.,** Synthesis of somatostatin by breast cancer cells and their inhibition by exogenous somatostatin and sandostatin, *Br. J. Cancer,* 59, 739, 1989.
55. **Klijn, J. G., Setyono-Han, B., Bakker, G. H., and Foekens, J. A.,** Effects of somatostatin analog (SMS-A) treatment (Sandostatin) in experimental and human cancer, *Eur. J. Cancer Clin. Oncol.,* 22, 727, 1986.
56. **Parmar, H., Bogden, A., Mollard, M., de Rougé, B., Phillips, R. H., and Lightman, S. L.,** Somatostatin and somatostatin analogues in oncology, *Cancer Treat. Rev.,* 16, 95, 1989.
57. **Lamberts, S. W.,** The role of somatostatin in the regulation of anterior pituitary hormone secretion and the use of its analogs in the treatment of human pituitary tumors, *Endocrinol. Rev.,* 9, 417, 1988.
58. **Camisa, C., Maceyko, R. F., O'Dorisio, T. M., Schacht, G. E., and Mekhjian, H. S.,** Treatment of psoriasis with long-term administration of somatostatin analog, 201-995, *J. Am. Acad. Dermatol.,* 21, 139, 1989.
59. **Märki, F., Bucher, U. M., and Richter, J. C.,** Multiple subcutaneous injections of somatostatin induce tachyphylaxis of the suppression of plasma insulin, but not glucagon in the rat, *Regul. Pept.,* 4, 333, 1982.
60. **Bloom, S. R.,** Somatostatin analogue treatment of endocrine tumors, in *Hormonal Manipulation of Cancer: Peptides, Growth Factors, and New (Anti) Steroidal Agents,* Klijn, J. G., Paridaens, R., and Foekens, J. A., Eds., Raven Press, New York, 1987, 451.
61. **Watson, D. M., Kelly, R. W., and Miller, W. R.,** Prostaglandins and prognosis in human breast cancer, *Br. J. Cancer,* 56, 367, 1987.
62. **Lathrop, A. and Loeb, L.,** Further investigations on the origin of tumors in mice. III. On the part played by internal secretion in the spontaneous development of tumors, *J. Cancer Res.,* 1, 1, 1916.
63. **Kaufmann, M., Jonat, W., Kleeberg, U., Eiermann, W., Jänicke, F., Kreienberg, R., Hilfrich, J., Albrecht, M., Weitzel, H. K., Schmid, H., Strunz, P., Schachner-Wünschmann, E., Bastert, G., and Maass, H.,** Goserelin, a depot gonadotrophin-releasing hormone agonist in the treatment of premenopausal patients with metastatic breast cancer, *J. Clin. Oncol.,* 7, 1113, 1989.
64. **Vickery, B. H., McRae, G. I., Sanders, L. M., Hoffman, P., and Pavlou, S. N.,** Studies with nafarelin and a long-acting LHRH antagonist, in *Hormonal Manipulation of Cancer Peptides, Growth Factors, and New (Anti) Steroidal Agents,* Klijn, J. G., Paridaens, R., and Foekens, J. A., Eds., Raven Press, New York, 1987, 281.
65. **Ruff, P., Derman, D. P., Weaving, A., and Bezwoda, W. R.,** Sequential hormonal therapy and sequential hormonal and chemotherapy for advanced prostate cancer, *Oncology,* 46, 288, 1989.
66. **Huggins, C. and Scott, W. W.,** Bilateral adrenalectomy in prostatic cancer, *Ann. Surg.,* 122, 1031, 1945.
67. **Judson, I. R.,** New endocrine agents, guidelines for future development, *Br. J. Cancer,* 60, 153, 1989.
68. **Ho, K. Y., Weissberger, A. J., Marbach, P., and Lazarus, L.,** Therapeutic efficacy of the somatostatin analog SMS 201-995 (octreotide) in acromegaly, *Ann. Int. Med.,* 112, 173, 1990.
69. **Silvestre, L., Dubois, C., Renault, M., Rezvani, Y., Baulieu, E-E., and Ulmann, A.,** Voluntary interruption of pregnancy with mifepristone (RU 486) and a prostaglandin analogue, *N. Engl. J. Med.,* 322, 645, 1990.

Chapter 4

HORMONE-LIKE SUBSTANCES (GROWTH FACTORS, INTERFERONS, INTERLEUKINS, PROSTAGLANDINS): CLINICAL AND THERAPEUTIC IMPLICATIONS

I. PROSPECTS IN CANCER: BIOLOGY AND TREATMENT

In the last decade a large class of substances called hormone-like substances were discovered and purified, and their role became increasingly significant in controlling cell differentiation and proliferation, and in tumor biology in general. These hormone-like substances encompass growth factors, interferons, interleukins, and prostaglandins, and are found in several human cancer cells as well as in their normal counterparts.[1-5] Compared to "classical" hormones, which are released by specific cell types (endocrine cells) in the circulation by endocrine mechanisms, hormone-like agents control cell proliferation by autocrine and paracrine mechanisms. They are released by multiple cell types under the influence of nonspecific stimuli, and by their own receptors exert a local control on their neighbor cells (paracrine mechanism) or on their own secreting cells (autocrine mechanism) (see Figure 1). Thus, there is a strong inter-relationship between hormones and hormone-like substances, and the success or failure of hormonotherapy in cancer patients depends largely on the presence of local growth factors. The action of hormones or hormone antagonists is counteracted at the cellular level in several instances by the occurrence of growth factors. There is ample evidence that differences in endocrine response of tumors, the hormone resistance or hormone "escape" phenomenon, are largely influenced by the presence of hormone-like agents. Comparison between classical hormones and hormone-like agents can be seen in Table 1.

The signals which trigger the synthesis of hormones and hormone-like substances come from the microenvironment (cell environment). There are also growth inhibitors. By inhibiting these responses, we can develop a new therapeutic strategy aimed at eventual medical intervention and prevention of proliferative diseases.[2] Genetic studies provide strong evidence for the existence of growth inhibitor genes ("antioncogenes") and suggest new strategies for cancer prevention and treatment, by directing drugs to growth factors and their receptors. The study of hormone-like substances is a rapidly emerging area that may provide opportunities for the discovery of new anticancer drugs, less toxic and more specific, and the autocrine/paracrine therapy will be an integral part of cancer treatment.[2-4] Most of the growth factors have been found to bind to specific receptors on cell membranes and to stimulate cell proliferation. The receptors for essential growth factors are an ideal target for potential anticancer agents, and they can serve as antigens for monoclonal antibodies which can act as pharmacologic agents to directly block the cell proliferation. Their location on the plasma membrane makes them readily accessible to antibody molecules. Antireceptor monoclonal antibodies have the potential to be unique reagents for antitumor therapy by blocking the function of a receptor for its growth factor, and also they can serve as convenient carriers of toxins, radionuclides, and drugs to specific targets. This chapter will deal with the clinical implications and potential therapeutic role as anticancer agents of: (1) polypeptide factors, (2) interferons (IFNs), (3) interleukins (ILs), (4) prostaglandins (PGs), (5) glandular extracts.

A. POLYPEPTIDE GROWTH FACTORS (GFs)

Current clinical investigations and therapeutic applications have focused on these five peptide growth factors: (1) epidermal growth factor or transforming growth factor-α (EGF/TGF-α), (2) transforming growth factor-β (TGF-β_1, β_2), (3) platelet-derived growth factor (PDGF), (4) tumor necrosis factor (TNF), and (5) colony-stimulating factors (CSF).

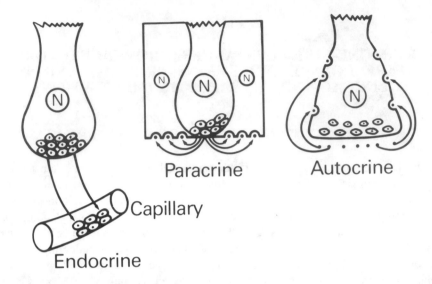

FIGURE 1.   Endocrine, paracrine, and autocrine mechanisms. (From Sporn, M. B. and Todaro, G. J., *N. Engl. J. Med.*, 303, 879, 1980. With permission.)

TABLE 1
Comparison between Classical Hormones and Hormone-Like Substances

Property	Classical hormones	Hormone-like substances
Origin of hormone	Endocrine cells	Multiple cell type
Control of production	Specific stimuli	Nonspecific signals
Transport of hormone	Circulation	Local diffusion
Mechanism of action	Endocrine, humoral	Autocrine, paracrine
Cell division	+ + +	+
Cell differentiation	+ + +	+ +
Cell proliferation	+	+ + +
Cell targets	Few cell types	Multiple cell types

1. Epidermal Growth Factors (EGF/TGF-α)

EGF is a structural homolog of transforming growth factor alpha (TGF-α). Both EGF and TGF-α bind to the EGF receptor and activate receptor-mediated tyrosine kinase activity. EGF has a molecular weight of 6.2 kDa and a membrane receptor of 180 kDa. It is now clear that human EGF is synthesized from a messenger that encodes 160 amino acids, and that this larger molecule is important with respect to cancer cells. EGF is secreted from a precursor of EGF called prepro-EGF. Prepro-EGF consists of around 1200 amino acids, and part of it is similar to the EGF receptor. Prepro-EGF is the source of urinary EGF (urogastrone, which is human EGF). Higher molecular weight peptides related to TGF-α are secreted in the urine of tumor-bearing patients, but not of controls; this may lead to the development of a diagnostic test for tumor as well as for progress of treatment. EGF is a potent mitogenic peptide. The EGF and TGF genes have been mapped to chromosomes 2 and 4, respectively. The receptor is a large glycoprotein of 175 kDa mol wt, with two domains, the first is an external EGF-binding domain of 62 amino acids, and the second is a cytoplasmic region of 542 amino acids that is homologous with other tyrosine kinases. The EGF receptor is the proto-oncogene of erb-B.[6] The EGF receptor is regulated by several ligand bindings and self-phosphorylation, and down regulation by ligand. However, EGF synthesis in normal cells was found only in the salivary gland and the kidney of the adult mouse.[7] Thus, both EGF and TGF-α bind to the same receptor to stimulate an intrinsic tyrosine kinase.

More than 40 companies are trying to commercialize EGF. Some applications are diagnostic; others involve clinical trials. EGF and TGF-α and their receptors are expressed in certain human cancers, such as: (1) lung cancer, (2) head and neck cancer, (3) bladder cancer, (4) breast cancer, and (5) colorectal cancer. Therefore, EGF and TGF-α will have clinical prognostic and therapeutic applications in cancer therapy. Expression of EGF-receptors (EGF-R) in high concentrations usually indicates a poor prognosis. Thus, EGF-Rs are significantly increased in invasive tumors (87.5%) as well as in poorly differentiated tumors. Since the biological effects on neoplastic cell proliferation require a long chain of molecular events, there will be several theoretical approaches and strategies to develop growth factor antagonists which can block each step; these include (1) the growth factor gene, (2) processing of the growth factor precursor, (3) release of growth factor from the plasma membrane to the extracellular space, (4) disruption of the growth factor ligand, (5) receptor antagonists, (6) blockage of signal transduction mechanism, and (7) interference with early gene expression and function. In the near future, biotechnology using recombinant DNA (rDNA) and cellular oncogenes, will play an important role in the pharmaceutical industry and will provide new therapeutic approaches for cancer treatment. Suramin, a β-naphtyl urea, has been found to be antagonistic to several growth factors (PGGF, EGF, TGF, FGF-β).

2. Transforming Growth Factors-β (TGF-β, TGF-B₁, TGF-β₂)

Transforming growth factor-β (TGF-β) appears to have a particularly important role in the repair process and in carcinogenesis. It is a homodimeric 25 kDa protein, has a multifunctional role in controlling the activities of other peptide growth factors, and is called a "panregulin". TGF-β is found in relatively high concentrations in platelets, T-lymphocytes, macrophages, and bone. Whether TGF-β stimulates or inhibits cellular proliferation depends on the type of target cell as well as the presence of other factors. TGF-β can control the effects of several other growth factors, such as PDGF, EGF/TGF-α, FGF (fibroblast growth factor), and interleukin-2 (IL-2). TGF-β has been a general mediator of negative growth control. Production of TGF-β is stimulated by antiestrogens (tamoxifen). Two TGF-βs were isolated from bovine demineralized bone and have been purified to homogeneity: one which induces embryonic rat mesenchymal cells to synthesize cartilage-specific proteoglycan (TGF-β₁) and the other, Type II collagen, which is now found to be identical to TGF-β₂. The inhibitory factors or chalones (meaning "inhibit") are basic glycoproteins which inhibit the cell cycle at the G_1-S, S-G_2, and G_2-M phases in the hairless mouse epidermis. Hormones and chalones intervene and act in the mitotic homeostasis of cancer cells as a negative feedback mechanism. TGFBs have been purified to homogeneity and most used sources include human placenta, human platelets, bovine kidneys, transformed murine L-929 cells, and most recently, porcine platelets and bovine bone.

Although TGF-β is a potent inhibitor of the growth of many cells, it exhibits a mitogenic activity for Schwann cells and osteoblasts. Potent inhibitory effects on many other epithelial cells have been demonstrated, such as bronchus, liver, skin, and intestine. TGF-β also inhibits the mitogenic action of insulin and hydrocortisone. It has been shown that both T- and B-lymphocytes synthesize and secrete TGF-β and also express receptors for TGF-β and subsequently prevent excessive immunoglobulin synthesis. Interestingly, in the case of MCF-7 breast cancer cells, which possess receptors for TGF-β, secretion of active TGF-β can be increased up to 20-fold by treatment of the MCF-7 cells with tamoxifen and its metabolite, hydroxytamoxifen. TGF-β is thus a hormonally regulated growth inhibitor with a negative feedback (negative autocrine action) on its producer cells.

The role of TGF-β in connective tissue synthesis by control of both matrix protein synthesis and proteolysis can be associated with a variety of connective tissue diseases, including atherosclerosis, pulmonary fibrosis, scleroderma, keloids, and rheumatoid arthritis.[3] In ovarian granulosa cells, TGF-β increases and decreases the effects of FSH on

TABLE 2
The TGF-β Family of Peptide Growth Factors

Factor	Source	Structure	Receptor(s) (280 kDa; 65,85 kDa)		Primary target organs
TGF-β$_1$	Platelets, placenta, kidney, bone, carcinomas	25 kDa, homodimer	+	+ +	Ubiquitous
TGF-β$_2$	Porcine platelets, bovine bone, human glioblastoma	25kDa, homodimer	+	−	Ubiquitous
TGF-β1.2	Porcine platelets	Heterodimer	+	−	Ubiquitous
Inhibin A	Embryonic reproductive structures	Heterodimers	?		Pituitary, gonads
Inhibin B					
Activin A	Embryonic reproductive structures	Homo- and heterodimers	?		Pituitary, gonads, bone marrow
Activin B	Embryonic reproductive structures		?		

receptors for LH, depending on the concentrations of TGF-β and FSH. It is likely that TGF-β blocks initiation of DNA synthesis at some step. Studies on the colorectal cell populations revealed that some are refractory to the inhibitory effects of TGF-β which may reside at the receptor or postreceptor level. Recently, a more rigorous purification of TGF-β has demonstrated the presence of multiple forms of the growth factor.[8] The original form, about which the most information is available, has been designated as TGF-β$_1$. It is a 25 kDa secreted protein consisting of two identical 112 amino acid subunits held together by disulfide bonds. The biologically active TGF-β is derived from a latent, precursor from that contains 390 amino acids per subunit and can be converted to the active protein either by acidification or proteolysis. The cDNA sequence of TGF-β has been recently resolved and, shows complete homology of the human, porcine, and bovine polypeptides. A second, less abundant type, TGF-β$_2$ is secreted by bovine bone and porcine platelets, and by a human glioblastoma cell line. TGF-β$_2$ also is a 25 kDa dimer; of identical subunits, approximately 70% identical to that found in TGF-β$_1$. Finally, a third form of TGF-β, designated TGF-β1.2, is a heterodimer containing a single TGF-β$_1$ monomer couplet to one TGF-β$_2$ monomer.[9] This last type has been demonstrated in porcine platelets in very low amounts. Multiple forms of the TGF-β receptors are present in most cells. Thus, a 280 kDa-receptor binds both TGF-β$_1$ and TGF-β$_2$ with equal and high affinity. (See Table 2).

From this class of proteins, only the TGF-βs are presently known to be modulators of many different cell types. Thus, TGF-β is unique among growth factors in that its effects on both cellular growth and differentiation are bifunctional: stimulatory and inhibitory, depending on cell type as well as the presence of other growth factors. TGF-β is also the modulator of the fibroblast growth factor (FGF). FGF exists under two closely related forms: basic (bFGF) and acidic (aFGF), which interact with common cell receptors. Interestingly, three oncogenes have been shown to be structurally related to FGF. The same oncogenes have been identified in Kaposi's sarcoma, which frequently occurs in patients with the acquired immune deficiency syndrome (AIDS). Both host and Kaposi's sarcoma oncogenes contain 206 amino acids, and the sequences of the oncogenes are approximately 45% identical with the sequence of bFGF and show less resemblance to the sequence of a FGF.[10] Both bFGF and aFGF are a family of 14 to 16 kDa growth factors and are composed of 155 amino acids. Our understanding of the importance of FGF-β as a principal mediator of embryogenesis, inflammation, wound healing, and carcinogenesis, is expanding. Thus, TGF-β can accelerate wound healing within 2 to 3 d at dose levels of less than 1 μg, and suppresses T- and B-lymphocytes, and subsequently, TGF-β can be used as an immunosuppressive agent. Studies using TGF-β as an anticancer drug are hampered because it is available only in small quantities, it is difficult to deliver it to target cells, and it has a very short half-life (only few minutes after intravenous administration).[10] Further progress in developing TGF-β analogs with a longer half-life and manufacturing it in large amounts by biotechnology with recombinant DNA (rDNA) should be fully explored.

3. Platelet-Derived Growth Factor (PDGF-1, PDGF-2)

Platelet-derived growth factor (PDGF), a potent mitogen for cells of mesenchymal origin, is released from human blood platelets upon their degranulation. It is a glycoprotein, a heterodimor of 30 to 32 kDa mol wt and consists of two polypeptide chains, PDGF-1 (or PDGF-A) of 14 to 18 kDa mol wt and PDGF-2 (or PDGF-B) of 16 kDa mol wt which are linked to each other by disulfide bonds, encoded by two different genes located on chromosomes 7 and 22, respectively. There is a 56% homology between the two mature PDGF chains. The PDGF (30 to 32 kDa) has mitogenic and chemotactic activity, is a potent vasoconstrictor, and stimulates synthesis of both matrix components and enzymes that degrade this matrix.[11] Human malignant epithelial cell lines were analyzed for expression or PDGF genes. Of the 12 cell lines tested, 9 derived from breast, lung, gastric, and ovarian carcinomas were found to express both PDGF-1 and PDGF-2 genes. Immunoprecipitation studies revealed that certain tumors produced PDGF-like proteins in addition to PDGF-1 and PDGF-2. Thus, breast, lung, and gastric carcinoma cells produced PDGF-like proteins that migrate as 30- and 32-kDa species under nonreducing conditions and as 15- and 16 kDa species under reducing conditions. Certain PDGF-like proteins produced by malignant epithelial cells may act by paracrine mechanisms, whereas, PDGF-like proteins produced by human malignant cells of mesenchymal origin osteosarcomas possess PDGF receptors and may act by autocrine mechanisms. Thus, PDGF may stimulate growth by an autocrine mechanism in mesenchyme-derived cells, whereas it may act by a paracrine mechanism is epithelial cells.

PDGF-like proteins have been found in many different types of cancers, including fibrosarcomas, osteosarcomas, and common epithelial cancers. PDGF was the first peptide growth factor to be directly implicated in carcinogenesis. PDGF may be involved *in vivo* in the processes of wound repair and in the etiopathogenesis of atherosclerosis. PDGF has been shown to induce fibroblasts to secrete growth factors, such as somatomedin C (a potent fibroblast growth factor) and the colony-stimulating factor (CSF), which are essential for the growth and differentiation of monocytes. The fibrosis, neovascularization, and inflammation seen in epithelial tumors may be related to the direct effect of PDGF on specific target cells. In addition to PDGF, sarcomas and gliomas may elaborate other factors, such as insulin growth factors (IGFs), which may cooperate with PDGF in the etiopathogenesis and progression of these tumors. Although anti-PDGF antibodies can effectively neutralize the PDGF-like activity associated with some of human tumor cell lines, the same antisera are ineffective or only partially effective in arresting the growth of these tumor cells.[12] It is now clear that the same growth factors that play a key role in the malignant transformation of cancer cells are physiologically expressed by inflammatory cells and particularly platelets, macrophages, and lymphocytes.

The therapeutic implications of growth factors will exceed the carcinogenic process, and may be beneficial in other processes such as inflammation, sarcoidosis, atherosclerosis, hepatic cirrhosis, wound repair, and rheumatoid arthritis. There is a synergic interaction between PDGF, TGFs (α and β), and IGFs (I, II). Insulin-like growth factors (IGF-I and IGF-II) are mitogenic peptide growth factors and they are identical with the somatomedins C and A, the endogenous mediators of growth hormone action; human IGF-I (somatomedin C) consists of 70 amino acids and IGF-II (somatomedin A) consists of 67 amino acids. IGF-I has a 7,600 mol wt and IGF-II has approximately a 7,500 mol wt. In addition to PDGF and FGF, other growth factors called angiogenic factors (angiogenin, tumor angiogenic factor TAF) are highly active in inducing capillary formation. Most growth factors produced by human mammary epithelial cells, such as EGF/TGF-α, IGF-I, and PDGF, are stimulated by estrogens, whereas TGF-β which exerts inhibitory effects is regulated by antiestrogens (tamoxifen). Growth factors do not enter into their target cells, but interact with specific receptors at the cell surface. This interaction activates mechanisms of "transmembrane signaling" which are required to transduce the mitogenic signal to the ultimate intracellular targets (enzymes, genes). The signal-transducing mechanism (known also as the cAMP-system) interacts upon activation with regulatory proteins called "G-proteins" which serve as signal amplifiers. Thus, a denylate cyclase is controlled by two different G-proteins, one of which (G_s) conveys stimulatory hormone signals and the other (G_i), inhibitory hormone signals.[12] The whole sequence of events starting with the interaction of a growth factor with its cellular receptor and resulting in cell division has been called the "mitotic cascade".

Recently, an interesting structural relationship between the erb-A oncogene and the nuclear receptors for thyroid and steroid hormones has been found. These nuclear hormone receptors interact with specific binding sites on DNA, enhancing the transcription of certain genes. This interaction is due to different "domains" in the receptor molecule. A high degree of amino acid sequence homology has been found for the DNA-binding domain of steroid and thyroid hormone receptors. A new protein called cyclin, which plays an important role in cell cycle and control of mitoses, has been identified. Cyclins are embryonic proteins which accumulate during each interphase. The transition from interphase to mitosis is induced by the appearance of a protein complex called maturation promoting factor (MPF) which induces cells to enter mitosis and meiosis. Cyclins have now been identified in many organisms as cyclin A and cyclin B. It is likely that some hormones (progesterone) may affect the cyclin synthesis and degradation.[13]

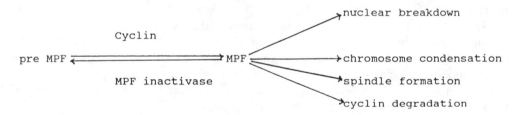

The discovery of cyclins is an important step in cell division, (mitosis and meiosis) which is the key point of neoplastic cell proliferation. The phenomenon of cell division may be affected by the interactions between cyclins and cytostatic factors which appear to stabilize MPF activity by blocking the degradation of cyclin. Interestingly, mammary epithelial normal and cancer cells can produce peptide growth factors, some of these having stimulatory activity, whereas others are inhibitory. Most of these factors are hormonally (estrogen) regulated. Other growth factors include MDGF-I, a 62-kDa peptide, which stimulates Type IV collagen production in the culture of mouse mammary epithelial cells. MDG-I (mammary-derived growth inhibitory factor) is structurally homologous to fatty acid and retinoid binding proteins.

More recently, a new peptide called mammastatin has been identified. Mammastatin is an inhibitory polypeptide factor of 47 and 65 kDa isolated from conditioned medium of normal human mammary cells (NHMC). It is decreased in neoplastic mammary cells. It inhibits both ER + and ER − cell lines, and it seems that it does not require an estrogen receptor for its action. Decreased production of mammastatin by transformed mammary cells may contribute to the loss of normal growth control cells.[14] Growth inhibitors, such as MDG-I, mammastatin, and TGF-β, appear superficially attractive as therapeutic agents, but have the disadvantage of cost of production. Thus, synthesis and availability of low molecular weight potent growth factor antagonists will allow the autocrine/paracrine method to be clinically tested, and the development of selective antagonists may have important therapeutic utility in the treatment of cancer patients.

4. Tumor Necrosis Factor (TNF)/Cachectin (TNF-α/TNF-β) (Lymphotoxin)

The term "tumor necrosis factor" was introduced to describe a serum protein produced after bacterial infections capable of causing hemorrhagic necrosis of animal tumors.[15] Cachectin is a macrophage-derived protein which can also induce a state of cachexia as it occurs in neoplastic disease. Thus, the identity of tumor necrosis factor (TNF) and cachectin was established. Tumor necrosis factor is part of a network of cell regulatory proteins collectively called cytokines which amplify immunologic effector functions and now include interleukin, interferons, colony-stimulating factor (CSF), lymphotoxin, and tumor necrosis factor (TNF). Among cytokines, TNF takes a special place in the context of cancer because its antitumor activity has engendered an enormous interest in the treatment of human cancer.

The story of TNF began a century ago with reports by Coley, who provided, in his opinion, convincing evidence that erysipelas infection produced a principal antagonist to sarcoma. During the progress of the erysipelas, most of the tumor disappeared, and the patient was seen 7 years later, without evidence of recurrence.[15] Studies regarding biosynthesis and chemical structure of TNF/cachectin revealed that it has a subunit molecular mass of 17 kDa.[16,17]

There are two tumor necrosis factors (TNFs): tumor necrosis factor alpha (TNF-α), which is macrophage-derived cytokine, and the lymphocyte-derived factor, which is called TNF-beta (TNF-β) or lymphotoxin. Human TNF-α is a nonglycosylated protein comprised of 157 amino acids and has a molecular weight of 17 kDa. TNF-β is a glycosylated protein comprised of 171 amino acids with a molecular weight of approximately 25 kDa.[18] Highly purified recombinant TNF-α and TNF-β (rTNF-α, rTNF-β) produced in bacteria are nonglycosylated molecules with a molecular weight of 17 and 18.6 kDa, respectively; they exert the same biologic activity as their natural counterparts.[16] The mature human protein is comprised of 157 residues, whereas the mature mouse protein is 156 residues long and the rabbit protein is only 154 residues in length. In all three mammalian species characterized to date, TNF/cachectin is synthesized as a prehormone. The prohormone sequence is composed of 79 amino acids in the mouse, 76 in the human, and 80 in the rabbit. The two TNF-α, -β proteins are 31% identical and 52% homologous to each other. Recombinant human TNF and mouse TNF cause acute hemorrhagic necrosis of murine and human tumor grafts in the mouse and have cytotoxic effects on susceptible murine and human cells *in vitro*.[16-18] Recombinant lymphotoxin has a molecular weight of 18,600 and appears to be the product of a single gene. Genetic manipulation of the primary structure has revealed that the carboxy-terminus of the cachectin molecule is particularly crucial for its bioactivity. Presently, the designation of TNF-α is used for macrophage-related TNF, and TNF-β for lymphocyte-related lymphotoxin.[16]

The action of TNF requires binding to specific cell surface receptors. Although TNF sensitivity could be controlled at the level of receptor expression, TNF resistance is determined at both receptor and postreceptor level. Despite the fact that the structure and function of TNF receptors are not yet known, the available data indicate that TNF-binding sites are comprised of a single class of membrane proteins of approximately 75 kDa which possess specific high affinity binding capacity for both TNF-α and TNF-β. However, there is a significant heterogeneity in the quantity of expressed membrane receptors, and some cell lines may carry between 100 and several thousands (up to 10,000) membrane receptors per cell, depending on the cell line. Since TNF receptors have been detected on TNF-sensitive as well as TNF-resistant cells, this suggests that the presence of TNF receptors per se cannot be the basis of its selective cytotoxicity.

However, in TNF-sensitive cells, the magnitude of response to TNF-α is proportional

TABLE 3
Physiologic Activities of TNF-α/Cachectin

Cell type	Cellular response
Neoplastic cells	Growth inhibition (cytostasis), cell death (cytotoxic), antiviral activity, HLA antigen expression
Activated T-lymphocytes	Enhancement of INF-γ production, expression of IL-2 receptors, HLA-antigen expression
Monocyte/macrophages, neutrophils	Cytotoxicity, phagocytosis
Hepatic cells	Stimulation of protein synthesis and responsiveness to glucagon
NK (natural killer) cells	Possible stimulatory effects
Bone marrow cells	Inhibition of colony formation (CSF)
Osteoblasts	Bone resorption
Fibroblasts	Proliferation, production of GM-CSF

to the number and concentration of TNF membrane receptors. The receptors for TNF-α can be up-regulated by both interferons and lectins. Up-regulation of receptors by interferons is accompanied by an enhancement of the biologic response, whereas up-regulation by lectins results in an antagonistic effect. Hence, two mechanisms control resistance to TNF-mediated cytostasis: down-regulation of receptor expression and post-receptor events. TNF can directly exert control of oncogene expression by affecting the myc-oncogene which is overexpressed in some carcinoma and leukemia cells. Cytostatis is preceded by a rapid down-regulation of myc transcriptional activity. Studies regarding the effects of TNF on the cell cycle revealed that the cytostatic effect is due to cell arrest in G_2-phase and was most pronounced at 4 h, with an increase in the number of cells in $G_2 + M$ and a decrease in G_1, indicating nearly total arrest in $G_2 + M$. This arrest was followed by a progressive cytolysis and at 24 h nearly all cells were lysed.[18] Using tumor necrosis factor-α (TNF-α), purified recombinant lymphotoxin, and gamma interferon (γ-INF) on proliferating human keratinocytes *in vitro*, it was revealed that cytostasis was dose dependent (up to 90% with TNF and 99% with γ-INF) and was maximal within 24 to 36 h. The tumoricidal activity of TFN has been demonstrated *in vivo* and *in vitro*. The mechanism of the antitumor activity of TFN is not yet known.

Thus, TNF is cytotoxic to certain tumor cells, whereas normal cells are resistant to its effects. The resistance of normal cells can often be overcome by treatment with inhibitors of transcription or translation, such as actinomycin D or cycloheximide, suggesting that normal (or nontransformed) cells produce a protein(s) that protects them from TNF-induced cytolysis. It has also been found that tumor necrosis factor-α enhances the cytolytic and cytostatic capacity of interleukin-2 (IL-2). Also synergistic cytotoxic and cytostatic effects have been observed between TNF and interferon-γ on human cancer cell lines.

TNF metabolism—At present, there is no information regarding the metabolism of TNF in man. In rabbits, the half-life was within few hours. In mice, the plasma half-life of ^{125}1-TNF-α was of the order of 6 to 7 min. After intravenous injection, TNF was cleared from the serum with a half-life of 15 to 30 min. Thus, in addition to its cytotoxic/cytostatic effects, it plays an important role in both humoral and cell mediated immune and inflammatory responses and probably in the regulation of neoplastic cell homeostasis. Therefore, TNF-α is a hormone-like polypeptide with pleiotropic activities, and it acts in conjunction with interleukin-1 and interferons. Recent studies demonstrated that both TNF-α and interleukin-1 (IL-1) are potent stimulants of ACTH secretion (ACTH secretagogues); however, the proximate target of TNF-α action appears to be peripheral (extrapituitary), whereas that of IL-1 appears to be the median eminence.[19] TNF also stimulates cortisol, epinephrine, glucagon, and bradykinin secretion. Some of the physiologic activities are described in Table 3. Therefore, the *in vitro* data suggest that TNA-α is an excellent candidate for cancer therapy in part due to its effects on some tumor cells producing either cell death (cytotoxic), or cytostasis. Second, TNF-α also fulfills all criteria of a typical immunomodulator, reaching multiple targets of the immune system.[18-22] The possible mechanism of antitumor action of TNF can at present be grouped into three categories: (1) direct cytotoxic action on cancer cells, (2) effects on tumor angiogenesis, and (3) activation of host antitumor mechanisms. So far, trials of recombinant tumor necrosis factor given systematically to patients with various types of cancer have yielded low response rates (<5%). *In vitro* studies showed that about one third of human epithelial cancer cell lines are very sensitive to the cytotoxic effects of TNF. Another third show cytostasis without lysis, and another third are relatively resistant to TNF. In contrast, the inhibitory activity of TNF against normal cells requires 100 to 10,000-fold higher concentrations, and this therapeutic advantage is superior to most classical cancer chemotherapeutic agents. The toxicity of TNF is dose related. It has been demonstrated that TNF is relatively cell-cycle-specific and inhibits tumor cells primarily during the G_2 period of the cell cycle. TNF also has a short plasma half-life (15 to 30 min) when administered i.v.[21] Refinements in recombinant DNA technology using *Escherichia coli* have facilitated the production on a large scale of a purified recombinant human TNF (rTNF) that are now available for clinical trials. *In vivo* antitumor effects occur in syngeneic murine tumor models and in human tumor xenografts in nude mice.[21]

Clinical trials—Clinical trials on Phase I and early Phase II of human recombinant TNF are now under way; recombinant human tumor necrosis factor (rTNF-α) in patients with advanced solid tumors has been used in a 30 min intravenous (i.v.) infusion on days 1 through 5, every 2 to 3 weeks, in daily doses ranging from 5 μg/m². Few clinical responses have been reported. Thus, large numbers of patients have been treated with recombinant TNF, but the question of therapeutic effect remains unanswered.[22] Combined treatment with rTNF-α and interleukin-2 resulted in a 100-fold stimulation of interferon (IFN). Thus, a combination of regimen of rTNF-α with low-dose interleukin (IL-2) or γ-INF may enhance the antiproliferative properties and may reduce some of the severe toxic effects previously reported in interleukin-2 clinical trials. Systemic side effects, including fever, chills, hypotension, and headaches, were mild. Hematologic toxicity was manifested by transient thrombocytopenia and leukopenia. Cachexia, characterized by anorexia and weight loss, is observed in tumor patients. Also one of the biochemical alterations associated with the response is hypertriglyceridemia. In dogs, similar changes were observed with elevated concentrations of catecholamines, glucagon, and glucocorticoid hormones.[16] Since some preclinical toxicologic studies showed that most primates including man, may experience hypotension, acute renal insufficiency, and, in some cases, disorders of intravascular coagulopathy after administration of rTNF, patients who had significant cardiac diseases, hemorrhagic diathesis, kidney disease, lipoprotein disorders, central nervous system metastases, or seizures should be excluded from participation in clinical trials. The most common side effects in clinical trials Phase I are fever and headache. Temperature higher than 38.5°C was seen in 50% after intravenous injection, and more than half of the patients complained of headache. Since TNF is a cell-cycle-specific agent that particularly affects cells in the G_2-period, it may act synergistically with other CCS agents such as fluorouracil (5-FU), dactinomycin, and doxorubicin. It has been postulated that TNF must first bind to a cell surface receptor, and then perhaps trigger the release of lysosomal enzymes that lead to lysis of the tumor cells. Until now, numerous Phase I and Phase II clinical trials have been reported with the single agent TNF, and generally, the overall response rate has been less than 5%. Thus, it is possible that cytokines, namely, TNF, with direct antitumor action are likely to synergize with direct antitumor action by different mechanisms, and they will have a promising role in treatment.

5. Colony-Stimulating Factors (CSFs)

Colony-stimulating factors (CSFs) or hematopoietic growth factors (HGFs) are a group of glycoproteins or polypeptide hormones that regulate myeloid proliferation and differentiation. Known collectively as "colony-stimulating factors (CSFs)", there are at least nine

TABLE 4
Hemopoietic Growth Factors (HGFs, Hemopoietins)

Hemopoietic growth factor	Molecular weight, (kDa)	*In vitro* effects
G-CSF	18—22	Stimulates growth of granulocyte colonies; activation of mature granulocytes
M-CSF	70—90	Stimulates the growth of monocytes colonies; activation of mature monocytes
GM-CSF	14—21	Stimulates growth of granulocyte; activation of mature granulocytes and monocytes
Erythropoietin (EPO)	34—39	Stimulates growth of erythroid and megakaryocyte colonies
IL-3	14—28	Stimulates early growth of granulocyte and erythroid cells
IL-1	15—20	Renders myeloid stem cells sensitive to "later" acting factors
IL-6	24—26	Renders myeloid stem cells sensitive to "later" acting factors
IL-7	17—18	Marrow stromal cells
IL-4 (BSF-1)	15—20	Stimulates mast cells, B-cell lymphocytes
IL-5	12—18	Stimulates eosinophils

distinct factors, such as macrophage-CSF (M-CSF), granulocyte-CSF (G-CSF), granulocyte macrophage-CSF (GM-CSF), eythropoietin (EPO), interleukin-1 (IL-1), IL-3, IL-4, IL-5, and IL-6. With the exception of erythropoietin, the precise *in vivo* role of the different factors is not yet fully understood,[23] Thus, in patients with infections or tumors associated with neutrophilia, CSF levels are elevated whereas normally the concentration of CSF is very low. Although CSFs have some overlapping activities, they have distinct molecular weights (see Table 4).

Interleukin refers to glycoprotein that mediates signal transfer between white cells. The word interleukin means "between white cells". This group of hormones, the hematopoietic growth factors (HGFs) are just entering their first clinical trials and may prove to be one of the most exciting areas in cancer treatment in the coming years.[24-28] Due to recent advances in biotechnology and genetic engineering, the genes for hematopoietic factors have been cloned, and purified proteins have been produced in recombinant forms. Hematopoietic growth factors (HGFs) are produced by cells common to all organs such as endothelial cells, fibroblasts, T-lymphocytes, and monocytes. Thus, there is a strong relationship between cell-cytokine interactions and the production of hematopoietic factors.[24] The CSFs (of HGFs) control the hematopoiesis by autocrine and paracrine mechanisms. Similar mechanisms of autocrine and paracrine stimulation may also contribute to transformation in acute mylogenous leukemia (AML). Chromosomal location of the gene for CSF or their receptors has been localized and chromosomal alterations are associated with malignant disease. Thus, the proto-oncogenic c-fms, possibly the CSF-receptors, and the human GM-CSF gene are located on chromosome 5, near the deletion site for the 5q-anomaly associated with leukemia. The multi-CSF molecule is a heterogenous mature protein of 14 to 28 kDa, and consists of 133 amino acids. The human GM-CSF gene which maps to chromosome 5q21 consists of 127 amino acids with a molecular weight of 14 to 35 kDa. The human G-CSF gene which maps to chromosome 17q11 to 17q22 and consists of 177 amino acids, the long form which is less active than the 174 amino acid form.

M-CSF is a heavily *N*-glycosylated 36 to 90-kDa homodimer. The human M-CSF gene is encoded by a single copy gene which is located on chromosome 5q33. There are three different forms of M-CSF: M-CSF-α which consists of 256 amino acids; M-CSF-β consisting of 554 amino acids; and M-CSF-gamma which consists of 438 amino acids. The human erythropoietin (EPO) gene has been localized to chromosome 7q11-7q22 and consists of 164 amino acids. The molecular weight of the natural EPO is 34 to 39 kDa. Interleukin-1 (IL-1) has two distinct proteins which are termed IL-1α (or hemopoietin-1) and IL-1β.

Similar to IL-1β, the IL-1α encodes a 31-kDa intracellular form and a 17-kDa extracellular form. Interleukin-4 (IL-4) encodes a protein of 153 amino acids, and is 129 amino acids long. Interleukin-5 (IL-5) encodes a protein of 134 amino acids with three N-glycosylation sites. The molecular weight of IL-5 is 18 kDa and 12 kDa for the nonglycosylated form. Interleukin-6 (IL-6), also referred to as IFN-β2, encodes a protein of 212 amino acids with a molecular weight of 23 to 29 kDa containing 32 hydrophobic amino acids in the N-terminal region. In contrast to IFN-β which is encoded by a gene located on chromosome 9, IL-6 is encoded by a gene assigned to chromosome 7. Interferon-gamma (IFN-γ) is encoded by a single gene located at chromosome 12. The native form of IFN-γ has a molecular weight of 45 kDa, and exists as a dimer with two major monomeric forms, with molecular weights of 20 and 25 kDa. Both the 20 kDa and 25 kDa forms are glycosylated. Recently, a minor species of IFN-gamma with a molecular weight of 15.5 kDa, and which is not glycosylated, was demonstrated. The action of these CSFs is, however, not confined to progenitor cells; thus, the action of GM-CSF on mature hematopoietic cells (neutrophils, eosinophils) involves increased expression of chemotactic receptors, enhanced phagocytic ability, inhibition of neutrophil migration. G-CSF and macrophage-CSF (M-CSF) are lineage-restricted CSFs. Hematopoietic growth and synergizing factors are also involved in specific immune responses as well. Like all polypeptide growth factors, the colony-stimulating factors (CSFs) bind to cell surface receptors prior to transmembrane signaling. Biologic effects of the CSFs can be achieved with 10% receptor occupation. While CSFs do not compete for binding to marrow cells, they have the ability to down-modulate each other with their own receptor. It appears that these factors render the most primitive cells sensitive to the "multi-CSF" and later acting factors, by stimulating division and maturation of the early cells, by up-regulating the receptors for the multi-CSF.[25,28] The clearance of metabolically-labeled [35]SGM-CSF injected into monkeys is multiphasic, with an initial half-life of 7 min and a second component of half-life of 80 to 90 min. The initial human studies in patients with HIV infections showed that GM-CSF caused a similarly rapid rise in circulating neutrophils, eosinophil and monocyte numbers, associated with increased bone marrow cellularity.[29] Human GM-CSF has also been shown to accelerate hemopoietic recovery in monkeys given total body irradiation. Interestingly, GM-CSF has been found to increase white cell counts in acquired immune deficiency syndrome (AIDS) patients in a dose-dependent manner. The maximum granulocytosis was observed at day 14 of treatment in patients with other hematologic deficiency. Granulocytic response to GM-CSF was usually biphasic. Increases of AGC (Absolute granulocyte counts) occurred 24 to 48 h after commencing treatment. The second increase was observed at day 4 to 5 of treatment. GM-CSF has also been reported to accelerate hematopoietic recovery following myelosuppressive therapy, in patients receiving chemotherapy for inoperable sarcomas. This agent, CG-CSF, also greatly extended the life of leukemic mice from 60 d in untreated animals to over 6 months in 80% of the G-CSF-treated animals. G-CSF may be useful as a stimulus of granulopoiesis in infected patients and is an effective agent against bone marrow suppression associated with radiation and chemotherapy. Recent analysis showed that hG-CSF (human G-CSF) is a mature protein of 174 amino acids. As compared to natural hG-CSF, recombinant hG-CSF (rG-CSF) lacks O-glycosylation, which may account for the difference in molecular weight of 18,800 for rG-CSF vs. 19,600 for hG-CSF.[30] At higher concentrations (500 U/ml) 10 to 20% macrophage colonies and additional mixed GM-colonies are detected on day 17 of culture. When G-CSF is combined with interleukin-1, the effects on bone marrow are further potentiated. Interleukin-3 (IL-3) given intraperitoneally to mice results in peripheral blood eosinophilia, neutrophilia, and monocytosis. Interleukin-1 (IL-1) has been reported to hasten granulocyte recovery after chemotherapy in mice when given in combination with G-CSF. Most interestingly, IL-1 given before sublethal total body irradiation has been reported to prevent severe myelosuppression. Both IL-1 (hemopoietin-1) and IL-6, act on very primitive hem-

TABLE 5
Potential Clinical Uses of CSFs to Stimulate Leukemic Cells

To increase differentiation of leukemic cells in myelodisplasia
  To induce leukemic stem cells into cycle (S-phase) before chemotherapy; to make them more susceptible to
    cycle specific agents
To stimulate mature phagocytic cell function
  Infection
  Neoplasia
Reduction of cancer treatment morbidity
Recovery following bone marrow transplantation
Burn patients
State of bone marrow failure
Radioprotective effect (IL-1)
To stimulate normal hematopoiesis
  Following chemo/radiotherapy (neutropenia)
  Aplastic anemia
  Anemia of chronic renal failure and anemia of chronic disease (erythropoietin)
  Adjunct to blood transfusion (erythropoietin)
  Porphyria cutanea tarda following hemodialysis (erythropoietin)
Management of infectious disease
Improvement of granulocyte procurement
Correction of platelet counts (combination therapy with IL-1, IL-3, or erythropoietin)
Management of granulocytopenia due to:
  Myelodysplastic syndrome (MDS)
  Aplastic anemia (AA)
  Cyclic neutropenia
  Solid tumors
  Kostmann's syndrome (congenital agranulocytosis)
  AIDS

opoietic cells and their precise effects are not fully understood, Erythropoietin (EPO), a glycoprotein hormone produced by the kidneys and released in response to tissue hypoxemia, is recognized as the primary regulator of erythropoiesis. It seems that the early events in the maturation of erythroid progenitor cells are probably controlled by T-lymphocytes. Many cases of aplastic anemia were associated with T-cell proliferation.[31] Innovative approaches to the treatment of red blood cell defects might include combination therapy: with infusions of gene-cloned EPO or interleukin-3 that will accelerate expansion of the erythroid cell pool. These specific approaches for stimulating erythropoiesis may eventually avoid the need for costly and risky red blood cell transfusion in many patients with severe refractory anemias. Thus, colony-stimulating factors (CSFs) have potential clinical applications in cancer therapy (see Table 5).

Clinical trials, Phase I and Phase II, have demonstrated that recombinant human granulocyte-macrophage CSF (rGM-CSF) and granulocyte CSF (rG-CSF) can increase the production of circulating leukocyte in patients with neutropenia. Clinical studies using cloned granulocyte colony-stimulating factor (G-CSF) in patients with MDS with pancytopenia and often lethal infections, by intravenous infusion for 6 d at different dosage levels (50 to 1,600 $\mu g/m^2$) showed in all 5 patients, an increase in both immature myeloid cells and mature granulocytes in the peripheral blood. Thus, in some cases of MDS, granulocytopenia can be improved by G-CSF.[32] Administration of GM-CSF to patients with aplastic anemia (AA), demonstrated only modest overall improvement of leukocyte counts. Administration of GM-CSF to children with Kostmann's syndrome produced only an increase in eosinophils. In a clinical trial using GM-CSF in severely leukopenic patients with AIDS at different doses of 1.0, 2.0, 4.0, or 8.0 $\mu g/kg$ given by i.v. bolus for almost 14 d, showed that by 7 d, all AIDS patients initially leukopenic had either normal or above normal total leukocyte counts.

TABLE 6
The Major Types of Interferons

Characteristics	Interferon-α	Interferon-β	Interferon-γ
Synonym	Leukocyte	Fibroblast	Immune
Cell/source	Monocyte/macrophage	Fibroblast/macrophage	T-lymphocytes
Molecular weight	20 kDa	26 kDa	17 kDa
Chromosome location	9	9	12
Number of genes (Subtypes)	>30	2	1
Main inducing stimuli	Virus	Virus	Antigen/mitogen
Cellular receptors	110 kDa	130 kDa	54 kDa
Effect on human leukocyte antigen expression	±	±	+ +

The use of recombinant human granulocyte macrophage colony-stimulating factor (rhGM-CSF) following autologous marrow transplantation for lymphoid malignancies, for 14 d of a 2-h infusion daily at doses up to 240 μg/m²/d, resulted in more rapid recovery of neutrophil and platelet counts. The use of recombinant human GM-CSF (rhGM-CSF) in patients on chemotherapy-induced myelosuppression at doses of 4 to 32 μg per kilogram of body weight per day induced a significant increase in leukocyte and granulocyte counts during the rhGM-CSF infusion. At doses of 250 μg/m and 30 μg/kg, respectively, both factors (GM-CSF and G-CSF) are well tolerated and seem to be clinically safe. The major clinical application will be the use of either one or both cytokines to improve supportive care in neutropenic patients following myelotoxic chemotherapy. Mild side effects usually were observed with GM-CSF treatment, including fever, myalgias, cephalalgia, nausea/vomiting, in 20 to 40% of patients without clear dose-response relation. Other side effects included bone pain, edema, dyspnea, and thrombosis. At higher doses more serious toxicity with GM-CSF were observed, such as the development of a "capillary-leak syndrome" (manifested by pericardial and pleural effusions) with pulmonary emboli.[32] Side effects encountered with G-CSF were similar to those reported in GM-CSF patients except serosal (pleural, pericardiac, and peritoneal) effusions. If the hematopoietic growth factors (HGFs) will be used (alone or in combination), the safety and efficacy of cancer chemotherapy, radiation therapy, and marrow transplantation will be significantly improved.

B. INTERFERONS (IFNS)

1. Classification (IFN-α, IFN-β, and IFN-γ)

Interferon was first described as a biological substance that inhibits viral replication and is elaborated by virus-infected cells.[33] This "interference" led to the term "interferon" and allows the measurement of the biological activity of interferons in terms of "antiviral units". Interferons are glycoproteins that are synthesized by a variety of cells in response to viral infection, immune stimulation, and certain chemical inducers. Although over 20 interferons have now been identified in humans, they can be classified into three groups: alpha, beta, and gamma.[34] Most of the subtypes belong to the alpha class, almost 20; two subtypes of beta (1 and 2) have been described; and there is only one gamma species. α-Interferon is originally secreted by leukocytes and β-interferon by fibroblasts. γ-Interferon, however, is secreted solely by T-lymphocytes. There are marked homologies between α- and β-interferons: they share the same cell surface receptor encoded on chromosome 21. γ-Interferon is a different molecule with stronger immunomodulatory effects, and its gene is on chromosome 12, the receptor is found on chromosome 6 and appears to be different from that of α- and β-interferons. Table 6 shows the major types of interferons.

The most biologically important is interferon-α-2. Interferon-α is more than 99% pure and can be produced from human lymphoblastoid cell lines, then purified by chromatography, and as recombinant interferon-α-2 (r-INFα-2); then again purified by chromatography (Roferon, interferon-α-2, Intron). The α- and β-interferons share approximately 30% homology in the amino acid sequences, but show no homology with γ-interferon. It is the anticancer potential of interferons that has led to the greatest recent interest in their clinical use. Interferons and related cytokines are pleiotropic effector molecules and exert a wide range of regulatory actions on normal cells, cancer cells, and host immune defense cells.[35] Since most, if not all, cells in the body have interferon receptors, it is not surprising that the mechanism of anticancer activity of interferons is not understood. However, it is likely to include the inhibition of cancer cell proliferation, oncogene suppression, and antiviral actions.

2. IFN Receptors

To exert their regulatory role on cells, IFNs must first interact with specific cell membrane receptors. Two distinct IFN cell-surface receptors are widely distributed in the body. IFN-α and IFN-β share a receptor which is thought to be about 110 to 130 kDa. The receptor for IFN-γ has now been cloned and has a molecular weight of approximately 54 kDa. The receptor genes for the INFα/β and γ receptors are located on chromosomes 21 and 6, respectively.[36,37] After binding to cell surface receptors, IFNs act rapidly by up-regulating some cellular genes and down-regulating others. Most IFN-induced genes are activated by all three types.

3. Mode of Action

The exact physiologic role of each of the interferons remains unclear. They exert both direct (cytotoxic) and immune (stimulatory) effects. Both effects result from interferon molecules binding to their cell surface receptors which trigger intracellular signals. At the cellular level, IFN appears to act by gene activation, which in turn is associated with decreased synthesis of a number of proteins, as well as the synthesis of new proteins. The enzymes which appear to inhibit viral replication may also be involved in the inhibition of tumor protein synthesis and possibly contribute to the prolongation of the cell cycle by inducing a reversible cytostasis. Thus, interferons exert cytostatic effects and others cytotoxic effects on cancer cells. Antitumor and antimetastatic activities can also be seen in mice deficient in T-lymphocytes and natural killer (NK) cells. The cell membrane is also altered as shown by increased expression of tumor-associated antigens, and human lymphocyte antigens (HLAs). In addition to those effects, interferons alter the immune system by stimulating the so-called "natural immunity", which includes the natural killer (NK) cell, and the lymphokine-activated killer (LAK) cell. IFNs also have other immunoaugmenting activities, including stimulation of interleukin-2 (IL-2) and tumor necrosis factor (TNF). IFN-γ appears to have a wider variety of immune stimulatory effects. Some actions of interferons are listed in Table 7. Thus, IFNs stimulate the immune system by enhancing the cytotoxicity of T-lymphocytes and NK cells, and increase phagocytosis by monocytes and neutrophils.

4. Clinical Use of Interferons

Within the past decade, interferons have undergone extensive Phase I and Phase II clinical trials in hematologic malignancies, lymphomas, and tumors of various other tissues. Most of clinical trials used interferon-α and recombinant α preparations. Thus, human lymphoblastoid interferon, HuIFN(Ly), and recombinant interferons (rIFNα2a and α2b or known as Roferon-A/Roche and Intron A/Schering) are used most frequently (Table 8).

Interferon-α-2a (Roferon-A) was also used for treatment of patients with cutaneous T-cell lymphoma (stages Ia to IVa) at dosage of 3 to 36 million IU i.m. daily for a 10-week period. At the end of treatment, 64% of patients had an objective antitumor response and another 27% of patients progressed from a partial to complete response with further treatment;

TABLE 7
Some Actions of Interferons (IFNs)

Function	IFN-α	IFN-β	IFN-γ
Cytostatic	+	+	+
Cytotoxic	+	±	+
Antitumor activity *in vivo*	+	+	+
Induce Class I-HLA	+	+	+
Stimulate B-cell proliferation	−	±	±
Oncogene expression	+	+	+
Stimulate T-cell growth	±	±	+
NK cell activity	+	+	+
LAK cell activity	+	+	+
Vaccine adjuvant property	±	±	+

TABLE 8
Therapeutic Activity of α-Interferon in Various Malignant Diseases (Phase-II Studies)

Type of tumor	Complete & Partial response (%)
Active	
Hairy cell leukemia (HCL)	80—90
Mycosis fungoides	70
Chronic myeloid leukemia (CML)	60—70
Non-Hodgkin's lymphoma	40—50
Carcinoid syndrome	47
Cutaneous T-cell lymphomas	>90
Moderately active	
Multiple myeloma	<50
Kaposi's sarcoma	30—40
Malignant melanoma	10—15
Renal cell cancer	15—20
Bladder cancer	>50
Ovarian cancer	18
Inactive	
Breast cancer	
Lung cancer	
Colon cancer	
Prostate cancer	
Active myelogenous leukemia	

altogether 91% had a favorable response.[38] Further studies are required for efficacy of interferons in patients with chronic lymphocytic leukemia (CLL), acute lymphocytic leukemia (ALL), Hodgkin's disease, myelodysplastic syndrome (MDS), astrocytoma, and osteogenic sarcoma.

At present, certain generalizations appear to emerge from the α-interferon trials:

1. Continuous dosing appears to be more effective than intermittent dosing.
2. Complete remission appears only on rare occasions; more often a partial remission can be seen.

3.   In many clinical trials, the median time to response has been 8 to 12 weeks. Thus, the response to interferon therapy is a slow process.
4.   Tumor size may play an important role in determining the potential activity, (more active in small tumors).
5.   A dose-response relationship is not yet established.
6.   For maintaining the effect a continuous or maintenance therapy is required.
7.   In many cases, after discontinuation of therapy, the effect persists for some time, but ends in recurrence in almost all patients.[39,40]

The clinical efficacy is generally seen at doses of 2 to 5 megaunits (equivalent to 20 to 50 μg) per m^2 daily or three times weekly. Such doses are usually well tolerated, with an influenza-like syndrome being the main side effect. An unexpected aspect of IFN-α therapy is the occurrence of antibodies that bind to, and in some cases, neutralize the IFN. However, the frequency and relevance of these antibodies is low and vary from 2 to 24% of patients.[35]

IFN-β, in the few clinical studies reported so far, gives no indication that it is of greater benefit than IFN-α. In a recent study, ten patients with hairy cell leukemia (HCL) were treated with recombinant beta-serine-interferon (rIFN-βser) at doses of 90×10^6 units s.c. three times a week and showed normalization of peripheral blood counts in 65%. rIFN-βser is a mutein that is tolerated at a dose five- to tenfold higher than IFN-α. Although α-interferon and β-interferons share approximately 40% amino acid homology, this indicates that rIFN-βser has activity in HCL.[41] INFγ is a more potent immunomodulator, also shows more potent antiproliferative activity then IFN-α or IFN-β, and interacts more closely with other cytokines.[42] This IFN-γ has been widely tested in patients with advanced cancer by i.v. infusion daily at doses of 0.1, 0.5, or 1 $mg/m^2/d$ followed by i.m. injections of recombinant (rIFN-γ) interferon-γ and can induce partial responses in few patients with chronic lymphocytic leukemia (CLL) and Hodgkin's disease. In chronic myeloid leukemia (CML) response rates of 38% have been reported. Interestingly, γ-interferon caused profound hormonal changes in patients with cancer, such as a significant elevation of ACTH, cortisol, and GH at 2 h after treatment.

Interferons (IFNs) have a limited clinical role as antiviral agents, such as the common cold and chronic hepatitis B, and may potentiate the activity of some vaccines. Clinical studies have been performed at the National Cancer Institute to document the dose and schedule for rIFN-γ administration. Two such Phase III trials, one in melanoma patients following the surgical excision of the primary lesion and the other in small cell lung cancer patients following induction of a complete response with chemotherapy and radiation therapy, have been conducted. Interferons augmented the effectiveness of the cytotoxic agents in leukemias, breast carcinoma, bladder carcinoma, and neuroblastoma in different animal tumor models. Further investigations are required to determine the effectiveness of combining interferons with hormones and vitamins, to design more effective and less toxic combination therapies. Phase II trials demonstrated a possible antitumoral activity of interferons in various solid tumors: malignant melanoma, renal cell carcinoma, ovarian adenocarcinoma, carcinoid tumor, and superficial bladder cancer.[43]

5. Toxicity and Side Effects of Interferons

Contrary to initial expectations, interferons have not proven to be an inoffensive treatment. Some general considerations can be drawn regarding the toxicity of INFs:

1.   Toxicity is strongly dose related. Doses over 50 million units are practically nontolerable; daily doses over 18 million units are only short-term tolerable. In practice, doses over 10 million U/d for long-term are nontolerable.
2.   The hematologic toxicity is relatively small and seldom dose limited.

3. By reducing the therapeutic dose of INF-α below 5 million/m^2/d, the side effects and toxicity will be less than 3%.

4. The severity and type of side effects are dependent on the underlying malignant disease.

5. Side effects of INF-α are almost reversible and practically not life threatening.

The side effects and toxicity of INFs can be described as early side effects (or acute toxicity) and later side effects (chronic toxicity).

Early side effects (acute toxicity)—Most patients taking doses above 1 million IU/m^2 usually develop fever, chills, myalgia, arthralgia, and cephalalgia. These symptoms often require acetaminophen and sometimes even meperidine hydrochloride (Demerol) for control. Also, most patients on their first exposure to IFN develop influenza-like symptoms (96%), such as myalgia and cough, which often requires dose reduction. Fatigue, perhaps reflecting CNS toxicity, is the most prevalent nonacute symptom. Other toxicities include myelo-suppression and vomiting.[40-44] At higher doses of interferon-α (more than 20 million/m^2) neurotoxicity is frequently encountered as manifested by psychosis, confusion, hallucination, and somnolence. Abnormal EEG (electroencephalographic) findings resembling those seen in diffuse encephalitis have been documented for rIFNα and more recently in Phase I studies of γ-interferon.

Later side effects (chronic toxicity)—Severe musculoskeletal pain occurs mainly in patients with CML and should be considered as a specific complication of this malignancy. Leukopenia, anemia, and sometimes occurrence of thrombocytopenia are seen. Cardiac toxicity remains questionable, although heart failure and arrhythmias have been associated with IFNs administration. Polyneuropathy is occasionally seen. Most of these effects are reversible. The incidence of antibodies is below 1% with natural IFN and between 0 to 10% with the use of recombinant (rIFN).[40] Therefore, with IFN-α, the type most widely used in clinical studies, doses of 1 to 9 million units (MU) are generally well tolerated, but doses of 18 million units or higher ($\geq$18 MU) caused moderate to severe toxicity. Doses $\geq$36 million units can induce severe toxicity and significantly alter the performance status of the patients. Thus, interferon is a biologic modifying agent, and in combination with other agents, can become the "fourth arm" of cancer therapy.

C. INTERLEUKINS (ILs)

1. Classification

Interleukins, which means "between white cells," are a large family of polypeptide hormones known also as cytokines, lymphokines, or interleukins; They are produced by several cell types (endothelial, fibroblasts, epithelial, T-cells, stromal cells, and hemopoietic cells), but mainly by the antigen-specific cells, especially T-cells. Currently, there are eight Interleukins and they exert pleiotropic effects on the immune cells, tumor cells, and hemopoietic cells. The characteristics, synonyms, cell source, and cell targets for each interleukin are described in Table 9.

Recently, it has been demonstrated that interleukins have potential therapeutic applications, which include infectious diseases, autoimmune disease, and cancers.[45-51] From all the interleukins, interleukin-2 (IL-2) is the most widely used in clinical trials for different cancers. Clinical and therapeutic investigations regarding their optimal dose, biologic mechanisms of response, toxicity, and resistance are still unresolved.

Production of recombinant human interleukins (rILS) are made by insertion of clone gene cDNA into *Escherichia coli*. These recombinant ILs are nonglycosylated and seem to be indistinguishable from those of natural molecules, which usually are glycosylated and synthesized by immune lymphocyte cells, or macrophages.

TABLE 9
Characteristics of Interleukins (ILs)

Interleukin	Synonyms	Molecular weight (kDa)	Sources	Cell targets
IL-1 (IL-1α, IL-1β	LAF (lymphocyte-activating factor) hemopoietin-1	17.5	Endothelial, epithelial, and macrophages	Lymphoid cells, hematopoietic cells
IL-2	TCGF (T-cell growth factor)	15.5	T-lymphocytes	T-cells, NK cells, thymocytes
IL-3	Multi-CSF	14—28	T-cells	Immature hemopoietic cells, pre-B cell line
IL-4	BSF-1	15—20	T-cells, mast cells	B-cells, T-cells, eosinophils, mast cells
IL-5	TRF, Eo-CSF (eosinophil growth factor)	12—18	T-cells	B-cells, eosinophils, thymocytes
IL-6	TFN-B$_2$, PGF (plasmocytoma growth factor)	26	Monocytes, T-cells, fibroblasts	B-cells, T-cells, fibroblasts
IL-7	Lymphopoietin-stromal cell factor	15—45	Stromal cells, thymocytes	Pre-B-cells, thymocytes
IL-8	Chemotactic factor	15—30	Monocytes, macrophages	Granulocytes

2. Biological Effects of Interleukins

Since the interleukins exert pleotropic effects on tumor cells, this suggests the existence of several specific cell surface receptors.[46-48]

a. Interleukin-1 (IL-1)

IL-1 is one of the key mediators of the body in response to inflammation, immunological reactions, and tissue injury. There are two species, IL-1α and IL-1β. The two forms have a low degree of homology (26%), but they have similar activities and share a common high-affinity receptor. There are three types of receptors. The first, isolated from a thymoma cell line, binds both forms, IL-1α and IL-1β, to this receptor. A second receptor has a higher affinity, and the third IL-1 receptor on the B-cell line or fibroblasts differs in binding properties from the thymoma receptor. Most cells have low numbers of receptors, and there is no clear correlation between the number per cell and the intensity of the biologic effect.[46] There is also a low-affinity receptor with a K_d of 300 to 500 pM and 15,000 sites per cell. The high-affinity receptors are rapidly internalized and bind to the nucleus, and the responsiveness to IL-1 is down-regulated.[45] The major systemic effects of Interleukin-1 are on CNS (fever, sleep, increasing ACTH, and neuropeptide secretion); hematology (lymphopenia, increase tumor cell killing, and increase growth factors synthesis); metabolism (increase synthesis of hepatic proteins and insulin); and vascular wall (increase leukocyte adherence, increase prostaglandin synthesis, and capillary leak syndrome). IL-1 exerts important immunologic effects by acting on T-lymphocytes, B-lymphocytes, and natural killer cells (NK cells). IL-1 has been reported to enhance granulocyte recovery, following chemotherapy in mice, and also can prevent the occurrence of myelosuppression when given subtotal body irradiation.[30] Therapeutic implications of IL-1 are mainly inflammatory and proliferative processes. IL-1 may have important therapeutic uses in injury and wound healing as well as in metastatic tumors, and some autoimmune disease. It may accelerate hematopoietic recovery after chemotherapy and radiation therapy.

b. Interleukin-2 (IL-2)

IL-2 is the first lymphocytotrophic hormone to be recognized and completely charac-

TABLE 10
Possible Antitumor Effects of Interleukin-2

Effect	Mechanism(s)	Comments
Cytotoxicity	Activation of NK, LAK, TIL cells	This phenomenon is dose and schedule related
	Activation of cellular proto-onco-genes (C-myb)	
Immunoaugmentation	Increased MHC Class I antigen expression, differentiation of B-cells to secrete immunoglobulin M	Adoptive immunotherapy of cancer
Induction of other cytokines (IFN, TNF, CSF)	T-cells, monocytes, macrophages	Recombinant TNF increases the cytotoxic and cytostatic capacity of rIL
Induction of hormones (ACTH, cortisol, GH)	Stress	Each of these hormones may mediate a number of effects and interfere with antitumor effect of IL-2

terized. IL-2, discovered as a T-cell growth factor (TCGF), has a molecular weight of 15.5 kDa and consists of 133 amino acids of glycoprotein acting as the second signal in T-lymphocyte mitogenesis. IL-2 is a true biological response modifier (BRM). IL-2 is also available as a recombinant protein (rIL-2), an *E. coli*-produced rIL-2, which is nonglycosylated, while natural human IL-2 (huIL-2) is a glycosylated protein. Recombinant IL-2 has the same biological effects as the natural molecule. Thus, IL-2 is secreted and synthesized by T-lymphocytes (Th1 subset) after their activation by antigen or mitogens.[47] The interaction of IL-2 with target cells occurs via a specific cell surface receptor. This receptor is expressed on T-lymphocytes and on activated B-lymphocytes, and macrophage/monocytes. It is a heterodimer composed of two independently regulated proteins that are associated noncovalently on the surface of activated T-lymphocytes (p75 and p55). Certain lymphoid cells, including natural killer (NK) cells, express one of these proteins, the p75 kDa or α-chain, which is responsible for internalization and biological effects. This protein p75 binds IL-2 independently, but at an approximately 100-fold lower affinity than the high affinity receptor. The second component p55 (also known as "TAC" antigen) is smaller and contains only 13 residues. While the p55 kDa molecule will bind IL-2, apparently no internalization and therefore no direct biological effects follow this binding.[52] It is known that high concentrations of IL-2 *in vitro* (100 to 1,000 U/ml) are required to produce activated NK cells and the other cells, such as lymphokine-activated killer (LAK) cells, which are a third and distinct population of lymphocytes; they are non-T, non-B "null" lymphocytes. It is postulated that higher doses of IL-2 may be necessary for the activation and maintenance of cytotoxicity of LAK-cell activity than for the proliferation of activated cytotoxic T-lymphocytes. Tumors responding through T-cell mechanisms would require lower doses of IL-2 than those responding through LAK-cell cytotoxicity. Also, combination of IL-2 with other cytokines, such as interferons (INF), CSF, tumor infiltrating lymphocyte (TIL) which are predominantly T-cells, will enhance significantly the response rates in animal tumors as well as in patients with metastatic melanoma.[46]

IL-2 exerts biologic effects on various normal and tumor cells (see Table 10). Cytotoxic activity is demonstrated on a wide range of tumor cells, including melanoma, renal cell carcinoma, squamous cell carcinoma, sarcomas, and pulmonary carcinomas. The antitumor effect of IL-2 was clearly demonstrated in methylcholanthrene-induced sarcomas and in pulmonary and hepatic metastases in mice, IL-2 markedly augments the effects of transferred LAK cells.[50] Thus, it appears that the antitumor effect for nonimmunogenic tumors is mediated primarily by LAK cells, and for weakly immunogenic tumors by T-cells as well

TABLE 11
Toxic (Side Effects) of IL-2 Therapy

Organ	Description	Management
Systemic	Chills, fever, diarrhea, vomiting, fluid retention	Antiprostaglandins (aspirin, indomethacin), antiemetics
Neuropsychiatric (CNS)	Euphoria, stupor, disorientation, coma, cerebral edema	
Dermatologic	Erythrodermia, oral mucositis	Steroids
Cardiopulmonary	Hypotension, atrial tachycardia, capillary leak syndrome, myocardial infarction	Vasopressors (Neosynephrine, dopamine)
Kidney	Oliguria, moderate dysfunction	No treatment required
Liver	Hyperbilirubinemia, increased alkaline phosphatase, moderate dysfunction	No treatment required
Hematologic	Anemia, thrombocytopenia, lymphopenia	Dose α schedule related, reversed rapidly after cessation of therapy
Endocrinologic	Increased ACTH, prolactin, GH, cortisol, hypothyroidism	Thyroxine
Vitamin deficiency	Vitamin C	

as LAK cells.[48] IL-2 has a short half-life (6 to 7 min). Antitumor activity may be increased by the use of IL-2 in combination with other cytokines or monoclonal antibodies. Recently, clinical trials have been performed at NCI as elsewhere using IL-2 alone, mainly recombinant interleukin-2 (rIL-2), or in combination with interferons, TNF, LAK cells, and TIL using different doses, schedules, and route of administration. Various types of tumors including melanoma, renal cell carcinoma, colorectal cancer, hypernephroma, and ovarian cancer, were treated with IL-2 alone or in combination. It appears from currently available data that only a minority of patients treated with IL-2 showed clinically significant responses, and only 5 to 10% achieved durable complete responses. However, more encouraging results were achieved, with at least a 50% reduction in tumor size in 20 to 30% of cases of advanced melanoma and renal cell cancer, following a combination therapy with LAK cells.[50] In a recent study conducted in 25 patients with disseminated cancer (renal cell carcinoma, melanoma, Hodgkin's lymphoma and CML, breast cancer, and colon cancer) who were treated with recombinant human interleukin (rIL2) by continuous infusion at a dose of $\geq 3.4 \times 10^6$ U/m^2/d for 6 d and the LAK cells transfused the following day; 9 patients (36%) had objective tumor regression. The current dosage used is 100,000/U/kg, three times a day intravenously for up to 14 d, given on alternate weeks of a 3-week cycle, with 1 week of rest. A study using a larger number of patients showed that combination of IL-2 + LAK produced a 27% response (complete and partial) in 74 patients with renal cell carcinoma, a 25% response in 68 patients with melanoma, and 8% response in 39 patients with colon cancer. More recently, a combination of rIL-2 and TIL was used in 28 patients with malignant melanoma, renal cell carcinoma, and non-small-cell lung cancer. The patients were treated with autologous expanded TIL and continuous infusions of rIL-2 at doses of 1 to 3×10^6 U/m^2/d; 29% of the patients with renal cell cancer and 23% of those with melanoma achieved tumor responses lasting 3 to 14 months. Thus, these early results in chemoresistant cancers indicate that adoptive immunotherapy can become, in the next decade, an important therapeutic modality in cancer treatment.[45,49,50]

The clinical toxicities of IL-2 therapy in humans are dose and schedule related; usually they are mild to moderate and only seldom require discontinuation of IL-2 therapy. There are systemic and organ toxic side effects (see Table 11). It was also shown that TIL cells are 100-fold more active than LAK cells in adoptive immune therapy.

c. Interleukin-3 (IL-3)

IL-3, or multi-CSF, is a glycoprotein of 14 to 15 kDa that regulates hematopoiesis. This factor consists of 133 amino acids with a chromosomal location of 5q and is produced by activated T-lymphocytes. IL-3 may act on pluripotent stem cells (PPSC). IL-3 has some therapeutic potential in diseases such as aplastic anemia. Clinical Phase I/II studies have begun recently, which suggest that IL-3 alone has no significant effects on neutrophil recovery in chemotherapy-induced myelosuppression.

d. Interleukin-4 (IL-4)

IL-4, a glycoprotein of 15 to 20 kDa, is 129 amino acids long and is a co-stimulator of B-cell proliferation. Thus, IL-4 is very important for immunoglobulin isotype regulation, particularly increasing the production of IgG$_1$ isotype in T-stimulated cells. IL-4 has a wide range of activities on B-cells, such as : (1) it increases expression of MHC Class II on B-cells, (2) it is important in clonal expansion of antigen-specific B-cells, and (3) by regulation of immunoglobulin isotype production it may modulate the humoral responses to antigenic stimuli. IL-4 is produced by a subset of helper T-cells (T$_H$2) that also produces IL-5 and IL-6.[46] IL-4 binds to a single high-affinity receptor on most T-cells, B-cells, mast cells, and epithelial cells, but the receptor number is generally low. In the mouse, IL-4 binds to a 65-kDa receptor, and in the human system, IL-4 binds to a 140-kDa polypeptide.

e. Interleukin-5 (IL-5)

IL-5, originally described as T-cell replacing factor (TRF), was subsequently found to have multiple effects on B-cells. It encodes a protein of 134 amino acids and has a molecular weight of 12 kDa (for the nonglycosylated form) and of 18 kDa (for the glycosylated form). Human recombinant IL-5 (rIL-5) has several effects on B-cells, including the induction of IgM and IgA synthesis.

f. Interleukin-6 (IL-6)

IL-6 is also referred to as B-cell stimulating factor-2 (BSF-2) or interferon-B$_2$. IL-6 encodes a protein of 212 amino acids and has some similarity to granulocyte colony-stimulating factor (G-CSF). It has been shown that some tumors, including cardiac myxomas, cervical cancers, and bladder carcinomas, produce large amounts of IL-6, and some patients with such tumors show evidence of autoimmune disease. Autoimmune disease disappeared after the tumor was removed. IL-6 exerts its multiple effects by binding to a specific receptor. IL-6 receptors (IL-6R) are found on various normal and tumor cells; the largest numbers are found on myeloma cells, and it is possible that autocrine secretion of IL-6 plays an important role in the pathogenesis of multiple myelomas.[46] Interestingly, the role of IL-6 as an autocrine growth factor for human multiple myelomas suggests the possibility that antagonists or antibodies to IL-6 could be used in the treatment of this tumor.

g. Interleukin-7 (IL-7)

IL-7, also referred to as lymphopoietin-1 stromal cell factor or pre-B-cell growth factor, encodes a large protein with a molecular weight of 15 to 45 kDa. It is primarily involved in the early stages of B-cell development or immature B-cells. IL-7 induces proliferation of immature thymocytes, with potential therapeutic implications in diseases such as aplastic anemia.

h. Interleukin-8 (IL-8)

Finally, a chemotactic factor, designated as Interleukin-8 (15 to 30 kDa) has been recently described. It is secreted by macrophages after stimulation with IL-1. This human monokine possesses neutrophil chemotactic skin reactive and granulocytosis-promoting activity.[46]

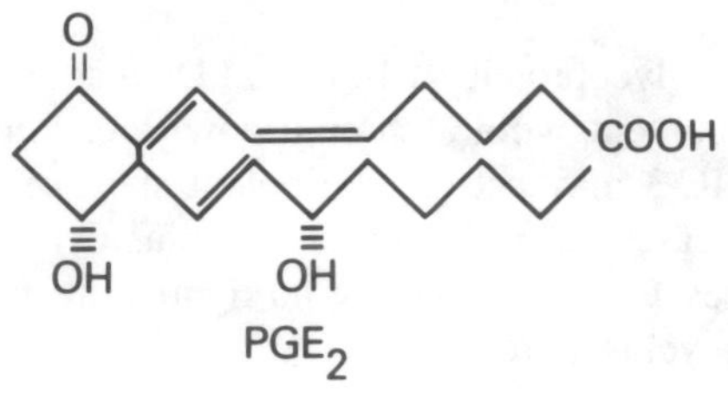

FIGURE 2.   Chemical structure of PGE_2.

D. PROSTAGLANDINS (PGs)
1. Classification (PGs)

Prostaglandins are tissue hormones, which are produced by cell membranes of many tissues and can act by endocrine as well as by autocrine and paracrine mechanisms. They exert pleiotropic effects, influencing most of major pathologic processes such as inflammation, reproduction, allergy, ulceration, immunity, and particularly cancer. Recent evidence that prostaglandins play an important role in control of proliferation has prompted numerous investigations on their possible association with cancer, as well as their therapeutic application for cancer therapy. The nomenclature of the prostaglandins (PGs) is based upon the prostanoic acid skeleton.[53] Interest in the prostaglandins and their derivatives (prostanoids, eicosanoids) began with the observation that human cancers synthesized very high levels of prostaglandins in comparison to normal tissue. Chemically, all prostaglandins have the basic prostanoic acid skeleton (See Figure 2). There are six "primary" prostaglandins (A, B, C, D, E, F), the cyclic endoperoxides (G, H, I_2), thromboxanes (TXA, TXB), and leukotrienes (LTA_4, LTC_4, LTD_4, LTE_4).

2. Biosynthesis

All prostaglandins (PG), cyclic endoperoxides (G, H, I_2), thromboxanes (TXA_2, TXB_2), and leukotrienes (LTA_4, LTE_4) are derived from arachidonic acid (AA), which is an essential fatty acid and a component of phospholipids found in all cell membranes. AA is known to be metabolized through multiple enzymatic pathways that yield numerous prostaglandins and metabolites. Interestingly, each step of this enzymatic process can be blocked by prostaglandin inhibitors (Figure 3). The body synthesizes some low levels of prostaglandins all the time. The terminal products formed depend upon a number of factors: (1) availability of free polyunsaturated fatty acids, (2) availability of PG-synthesizing enzymes, and (3) presence of cofactors. Prostaglandins are released into circulation and then rapidly metabolized; 90% are broken down during the first passage through the lung. However, the breakdown of PGs can be retarded to some extent by various synthetic substitutions to the prostaglandin molecule, such as methylation of the 15 or 16 carbon in the fatty acid chain. These substitutions have raised the half-life of the prostaglandins from 4—7 min to 2—4 h, and they also can be absorbed orally.[53] By using radioactive labeled prostaglandins, such as [^{3}H]-PGE_2, [^{3}H]-PGD_2, and [^{3}H]-$PGF_{2\alpha}$, it was found that there are high and low affinity receptors in several cells such as in rat liver, bovine thyroid, hamster adipocyte, human adipocytes, mammary carcinoma, and human polymorphonuclear neutrophils (PMN). These are plasmalemmal receptors. LTB_4 is also involved in glucocorticoid cell growth inhibition and may offer a new approach to increase the therapeutic efficacy of glucocorticoid therapy in leukemias and lymphomas.[57]

3. Prostaglandins and Cancer

A considerable volume of research indicates that PGs are possibly involved in tumor promotion, tumor metastasis, tumor transplantation, osteolysis, and hypercalcemia.[54-57] Early

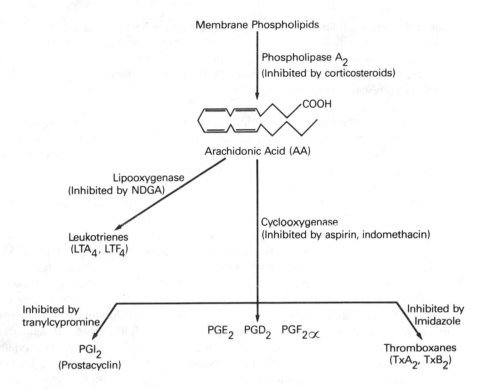

FIGURE 3. Biosynthesis of prostaglandins and their selective inhibition. (NGDA — nordihydro-guaiaretic acid.)

studies showed that high levels of PGE-like material in breast tumors were associated with poor postoperative survival and with the presence of bone metastases.[58,59] However, a recent study showed no significant relationship between levels of prostaglandins E_2 and $F_{2\alpha}$ in human breast cancer, presence of estrogen receptors (ER), lymph node metastases, and disease-free interval following primary treatment. Thus, it seems unlikely that the level of these particular prostaglandins within breast carcinomas plays a fundamental role in the prognosis of the disease.[58] Some authors found that prostacyclin (PGI₂) had a beneficial influence against pulmonary metastases of B_{16} amelanotic melanoma tumors in mice.[56]

Most of the proposed mechanisms to explain the ability of tumor prostaglandins to promote growth and metastasis involve interactions between: (1) tumor cells and homeostatic elements, (2) immunomodulators (namely immunosuppressors), and (3) interaction of prostaglandins with growth factors and hormones (EGF, PDGF, insulin). Thus, it is likely that prostaglandins may act as direct growth factors in an autocrine and paracrine manner for cancer cells.

In previous experiments, we found that prostaglandins (PGE₂ and PGF₂ₐ) markedly enhanced the epidermal carcinogenesis (squamous cell carcinomas) in mice induced by methylcholanthrene (MCA). PGs also increased DNA, RNA, and protein synthesis of epidermal cancer cells. These findings indicate that PGs are not directly carcinogens, but act mainly as cocarcinogens.[54] Administration of PGE₂ and PGF₂ₐ markedly increase DNA, RNA, and protein synthesis and are accompanied by changes in the ultrastructural and cell surface morphology of precancerous cells. PGs might act as cocarcinogens or tumor promoters by affecting DNA, RNA, and protein synthesis of precancerous cells. Concomitant administration of both PGE₂ and PGF₂ₐ to syngeneic mice transplanted with squamous cell carcinomas from the same species (allograft) markedly increased (by approximately 87%) the transplantability and cellular atypicality of these tumors. Thus, prostaglandins might play an important role in tumor transplantation and cellular immune-host defense mechanisms.[55] The mechanisms of prostaglandins in cancer development is more complex. Some prostaglandins such as PGE_2 and $PGF_{2\alpha}$ exert stimulatory effects on different types of tumors, whereas others, such as PGD_2 and prostacyclin (PGI_2), exert a cytoprotective activity and are powerful antimetastatic agents.[56]

4. Prostaglandins and Prostaglandin-Synthesis Inhibitors in Cancer Treatment

While the experimental evidence regarding the role of prostaglandins and their analogs in tumor growth and metastasis is considerable, only a few clinical trials have been initiated for cancer treatment. Since certain studies demonstrate *in vitro* and *in vivo* inhibitory effects of prostaglandins on several tumor cells (neuroblastoma, mammary carcinoma), these findings suggest a potential use of prostaglandins in the treatment of human cancers, particularly neuroblastoma. Prostaglandin synthetase or cyclooxygenase inhibitors, such as aspirin and indomethacin, were found to reduce the growth of tumors induced in mice by Moloney sarcoma virus. Thus, aspirin and other nonsteroidal anti-inflammatory drugs (NSAIDs) block the biosynthesis of PGs and thromboxane A_2. Aspirin inhibits it irreversibly, whereas other NSAIDs act reversibly. A prostaglandin synthesis inhibitor, called flurbiprofen, induces significant inhibition of tumor growth and increases survival rates of mice with tumors. However, a recent clinical study used benorylate (a cyclooxygenase inhibitor) in 161 patients with primary breast cancer and no detectable metastases; after a followup of $\geqslant 9$ years, no difference in survival, disease-free interval, or incidence of bone metastases for the benorylate vs. placebo group was seen.[59] Increased concentrations of LTB_4 in hamster and human squamous cell carcinoma of the oral cavity suggests that LTs can protect cancerous tissue against radiation therapy. Prostaglandin synthesis inhibitors were used as well as glucocorticoids, calcitonin, and mithramycin in treatment of hypercalcemia with increased bone resorption in cancer patients.

In summary, prostaglandins and the prostaglandin synthesis inhibitors may play an important role in cancer therapy and can act by: (1) direct cytotoxic activity, (2) immunomodulation, (3) controlling the transformation of rate of preneoplastic cells into neoplastic cells, and (4) interaction with other growth factors (EGF, PDGF) and hormones (insulin, calcitonin).

E. GLANDULAR EXTRACTS (OPOTHERAPY)
1. General Considerations

Before the modern era of hormones, several glandular extracts (opotherapy) were used to treat cancers. In France, Naamé successfully treated several types of cancers by using glandular extracts or opotherapy. He treated uterine cancer by mammohypophyseal and thyro-mammary extracts, breast cancer by thyro-ovarian extracts, and several types of epithelioma with thyroid and pancreatic extracts in combination.[60] At the same time, Engel[61] showed that tumor growth is under strong hormonal control. Using various glandular extracts (called optonen), such as hypophyseal (hypophysis opton), thymus (thymus opton), and thyroid (thyroid opton), he reported that glandular extracts exert an important role in development and transplantation of mouse carcinoma. Interestingly, he assumed that the cancer treatment and cancer prevention would be possible, controlled by hormones and glandular extracts. Thymus extract (thymus opton) exerts the strongest tumor inhibitory effect, whereas ovarian and testicular extracts have no effect. Later, it was found that thymus and pineal extracts exerted important antitumor and antiproliferative activities. Hence, the thymus and the pineal gland are involved in the regulation of cancer development, and they are oncostatic glands. Melatonin, the main pineal hormone, has been shown either to counteract pinealectomy-induced tumor stimulation, or to induce tumor regression in animals (see Chapter 2).

2. Pineal Extract

Pineal extract induced regression of spontaneous mammary carcinoma, Ehrlich carcinoma in mice, and Walker carcinosarcoma, which exhibit extensive necrosis after treatment with pineal extract as compared to untreated animals.[61]

3. Thymic Hormones (Thymosins)

Thymic peptide hormones play a necessary role in the regulation of the immune system by acting on T-cell differentiation. Until now, a family of biologically active, acidic polypeptides, called thymosins, have been isolated from calf thymus, and their amino acid sequences have been determined. These are: thymosin-α, thymosin-β_4, thymopoietin, thymosin-5, and thymulin. Recently, thymosin-β_4 was isolated from a human medullary thyroid carcinoma (MTC) and has the same amino acid sequence to that isolated from calf thymus, e.g., 43 amino acid residues. Most of thymosins have a molecular weight of 5 to 15 kDa. Recently, it has been shown that thymulin secreted by thymic epithelial cells is under hormonal control, such as hypothalamic-releasing factors, pituitary hormones (TSH, ACTH, FSH), and prolactin (PRL). Prolactin induced a specific increase in thymulin synthesis and secretion. Bromocriptine that inhibits PRL secretion significantly decreases the thymulin secretion.[62] Clinical trials using thymosin fraction V showed some direct antitumor effect in patients with renal cancer. Some effects for immunomodulation in cancer patients and AIDS were found following treatment with thymic humoral factor (THF), a peptide hormone isolated from calf thymus.[63] Despite the fact that the glandular extracts were used on an empirical basis, they suggested that cancer is a systemic disease which can be treated and prevented by hormones and glandular extracts.

II. COMMENTS AND CONCLUSIONS

Recent advances regarding the discovery of new biologically active agents with hormone-like properties called cytokines expanded our knowledge in the field of cancer biology and therapy. Thus, a new form of cancer therapy called cytokinetherapy emerged and will soon become the "fourth arm" of cancer therapy.[35,48] Cytokines are secreted glycoproteins that interact with specific cellular receptors, and their biologic activities are similar to those of polypeptide hormones. Cytokines form a parallel network of intercellular signals which can trigger a series of events called "cytokine cascade". These signals are transduced at the cell surface through specific receptors by interactive effects with G-proteins. The clinical response of cytokines is mainly due to their binding to specific cell surface receptors and relate to their receptor-binding capacity. Using [^{125}I]-labeled-α, -β, or -γ interferons to mass cell populations and electron microscopic autoradiographic techniques, it was postulated that interferons as other cytokines act by two mechanisms: specific receptor-mediated endocytosis and bulk pinocytosis.[37] Thus, they bind to plasma membrane receptors and are transported into coated vesicles, then into receptosomes, and finally into the nuclear envelope, penetrating through nuclear pores into the nucleus. Here, by combining with nuclear chromatin they can trigger the synthesis of new proteins. Other modes of transport of the cytokine-receptor complex include a direct transport to lysosomes or bulk pinocytosis.

Cytokines are autocrine/paracrine factors that modulate important physiologic functions such as the specific (antibody formation) and nonspecific host defense mechanisms. Recent advances in molecular biotechnology have led to the manufacture on a large scale of various recombinant cytokines, including r-INF, r-IL, and recombinant erythropoietin (rEPO), and subsequently to use in clinical trials. Thus, treatment of anemia of chronic renal disease with recombinant human erythropoietin at a dose of 50 to 150 units/kg/body weight showed favorable results, without affecting renal function in all 17 patients. Increased hematocrits and appetite were also observed.[64]

Recently, biologic response modifiers or "biomodulators" have emerged as an important new class of agents for cancer treatment. Generally, biomodulators are agents which: (1) enhance the host's antitumor response directly; (2) decrease suppressor mechanisms and indirectly increase the host's immune response; (3) increase the ability of the host to tolerate damage by cytotoxic and radiation therapy; (4) by changing the tumor cell membranes increase their immunogenicity, alter their metastatic capacity, and make them more susceptible to killing by cytotoxicity or radiation; and (5) promote the maturation of the "primitive" tumor cells.

Another intriguing aspect of cytokine therapy is the resistance to various cytokines. In many aspects, there are analogies with hormone resistance. It is a general assumption that the responsiveness or resistance to cytokine administration is mainly dependent on the presence or absence of specific cell surface receptors. In the case of responsive cells, the correlation between the number of receptors can be precisely correlated to the clinical response. There are, however, many cell lines which respond poorly to cytokines or not at all.[37] Most of these resistant cell lines have receptors, and the cytokines bind to these receptors, but produce no biologic effect. It is possible that the presence of "defective" receptors or post-receptor level events are taking place. Further studies are necessary to explain and overcome the cytokine resistance and the clinical response of patients. Receptor status does not play a crucial role in patient selection for cytokine therapy and for prediction of the response rate or overall survival, as it does in hormonotherapy.

The presence of growth factors can also render some neoplastic cells more resistant to hormone therapy. They can incrase the sensitivity of tumor cells to antiestrogens, such as TGF-β does in tamoxifen treatment. These growth factors can be produced by tumor cells themselves or can originate in the stromal tumor cells and act by paracrine or autocrine mechanisms (see Figure 4).[65] Recent evidence indicates that TGF-β is a potent antiproliferative agent for most epithelial cells. Development of pharmacologic agents that can enhance TGF-β secretion in premalignant epithelia offers a new approach to chemoprevention and cytokine therapy of cancer. Both tamoxifen and retinoids may also act by a mechanism that involves TGF-β. Recent data indicate that TGF-β is a potent immunosuppressive *in vitro* and *in vivo*. Thus it is 10,000 to 100,000 times more potent (on a molar basis) than cyclosporine in suppressing the lymphocyte proliferation and function. It can act as an autocrine "stop" signal by inhibiting the action of interleukins and tumor necrosis factor (TNF). Clinical trials using recombinant cytokines (rINF, rILs), which allow the use of a larger number of patients to estimate the adequate dosage, route of administration, and schedule, should be performed. For instance, the administration of "depot-preparation" of hematopoietic growth factors (HGFs) will shorten the treatment courses and period of hospitalization. Colony-stimulating factors (CSF) are also promising drugs in the treatment of myelosuppression that follows combination chemotherapy in cancer patients and autologous bone marrow transplantation; they also reduce the toxicity of AZT in AIDS patients.[66-68]

Studies on interleukines, particularly IL-3, which stimulates stem cell differentiation at its earliest stage, will be helpful in reducing bone marrow transplants (over 5,000 per year), mainly in cancer patients receiving chemotherapy and in AIDS patients. Use of recombinant human erythropoietin (rhEPO) in anemia due to kidney failure, particularly those with renal cancer, will reduce significantly the required transfusions for these cancer patients. This group of cytokines, is likely to have a major role, not only in oncology but in general medicine. More recently, IL-6 has been shown to act as a possible autocrine growth factor for human multiple myeloma[5], and it has been proposed that the underlying pathologic process in Kaposi's sarcoma is autocrine secretion of cytokines with the properties of basic fibroblastic factor (bFGF) and angiogenesis factor. Some of cytokines, including IL-7, TGF-β originate from stromal cells, and by a paracrine mechanism, can counteract the effect of hormones on tumor cells (Table 12). The role of stroma cells of many tumors is believed

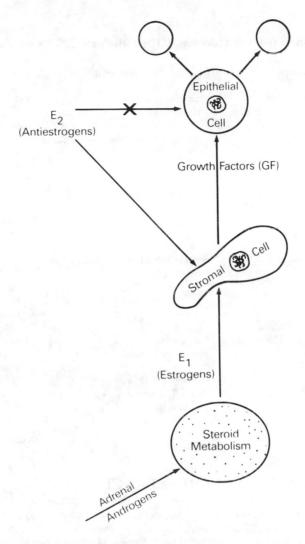

FIGURE 4. Interactions between growth factors, antiestrogens, and stromal tumor cells.

to play an important role in oncogenesis. The effect of certain hormones or antagonists on cancer cells is inhibited or antagonized by growth factors synthesized in the stromal cells and acts by a paracrine action. Although we do not fully understand at present the modus operandi of growth factors or cytokines at cellular and molecular levels, this will be an exciting field in cancer biology and will open new rational approaches to cancer therapy.

TABLE 12
Hormone-Like Substances and Their Biologic Effects on Cancer Cells

Substances	Function(s)	Cell producer
Interleukins (ILs)	Immunomodulation	T-cells
IL-1, IL-2, IL-3, IL-4, IL-5, IL-6,	Cell homeostasis	Monocytes
IL-7, IL-8		Stromal cells
Interferons (IFNs)	Antiviral activity, immunomodulation	
INF-α		Leukocytes, macrophages
INF-β		Fibroblasts
INF-γ		T-cells
Growth factors (GFs)	Cell growth, cell proliferation	
EGF		Epidermal cells
TFG-β		Tumor cells
FGF		Fibroblasts
PDF		Platelets
Colony-stimulating factors (CSPs)	Stem cell differentiation and proliferation	
G-CSF		Fibroblasts
M-CSF		Stromal cells
GM-CSF		Monocytes
EPO		Kidney cells
Tumor necrosis factors (TNFs)	Cell toxicity	
TNF-α/cachectin	Immunomodulation	Macrophages
TNF-β/lymphotoxin		T-cells
Prostaglandins (PGs)	Immunomodulation	Many cell types
PGE$_2$, PGF$_{2\alpha}$,	Cell differentiation	
PGI$_2$, PGA	Cell toxicity (?)	

REFERENCES

1. **Neal, D. E.,** Growth factors and tumor biology, in *The New Endocrinology of Cancer,* Waxman, J. and Coombes, R. C., Eds., Edward Arnold, London, 1987, chap. 2.
2. **Greig, R., Dunnington, D., Murthy, U., and Anzano, M.,** Growth factors as novel therapeutic targets in neoplastic disease, *Cancer Surv.,* 7, 653, 1988.
3. **Sporn, M. B. and Todaro, G. J.,** Autocrine secretion and malignant transformation of cells, *N. Engl. J.Med.,* 303, 878, 1980.
4. **Roberts, A. B. and Sporn, M.B.,** Principles of molecular cell biology of cancer: growth factor related to transformation, in *Cancer: Principles and Practice of Oncology,* DeVita, V. T., Hellman, S., and Rosenberg, S. A., Eds., Lippincott, Philadelphia, 1989, 67.
5. **Steel, C. M.,** Peptide regulatory factors and malignancy, *Lancet,* 2, 30, 1989.
6. **Thompson, D. M. and Gill G. N.,** The EGF receptor: structure regulation and potential role in malignancy, *Cancer Surv.,* 4, 767, 1985.
7. **Waterfield, M. D.,** Epidermal growth factor and related molecules, *Lancet,* 1, 1243, 1989.
8. **Knecht, M., Feng, P., and Catt, K. J.,** Transforming growth factor-beta: autocrine, paracrine, and endocrine effects in ovarian cells, *Semin. Reprod. Endocrinol.,* 7, 12, 1989.
9. **Gospodarowicz, D.,** Fibroblast growth factor: involvement in early embryonic development and ovarian function, *Semin. Reprod. Endocrinol.,* 7, 21, 1989.
10. **Sporn, M. B. and Roberts, A. B.,** Transforming growth factor-β: multiple actions and potential clinical applications, *JAMA,* 262, 938, 1989.
11. **Sariban, E., Sitaras, N. M., Antoniades, H. N., Kufe, D. W., and Pantazis, P.,** Expression of platelet-derived growth factor (PDGF)-related transcripts and synthesis of biologically active PDGF-like proteins by human malignant epithelial cell lines, *J. Clin. Invest.,* 83, 1157, 1988.
12. **Ross, R., Raines, E. W., and Bowen-Pope, D. F.,** The biology of platelet derived growth factor, *Cell,* 46, 155, 1986.

13. **Murray, A. W. and Kirschner, M. W.,** Cyclin synthesis drives the early embryonic cell cycle, *Nature (London),* 339, 275, 1989.
14. **Ervin, P. R., Kaminski, M. S., Cody, R. L., and Wicha, M. S.,** Production of mammastatin, a tissue-specific growth inhibitor, by normal human mammary cells, *Science,* 244, 1585, 1989.
15. **Coley, W. B.,** The treatment of malignant tumors by repeated inoculations of erysipelas; with a report of ten original cases, *Am. J. Med. Sci.,* 105, 487, 1893.
16. **Beutler, B. and Cerami, A.,** Cachectin (tumor necrosis factor): a macrophage hormone governing cellular metabolism and inflammatory response, *Endocrinol. Rev.,* 9, 57, 1988.
17. **Sherry, B. and Cerami, A.,** Cachectin/tumor necrosis factor exerts endocrine, paracrine, and autocrine control of inflammatory responses, *J. Cell Biol.,* 107, 1269, 1988.
18. **Pfizenmaier, K., Krönke, M., Scheurich, P., and Nagel, G. A.,** Tumor necrosis factor (TNF) alpha: control of TNF-sensitivity and molecular mechanisms of TNF-mediated growth inhibition, *Blut,* 55, 1, 1987.
19. **Sharp, B. M., Matta, S. G., Peterson, P. K., Newton, R., Chao, C., and McAllen, K.,** Tumor necrosis factor-α is a potent ACTH secretagogue: comparison to interleukin-1β, *Endocrinology,* 124, 3131, 1989.
20. **Selby, P., Hobbs, S., Viner, C., Jackson, E., Jones, A., Newell, D., Calvert, A. H., McElwain, T., Fearon, K., Humphreys, J., and Shiga, T.,** Tumor necrosis factor in man: Clinical and biological observations, *Br. J. Cancer,* 56, 803, 1987.
21. **Frei, E. and Spriggs, D.,** Tumor necrosis factor: still a promising agent, *J. Clin. Oncol.,* 7, 291, 1989.
22. **Sherman, M. L., Spriggs, D. R., Arthur, K. A., Imamura, K., Frei, E., and Kufe, D. W.,** Recombinant human tumor necrosis factor administered as a five-day continuous infusion in cancer patients: phase I toxicity and effects on lipid metabolism, *J. Clin. Oncol.,* 6, 344, 1988.
23. **Devereux, S. and Linch, D. C.,** Clinical significance of the haemopoietic growth factors, *Br. J. Cancer,* 59, 2, 1989.
24. **Griffin, J. D.,** Hemopoietins in oncology: factoring out myelosuppression, *J. Clin. Oncol.,* 7, 151, 1989.
25. **Herrmann, F., Lindemann, A., and Mertelsmann, R.,** Polypeptides controlling hematopoietic blood cell development and activation: clinical results, *Blut,* 58, 173, 1989.
26. **Morstyn, G. and Fox, R.,** Colony-stimulating factors: twenty years from discovery to clinical trials, *Aust. N.Z. J. Surg.,* 58, 275, 1988.
27. **Groopman, J. E.,** Clinical applications of colony-stimulating factors, *Semin. Oncol.,* 15, 27, 1988.
28. **Laver, J. and Moore, M. A.,** Clinical use of recombinant human hematopoietic growth factors, *J. Natl. Cancer Inst.,* 81, 1370, 1989.
29. **Groopman, J. E., Mitsuyasu, R. T., DeLeo, M. J., Oette, D. H., and Golde, D. W.,** Effect of recombinant human granulocyte-macrophage colony stimulating factor on myelopoiesis in the acquired immune deficiency syndrome, *N. Engl. J. Med.,* 317, 593, 1987.
30. **Neta, R., Douches, S., and Oppenheim, J. J.,** Interleukin 1 is a radioprotector, *J. Immunol.,* 136, 2483, 1986.
31. **Mangan, K. F.,** Stimulating red blood cell production with immunomodulating agents, *JAMA,* 259, 727, 1988.
32. **Kobayashi, Y., Okabe, T., Ozawa, K., Chiba, S., Hino, M., Miyazono, K., Urabe, A., and Takaku, F.,** Treatment of myelodysplastic syndromes with recombinant human granulocyte colony-stimulating factor: a preliminary report, *Am. J., Med.,* 86, 178, 1989.
33. **Isaacs, A. and Lindenmann, J.,** Virus interference. I. The interferon, *Proc. R. Soc. Lond. Biol.,* 147, 258, 1957.
34. **Goldstein, D., and Laszlo, J.,** The role of interferon in cancer therapy: a current perspective, *CA,* 38, 258, 1988.
35. **Balkwill, F. R.,** Interferons, *Lancet,* 1, 1060, 1989.
36. **Hochkeppel, H. K.,** Recent developments in interferon research, *Experientia,* 45, 500, 1989.
37. **Grossberg, S. E., Taylor, J. L., and Kushnaryov, V. M.,** Interferon receptors and their role in interferon action, *Experientia,* 45, 508, 1989.
38. **Olsen, E. A., Rosen, S. T., Vollmer, R. T., Variakojis, D., Roenigk, H. H., Diab, N., and Zeffren, J.,** Interferon alfa-2 in the treatment of cutaneous T cell lymphoma, *J. Am Acad. Dermatol.,* 20, 395, 1989.
39. **Figlin, R. A.,** Biotherapy with interferon — 1988, *Semin. Oncol.,* 15, 3, 1988.
40. **Schwarzinger, I., Bettelheim, D., and Lechner, K.,** Interferon therapie bei hämatologischen neoplasien, *Wien, Klin. Wochenschr.,* 100, 497, 1988.
41. **Glaspy, J. A., Marcus, S. G., Ambersley, J., and Golde, D. W.,** Recombinant beta-serine-interferon in hairy cell leukemia compared prospectively with results with recombinant alpha-interferon, *Cancer,* 64, 409, 1989.
42. **Jaffe, H. S. and Herberman, R. B.,** Rationale for recombinant human interferon-gamma adjuvant immunotherapy for cancer, *J. Natl. Cancer Inst.,* 80, 616, 1988.

43. **Dorval, T. and Pouillart, P.,** Interferons dans le traitement des tumeurs solides. Revue générale, *Bull. Cancer,* 75, 885, 1988.

44. **Jones, G. J. and Itri, L. M.,** Safety and tolerance of recombinant interferon alpha-2a (Roferon-A) in cancer patients, *Cancer,* 57, 1709, 1986.

45. **Dinarello, C. A.,** Biology of interleukin 1, *FASEB J.,* 2, 108, 1988.

46. **O'Garra, A.,** Interleukins and the immune system, *Lancet,* 1, 943, (part 1), 1003 (part 2), 1989.

47. **Oldham, R. K., Maleckar, J. R., Yanelli, J. R., and West, W. H.,** IL-2: a review of current knowledge, *Cancer Treat. Rev.,* 16 (Suppl. A), 5, 1989.

48. **Lotze, M. T. and Rosenberg, S. A.,** The immunologic treatment of cancer, *CA,* 38, 68, 1988.

49. **Parkinson, D. R.,** Interleukin-2 in cancer therapy, *Semin. Oncol.,* 15, (Suppl. 6), 10, 1988.

50. **Rosenberg, S. A.,** Cancer therapy with interleukin: immunologic manipulations can mediate the regression of cancer in humans, *J. Clin. Oncol.,* 6, 403, 1988.

51. **Herberman, R. B.,** Interleukin-2 therapy of human cancer: potential benefits versus toxicity, *J. Clin. Oncol.,* 7, 1, 1989.

52. **Smith, K. A.,** Interleukin-2: inception, impact, and implications, *Science,* 240, 1169, 1988.

53. **Oates, J. A., Fitzgerald, G. A., Branch, R. A., Jackson, E. K., Knapp, H. R., and Roberts, L. J.,** Clinical implications of prostaglandin and thromboxane A_2 formation, *N. Engl. J. Med.,* 319, 689, 1988.

54. **Lupulescu, A.,** Enhancement of carcinogenesis by prostaglandins, *Nature (London),* 272, 634, 1978.

55. **Lupulescu, A.,** Effects of prostaglandins on tumor transplantation, *Oncology,* 37, 418, 1980.

56. **Honn, K., Cicone, B., and Skoff, A.,** Prostacyclin: a potent antimetastatic agent, *Science,* 212, 1270, 1981.

57. **Feuerstein, G. and Hallenbeck, J. M.,** Leukotrienes in health and disease, *FASEB J.,* 1, 186, 1987.

58. **Watson, D. M., Kelly, R. W., and Miller, W. R.,** Prostaglandins and prognosis in human breast cancer, *Br. J. Cancer,* 56, 367, 1987.

59. **Powles, T. J.,** Prostaglandins and cancer: clinical approaches, in *Prostaglandins in Cancer Research,* Garci, E., Paoletti, R., and Santoro, M. G., Eds., Springer-Verlag, Berlin, 1987, 184.

60. **Naamé, O.,** Cancer et opothérapie, *Gaz. Hôp.,* (Paris), 94, 170, 1921.

61. **Engel, D.,** Experimentelle studien über die Beeinflussung des Tumor Wachstum mit Abbauprodukten (Abderhaldenschen optonen) von Endokrinen Drüsen bei Maüsen, *Z. Krebsforsch.,* 19, 339, 1922.

62. **Dardenne, M., Savino, W., Gagnerault, M-C., Itoh, T., and Bach, J-F.,** Neuroendocrine control of thymic hormonal production. I. Prolactin stimulates *in vivo* and *in vitro* the production of thymulin by human and murine thymic epithelial cells, *Endocrinology,* 125, 3, 1989.

63. **Trainin, N., Burstein, Y., Ben-Efraim, S., Goebel, F. D., and Handzel, Z. T.,** The use of THF, a thymic hormone for immunomodulation in cancer and AIDS, in *Novel Approaches in Cancer Therapy,* Lapis, K. and Eckhardt, S., Eds., Akad. Kiadó, Budapest, 1987, 253.

64. **Eschbach, J. W., Kelly, M. R., Haley, N. R., Abels, R. I., and Adamson, J. W.,** Treatment of the anemia of progressive renal failure with recombinant human erythropoietin, *N. Engl. J. Med.,* 321, 158, 1989.

65. **Leake, R.,** The molecular endocrinology of steroid hormones and their relation to cancer cell proliferation, in *The New Endocrinology of Cancer,* Waxman, J. and Coombes, R. C., Eds., Edward Arnold, London, 1987, 37.

66. **Anderson, K. E., Goeger, D. E., Carson, R. W., Lee, S. K., and Stead, R. B.,** Erythropoietin for the treatment of porphyria cutanea tarda in a patient on long-term hemodialysis, *N. Engl. J. Med.,* 322, 315, 1990.

67. **Appelbaum, F. R.,** The clinical use of hematopoietic growth factors, *Semin. Hematol.,* 26, 7, 1989.

68. **Groopman, J. E.,** Status of colony-stimulating factors in cancer and AIDS, *Semin. Oncol.,* 17, 31, 1990.

Chapter 5

VITAMINS — VITAMIN THERAPY

I. OVERVIEW OF VITAMIN ROLE IN CANCER THERAPY

The profound effect of vitamins on cell growth and differentiation led, shortly after their discovery, to the hypothesis that they might play a role in cancer development, prevention, and treatment. In recent years, there has been considerable interest regarding the role of vitamins in the process of carcinogenesis and prevention of cancer. Since it is known that the development of cancer is accompanied by a loss of cellular differentiation, and certain vitamins (A, C, E) are essential for normal as well as neoplastic cell growth and differentiation, this was a rational basis for the use of vitamins in cancer treatment.

Recent data from experimental and clinical investigation strongly suggest that vitamins are a new class of substances exerting a preventive and a therapeutic effect both in certain animal tumor models and in certain clinical conditions of preneoplastic and neoplastic lesions. Due to their particular physiologic mechanism of action, vitamins offer a new approach to cancer therapy, which is different from those of surgery, radiation therapy, conventional chemotherapy, and immunotherapy. Since the discovery of vitamins more than a century ago and the recognition that vitamins are an essential growth factor, the elucidation of their mechanism(s) of action has been a challenging problem to physiologists, biochemists, and cancer cell biologists.[1-3]

Significant therapeutic advances have also occurred with vitamins in some drug-resistant cancers and several others that have become refractory. It has been postulated that certain vitamins exert their antitumor effects by a mechanism similar to hormones, acting as pro-hormone, or hormone-like substances. Others act by paracrine and autocrine mechanisms similar to growth factors. Thus, a close relationship between hormones, growth factors, and vitamins has been demonstrated. (See Figure 1).

Thus, vitamin therapy, hormonotherapy, and cytokine therapy will be new and promising strategies for treatment of cancer patients, and will dominate the pharmacology and experimental therapeutic research in coming years. Studies regarding the effects of hormones, growth factors, and vitamins have indicated some identical intracellular pathways at cellular and molecular levels that will play a paramount role in cell growth, differentiation, and cell proliferations which are the cornerstones of carcinogenesis. The therapeutic use of new synthetic vitamin analogs, with more potent, less toxic, and long-lasting effects will open a fascinating field in cancer biology and therapy. Wolbach and Howe[4] were the first to report a relationship between Vitamin A and cancer in their 1925 study on the effects of Vitamin A deprivation and restoration on rat epithelial carcinogenesis. Studies of normal and cancer cells in culture as well as *in vivo* (in different animal tumor models) have shown that Vitamins A, C, and E can exert antiproliferative effects which are frequently accompanied by maturation and cell differentiation. The extent of the effect on cellular growth and differentiation depends both on the vitamins as well as the source of the cell. These *in vitro* and *in vivo* models are useful in elucidating the mechanisms and the process by which cancer cells acquire resistance to vitamins, becoming vitamin-resistant. The isolation of vitamin-resistant clones should help the understanding of the cellular and molecular mechanisms by which resistance to vitamins occur.[5] Numerous laboratory studies have confirmed that combinations of vitamins are more effective in chemoprevention and treatment than any single vitamin.[5,6] At present, it is not certain whether a specific vitamin is needed to prevent a specific type of cancer, or cancer as a group. From experimental and epidemiological studies, it appears that there is, in human populations, an inverse relationship between serum and tissue levels of Vitamins A, C, and E and certain cancers.

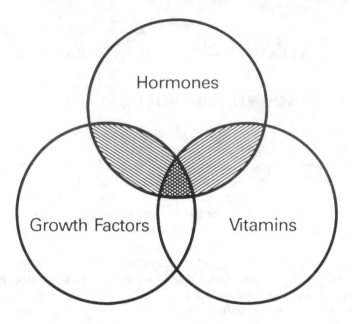

FIGURE 1.   Diagram showing the relationship between hormones, vitamins, and growth factors.

TABLE 1
Daily Vitamin Requirements

Vitamin	Synonym	Adults	Children and adolescents
Vitamin A (IU)	Retinol	3000	2300
Vitamin B_1 (mg)	Thiamin	3.0	1.2
VitaminB_2 (mg)	Riboflavin	3.4	1.6
Vitamin B_6 (mg)	Pyridoxine	4.0	1.0
Niacin (mg)	Vitamin P-P	40.0	17.0
Biotin (μg)	Vitamin H	60	20
Vitamin B_{12} (μg)	Cyanocobalamin	5	1
Vitamin C (mg)	Ascorbic acid	100	80
Pantothenic acid (mg)	B complex	15	5
Vitamin D (IU)	Calciferol	300	400
Vitamin E (IU)	Tocopherol	20	7
Folic acid (μg)	Vitamin M	400	140
Vitamin K_3 (mg)	Menadione	70—140	200

At present, vitamin preparations are used extensively in the practice of medicine. However, it is important to distinguish between the role of vitamins used as dietary supplements and vitamins used as therapeutic agents. Vitamins are essential organic substances, usually supplied by food, which are required by man in amounts ranging from micrograms to milligrams per day (See Table 1). There are four fat-soluble vitamins (A, D, E, and K), and nine water-soluble vitamins (thiamin or B_1, riboflavin or B_2, niacin or Vitamin P-P, pantothenic acid, folic acid, biotin, and Vitamins B_6, B_{12}, and C), and all are essential for the normal growth, development, and maintenance of the human body. Most of them are also essential for the cell growth, division, and proliferation. They play an important role in the immune defense system as well as in the immune host defense. Their chemical configuration is already established (See Figure 2).

However, vitamins, vitamin analogs, and vitamin mixtures have been used and misused

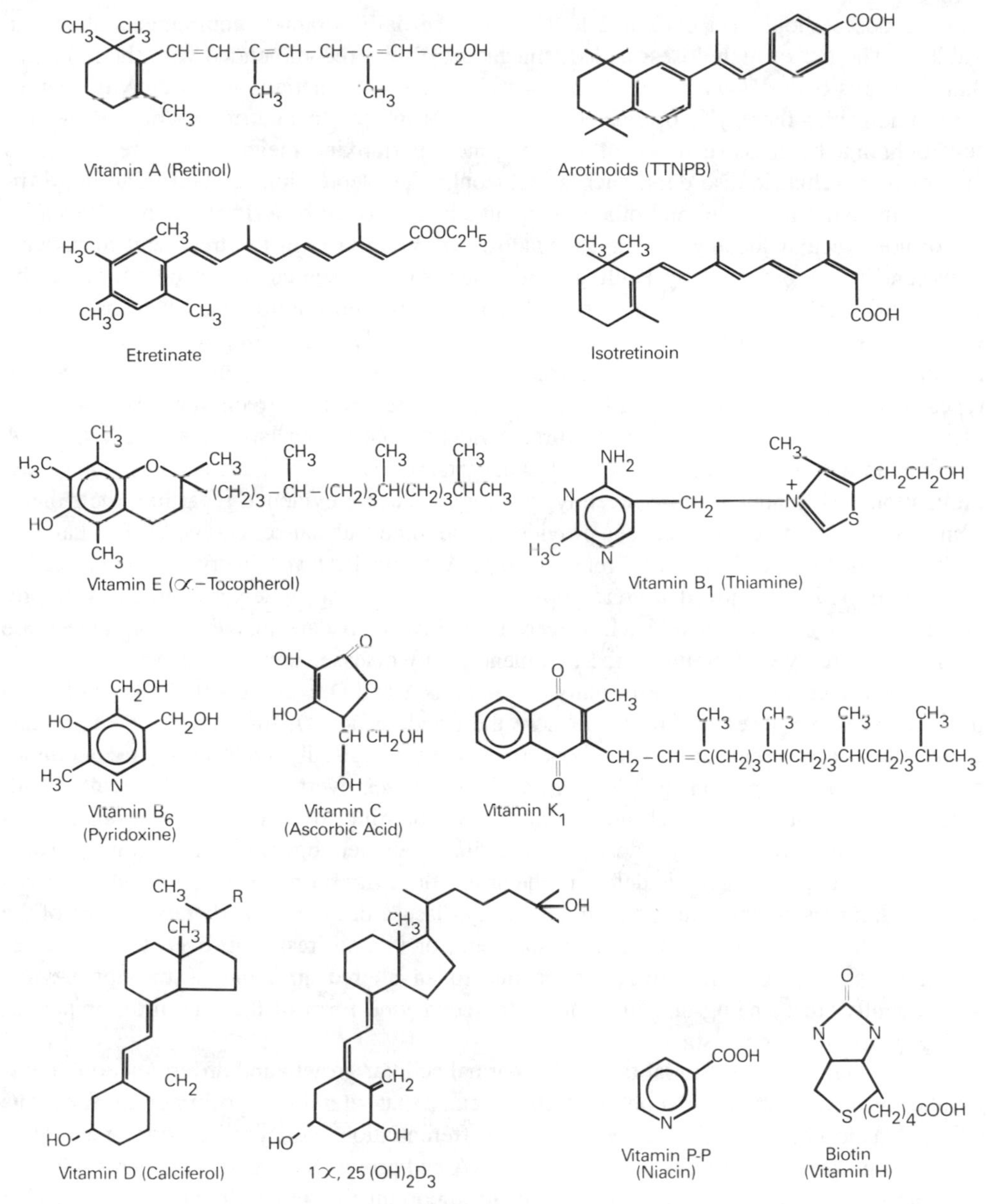

FIGURE 2. Chemical configuration of commonly used vitamins and their analogs in cancer treatment and prevention.

in treatment of various diseases, including malignancies, for a long time. Hence, it is important for practitioners to have more knowledge regarding their pharmacology, physiology, and mechanism of action at cellular and molecular levels, in order to have a more rational and scientific basis for their use in cancer treatment. Undesirable effects ranging from trivial to major, have been reported in association with use of inappropriately high doses (megadoses) of vitamins. Severe illness has resulted from the excessive use of vitamins, and particularly vitamins A, E. C, and B_6, are abused more commonly than others. Higher doses are required during pregnancy and lactation. For this reason, vitamin supplements are often prescribed for pregnant and lactating women.[7]

The decision to employ vitamins in therapeutic amounts clearly rests with the physician, and the doses should not exceed 2 to 10 times the daily vitamin requirements shown in Table 1. The use of high doses, called "megadose," was recommended with the inference that "more is better", which clearly is not the case. A new therapy with megavitamins, or "orthomolecular therapy", originated in the 1950s in the psychiatric practice of treating schizophrenia by massive doses of niacin. Later, pyridoxine megadoses were used in a variety of psychiatric disorders, such as schizophrenia, depression, autism, learning difficulties, mental retardation, and others, without any confirmed beneficial results.[8] Recently, the orthomolecular therapy of using megadoses of Vitamin C in the treatment of patients with cancer was proposed by Pauling.[9] However, such claims could not be confirmed by subsequent clinical trials, and the original reports remained controversial.[10] Thus, several vitamins have been proposed as anticancer agents, namely, preventing the development of different types of cancers. Although epidemiological studies have suggested that certain types of cancer are associated with a low intake of yellow and green vegetables and low plasma Vitamin A levels, there is no direct evidence that taking large doses of Vitamin A or carotene will prevent cancer in man.[11] Other vitamins (E, D, K) have been used in cancer prevention and treatment more recently, but no conclusive evidence regarding their therapeutic beneficial effects has yet been provided. Also, other substances claimed to be vitamins, such as pangamic acid (wrongly referred to as Vitamin B_{15}) and laetrile (wrongly called Vitamin B_{17}), have enjoyed a great popularity and are being widely promoted as helpful agents against cancer. There is, however, no evidence to date that these substances are vitamins or are even effective in the treatment of any disease, including cancer.

Toxic effects of vitamins, especially of Vitamins A and D, were reported after prolonged uses of excessive doses (ten times or more the standard doses); for Vitamin A the effects include dry, scaly skin, stomatitis, bone pain, hyperostosis, hypercalcemia, pseudotumor cerebri, and hepatosplenomegaly. Vitamin D also causes overt toxic reactions called "idiopathic hypercalcemia" which include anorexia, vomiting, hypertension, and renal insufficiency.[12] Furthermore, large doses of Vitamin A are teratogenic.[13] Interestingly, some patients may express a genetic defect in the absorption, transport, or metabolism of a given vitamin and present with a nutritional deficiency disease despite usual dietary intakes of the vitamins. Also, these patients are nonresponders, or vitamin resistant, even to large doses of vitamins. This genetic defect can be due to an altered structure of the apoenzyme; subsequently, the binding and function of the coenzyme form of the vitamin is impaired, and they are vitamin-resistant.[14]

Since vitamins are essential factors for normal cellular growth and differentiation, a vast number of *in vitro* and *in vivo* observations revealed that vitamins exert important functions on neoplastic cell physiology, such as cell differentiation, cell proliferation, membrane structural properties, antioxidant properties, DNA and protein synthesis, collagen synthesis, and immune functions. Thus, vitamins play an important role in carcinogenesis. They also exert significant antiproliferative and differentiation-inducing effects, as well as potent antitumor activity. These laboratory data prompted several epidemiologic and clinical studies regarding the role of vitamins in cancer treatment and chemoprevention. Great hopes were raised for the therapeutic beneficial effects of vitamins in various types of cancers, since they are less toxic and act in certain ways similar to hormones and growth factors, also being biologic modifiers. There are, at present, a multitude of vitamins and their synthetic analogs, including over 2000 synthetic only retinoids available for testing *in vitro* and *in vivo* for their anticancer action.[15] Significant advances have been made in human cancer prevention, such as dermatologic cancers (keratoacanthoma, basal cell carcinoma), actinic keratosis, other premalignant conditions (oral leukoplakia, bronchial metaplasia, laryngeal papillomatosis, cervical dysplasia, myelodysplastic syndrome), benign neoplastic breast disease, and urinary bladder cancer. Also, important therapeutic advances with vitamins have been made in certain refractory malignancies, including squamous and basal cell carcinoma, lymphoma, neuroblastoma, mycosis fungoides, melanoma, and acute promyelocytic leukemia.

Since vitamins have synergistic effects with hormones, growth factors, DNA synthesis inhibitors, and biologic modifiers, they should be used as adjuvants for chemotherapy, radiation therapy, and immunotherapy. Certain vitamins act as immunoaugmentators (A, D, C), and increase the effects of chemotherapy in metastatic breast cancer.[16] Despite a plethora of laboratory data showing the important role of vitamins in controlling cancer incidence and development, the clinical work is just beginning. Vitamin therapy is in the same stage as hormonotherapy was two decades ago (the prereceptor era). At present, the selection of patients for vitamin therapy is based only on clinical status. More objective criteria, such as biologic markers, vitamin receptors, DNA content, and enzyme activity should be used in order to predict the prognosis and therapeutic effects of vitamins in cancer patients.

Several clinical trials have clearly indicated that natural vitamins at clinically tolerable doses have only limited activity against human cancers; therefore, work should be focused on the synthetic derivatives with higher therapeutic activity. As compared to cytostatics, vitamins have no genuine carcinogenic activity. In combination with chemotherapy and radiotherapy, they reduced the toxic effects and improved the quality of life. Patients with cancer will profit from a diet rich in vitamins and micronutrients.[17] A serious drawback of chemotherapy and radiotherapy is that often the cytostatic drugs used, as well as the radiation, have a mutagenic and carcinogenic potential and are poorly tolerated. The disadvantage of these treatments is their indiscriminate action against cancer and normal cells. Both Vitamin C and Vitamin E can inhibit mutagenesis and carcinogenesis *in vitro*. Each of the vitamins has been shown to inhibit tumor cell growth and carcinogen-induced DNA damage.[18] Since cancer is the second leading cause of death (22.1%) as compared to heart diseases (37.0%) in the U.S. it is concluded that the potential usefulness of vitamins in the treatment and prevention of cancer should not be ignored.

Vitamins are involved in the regulation of growth, differentiation, and function of a wide range of normal as well as malignant tissues. They exert significant antiproliferative and antitumor activities and play an important role in normal cell biology as well as in cancer biology. It remains unclear how certain vitamins can exert strong antitumor action in animal tumor models or in human cancer cell lines, but be less active in the same human cancers. The difference in vitamin sensitivity of the same type of cancer may be related to species-specific sensitivity, presence of receptors, or host immune defense system. The development of newer synthetic vitamin analogs with a greater specificity in their antineoplastic effects, lower doses, and less toxicity are obviously needed.

A. VITAMIN A (RETINOL) AND ITS SYNTHETIC ANALOGS (RETINOIDS) IN CANCER TREATMENT

Vitamin A (retinol) is a fat-soluble vitamin which is essential for normal and neoplastic cellular growth and differentiation. The word "retinoids" is a generic term that includes both naturally occurring compounds with Vitamin A activity and synthetic analogs of retinol. Different retinoids can display some, but not necessarily all, of the biologic activities of Vitamin A (retinol). One international unit of Vitamin A is defined as 0.3 µg of all trans-retinol. For nutritional and therapeutic purposes, a better term is "retinol equivalents", which is used to convert all sources of Vitamin A and carotenoids from the diet into a single unit; thus 1 µg all transretinol equals 1 retinol equivalent, and 1 µg of retinol is assumed to be biologically equivalent to 6 µg of β-carotene.

Although β-carotene can be converted into retinol, and both are often loosely classified as Vitamin A, they are two different substances in relation to cancer. Also, the dietary sources of retinol and β-carotene are certainly different. Retinol is derived from animal foods, the main sources being liver, dairy products, and vitamin supplements. The mean

TABLE 2
Difference between Retinol and β-Carotene

	Retinol (Vitamin A)	β-Carotene (Provitamin A)
Source	Animal foods	Vegetable foods
Serum level	Under homeostatic control (feedback mechanism)	Not under homeostatic control
Transport		
In vivo	Bound to RBP	In LDL
Carcinogenesis		
In vivo	Yes	Little
In vitro	Yes	No
Action	Hormone-like	Antioxidant
Toxicity	Yes (high doses)	No

daily intake of retinol is 1600 μg. β-Carotene, in contrast, is derived almost entirely from vegetable foods, namely, carrots and green vegetables. Their transport in blood is also different, retinol is bound to a specific carrier protein or retinol-binding protein (RBP), while β-carotene is carried in low-density lipoproteins (LDL). Usually, ingested Vitamin A is absorbed in the circulation and stored in the liver, and is regulated by a feedback mechanism (homeostatic control), while β-carotene is not under homeostatic control There is considerable evidence regarding the role of Vitamin A (retinol) in carcinogenesis (animal models and *in vitro*), while there is little or no evidence for the β-carotene.[18] Vitamin A (retinol) and most retinoids bind to specific cell surface receptors and act similar to steroid hormones (steroid-like) or hormone-like, while β-carotene acts mainly as an antioxidant. Retinol is toxic in high doses, whereas β-carotene is not. Hence, β-carotene is a provitamin which is enzymatically converted to Vitamin A *in vivo* (See Table 2). However, in most epidemiological studies the term Vitamin A also includes β-carotene. At present, there are more than 2,000 retinoids or synthetic Vitamin A analogs, and most of them have already been tested for their role in cancer treatment and prevention.

The impact of Vitamin A and retinoids in carcinogenesis is of considerable interest. The experimental and clinical evidence that Vitamin A exerts an anticancer effect applies mainly to retinol and the other natural and synthetic retinoids which prevent or delay cancer in animals and inhibit malignant progression in cultured cells.[19] In the past several years, many investigations have confirmed that retinoids inhibit the phenotype expression of cancer in humans and animals, regardless of the underlying initiators or promoters.[20] Earlier studies (1941) first associated Vitamin A deficiency with established human malignancy, and further supported a link between Vitamin A and cancer.[21] Recognition that Vitamin A deficiency induced hyperkeratosis of the skin in humans and squamous metaplasia in animals spurred an initial interest in treating cancer patients with this new wonder drug.[22] Most pharmacologic preparations of Vitamin A and β-carotene come from vegetable foods (yellow and green vegetables) or animal foods (milk, eggs, butter). Until now, substantial clinical investigations have been limited to only four retinoids: Vitamin A (retinol) and its esters, isotretinoin, etretinate, and arotinoids (See Figure 2). The basic structure of the retinoid molecule consists of a cyclic end group, a polyene side chain, and a polar end group (See Figure 2). By modifying any part, different therapeutic ratios can be achieved. Thus, the arotinoid TTNPB is less toxic and over 1000 times more potent than retinol, and is now entering clinical trials.

This section will describe the major biologic effects and their mechanism of action, and the clinical activity of retinoids as therapeutic and preventive anticancer agents.

1. Biologic Effects and Their Mechanism of Action

Although β-carotene can be directly absorbed in small amounts via lymphatic chylomicrones, it is mostly converted to retinol during absorption through the intestinal mucosa, where it and preformed Vitamin A (obtained from animal sources) are transported in the plasma by lipoproteins. Uptake by the liver appears to occur primarily by receptor-mediated endocytosis. There is evidence that apolipoprotein E plays a part in this uptake process.[23] Hepatic Vitamin A (mostly retinyl palmitate) normally represents over 90% of the body's total reserves of Vitamin A. In the liver, Vitamin A is stored in hepatic parenchymal cells, namely, in the fat-storing cells, which play an important role in Vitamin A storage in both normal and hypervitaminotic conditions. These cells represent a small proportion of hepatic nonparenchymal cells and have been referred to in the literature by various names, such as "lipocytes", "Vitamin A storing cells", and "Ito cells". These fat-storing cells contain numerous small lipid droplets.[24] When large doses of Vitamin A are given, the fat-storing cells become larger, and the number and size of fat-droplets increase considerably. It appears that the retinol (Vitamin A), after its uptake, is transferred from parenchymal cells to fat-storing cells for storage (as retinyl ester).

Thus, the mammalian liver has a remarkable capacity to store varying amounts of Vitamin A over a wide range of dietary intakes. Whereas Vitamin A is mainly stored in the liver, carotenoids are stored in several tissues, primarily in fat and liver. The parenchymal cell is the major cell type involved in the hepatic uptake and storage of retinol (as retinyl ester), and also is the cell type responsible for mobilization of retinol from the liver. After storage, the retinyl esters are hydrolyzed into retinol and released from the liver in a highly regulated manner. Retinol is transported in the blood as a complex consisting of retinol-binding protein (RBP), transthyretin (also called prealbumin), and thyroxine. Other retinoids have different routes of absorption, storage, and transport. Thus, retinoic acid is absorbed primarily by the venous portal route and is rapidly metabolized to by-products before elimination through both hepatic and renal routes.

It is possible that relative absence of hepatotoxicity of retinoic acid may be due to its tendency to avoid hepatic storage. Since retinoic acid and other acidic retinoids circulate bound to albumin rather than to RBP, it is likely that retinoic acid is not delivered to tissue by a specific, receptor-regulated process. Thus, unlike the plasma retinol concentration, the plasma level of an acidic retinoid should correlate well with the risk and occurrence of toxicity and should provide an accurate means of assessing and monitoring toxicity in clinical trials.

Naturally occurring Vitamin A plays a vital role in vision, growth, reproduction, and epithelial cell differentiation and proliferation.[25] Thus, Vitamin A exerts multiple functions, some of them similar to that of hormones (e.g., steroid hormones) or growth factors (paracrine mechanism).[26,27] Metaplastic changes in the epithelium along with increased cell division and nucleic acid synthesis occur in Vitamin A deficiency.[4,28] Vitamin A deficiency also enhances the effect of chemical carcinogenesis on epithelial tissues. Vitamin A replacement frequently induces a reversion of these premalignant and malignant changes to normal.

In the last several years, it has been shown that Vitamin A and retinoids block the phenotypic expression of cancer in humans and animals.[29,30] In addition to inhibiting cancer development, retinoids show antiproliferative and differentiation-inducing activity in *in vitro* cultures of cells and in human tumor biopsies grown in semisolid medium.[31]

In general, the antiproliferative activity of retinoids occurs in a broad range of transformed cell types, and is a reversible phenomenon. It takes effect after 2 to 3 d of cell exposure to the retinoid and requires about the same amount of time to be reversed, which suggests a cell cycle specific inhibition. Retinoids inhibit proliferation of many cancer cell lines with accumulations of cells in the G_1-phase of the cell cycle, thus slowing their entry into the S-phase.[32] In another study, after 24 h of retinoid exposure, cultured human breast carcinoma cells accumulated in the S-phase. However, after 4 to 7 d, the cells accumulated in the resting phase. Thus, it seems that in most cells, there is a retinoic acid-sensitive G_1 restriction point. It is possible that the arrest of G_1 growth may be regulated separately from differentiation in the HL-60 human promyelocytic cell line.[33]

In our study using Vitamin A (retinol) in chemically induced (by 3-methylcholanthrene) squamous cell carcinomas in mice and basal cell carcinomas in rats, the DNA radioactivity and autoradiographic studies with [³H]-thymidine showed a marked inhibition of DNA synthesis in the epithelial neoplastic cell nuclei. Since no papillomas occurred in both rats and mice treated with MCA alone, this suggests that retinol may act by diverting or shunting the inhibited cells into a dormant (latent) pool or G_0-phase.[30] A moderate inhibition of DNA synthesis was also found in chemically induced mammary tumors by DMBA or NMU in the female inbred SD rats.[34] The antiproliferative activity of retinoic acid and retinyl acetate in 31 different cell lines was studied; although responses in each line differed somewhat from one another, growth was inhibited in >60% of the cell lines.[35] The response pattern varied within different cell types, the same cell types, or even in different subclones, which may be related, in part, to differences in cellular retinoid metabolism and stage of transformation.[36]

It has also been shown in murine melanoma S_{91} cells that a small subset of drug-resistant cells may escape retinoid suppression even within "sensitive" cell lines.[37] In both antiproliferation and differentiation, retinoic acid and its analogs have been consistently more active than retinol, retinyl esters, and retynaldehyde.[38] It has been demonstrated that the terminal carboxyl group present in retinoic acid (see Figure 2), but not in retinol, is essential for the potency of synthetic retinoids as inducers of differentiation in HL-60 and F_9 cell lines.[39]

Recently, it has been shown in both normal and leukemic HL-60 and KG-1 human cell lines exposed to ten structurally different retinoids, that retinoic acid derivatives with a carboxyl group were significantly more active for both stimulation of normal hematopoiesis as well as inhibition of clonal growth of leukemic cells, than were retinoids with a carboxyl moiety.[40] This observation suggests that an important common structural requirement for the normal or abnormal hematopoiesis may exist. The structure-function relationship of retinoids is demonstrated by the abolition of biologic activity resulting from moving the carboxyl group of an arotinoid (TTNPB) from the para to the meta position on the benzene ring.[41] Also, another synthetic analog, retinamide (4HPR), has a high therapeutic potential against chemically induced rat mammary tumors, urinary bladder, and hamster trachea; however, it has limited activity in hematopoietic cells such as HL-60 and KG-1. Combined treatment of retinamide with ovariectomy enhanced inhibition of rat mammary tumors.[42] Evaluation of structure-function relationship of various retinoids *in vivo* and *in vitro* will be very important for chemical trials.

Furthermore, the antiproliferative and differentiating effects of retinoids may be biphasic, with high concentrations producing effects completely opposite to those of low concentrations, and the effect of early exposure differing markedly in effect from late exposure, all in the same experimental system. Retinoids are effective inhibitors of chemical carbinogenics in the skin, mammary gland, esophagus, respiratory tract, pancreas, colon, and urinary bladder of experimental animals. Modification of the basic retinoid structure has produced retinoids with increased anticancer activity and reduced systemic toxicity. Combining retinoid treatment with other modulators of carcinogenesis results in a synergistic inhibition of tumor growth. Retinoids in combination with hormones are much more effective in inhibiting mammary carcinogenesis than is either treatment alone. This combination also inhibits mammary tumor recurrence following surgical removal of the primary tumor. Thus, in rats with mammary carcinoma induced by 7,12-dimethylbenz(α)anthracene (DMBA) and treated with 2.5 mg of retinyl acetate/d 52% had less cancer than those receiving a placebo diet.[43] Combined hormonal manipulation with retinoids is more effective than each treatment alone. Either ovariectomy or bromocriptine (a pituitary prolactin inhibitor) plus retinyl acetate or 4-HPR is significantly more effective in cancer treatment than either treatment alone.[42] Also, combining 4-HPR (a retinamide) or retinyl acetate with the antiestrogen tamoxifen is synergistic in preventing rat mammary carcinogenesis.

Interestingly, retinoids can play a role in altering drug resistance by inactivating selectively the phosphorylation of certain surface proteins, including P_{150} which is associated with drug resistance. Retinoids are also active against certain hormone-resistant transformed cells.[44]

2. Mechanisms of Action of Vitamin A and Retinoids

Despite extensive investigations, the complex mechanism(s) of action which cause the diverse changes modulated by retinoids on cancer cells remains incompletely understood. Research, however, indicates a possible basic mechanism of action which makes it possible to postulate a unifying concept of retinoid anticarcinogenic activity.[45] This involves the action of the protein kinase-C (PK-C) cascade system, to account for retinoid's different biologic effects. Thus, the major biologic effects include regulation of enzyme synthesis, membrane function, growth factors, binding proteins, genomic and postgenomic expression, extracellular effects, immunological activity, and the PK-C cascade system.

a. Retinoids Have Prominent Effects on Several Enzyme Systems

The enzyme systems affected by retinoids include the ornithine decarboxylase (ODC), transglutaminase (TG), and cAMP-dependent and cAMP-independent protein kinases which appear to be widely involved in the pattern of cellular and molecular responses. The induction of ODC is a G_1-specific transcriptional event, which is correlated with tumor promotion and may be obligatory for progression through the cell cycle in normal and cancer cells. In most experimental systems, the inhibition of ODC by retinoic acid is directly correlated with growth inhibition, differentiation, and the accumulation of cells in the G_1-phase.[45] It is likely that retinoids decrease the synthesis of ODC. Retinoids also induce a soluble TG that may trigger the antipromotion activity of retinoids in skin carcinogenesis by antagonizing the phorbol ester-induced increase in epidermal TG.[46] Retinoids also affect the calcium cAMP intracellular regulatory mechanism. There is a direct correlation between the degree of retinoic acid-induced differentiation and the activity of cAMP in cell culture. Retinoid effects were also apparent when agents that elevated cAMP levels acted synergistically with retinoids in inducing differentiation. They also may stimulate alkaline phosphatase. The anticarcinogenic activity of retinoids may also be derived in part from their major effects on other enzyme systems. Thus, a change in tyrosine phosphorylation is one of the earliest events in chemically induced carcinogenesis and is also involved in the control of certain growth factors. Inhibition of the tyrosine phosphorylation in transformed cells by retinyl acetate could be an important part of its chemopreventive activity.[47] Retinoids also inhibit certain cytochrome P-450 isoenzymes required for activation of cutaneous precarcinogenesis (DMBA). Vitamin A also inhibits TPA-induced epidermal glutathione reductase activity in mice, and regulates acetyl cholinesterase in human neuroblastoma cell lines.[48] Thus, retinoids affect other enzymes which may play a role in their anticarcinogenic activity.

b. Retinoids Influence Synthesis and Distribution

Retinoids influence the synthesis and distribution of membrane glycoproteins, glycolipids, proteoglycons, and glycosaminoglycons.[3] The synthesis, distribution, and binding of cell-associated fibronectins, a large surface glycoprotein which is quantitatively reduced in neoplastic cells, is altered by retinoid exposure.[49] Increased release of fibronectin may be a required event for tumor promotion and transformation. Retinoic acid antagonizes TPA-induced fibronectin release in promotable clones of human lung fibroblasts and a JB_6 mouse epidermal cell line.[49] Retinoids also modulate the number of specific surface receptors, such as insulin-binding sites on human histiocytic lymphoma cell lines and specific $1\alpha,25$-dihydroxy vitamin D_3 receptors in osteosarcoma cells, which are associated with the induction of differentiation.[50] Thus, cell membrane glycoconjugate alterations affect cell-to-cell interactions, including cell adhesion, contact inhibition, migration, differentiation, growth, and transformation. All these interactions may affect tumor behavior.[51] However, retinoic acid regulates the production of specific glycoconjugates in transformed cells independently of its effects on cell differentiation. In addition to these specific biochemical effects, retinoids stimulate the synthesis of gap junctions and enhance intercellular communications. Retinoic acid can restore density-dependent contact inhibition of growth to transformed mouse cells. It is well demonstrated that anchorage-independent growth is highly correlated with neoplastic growth *in vivo* and retinoids inhibit this property in a wide variety of transformed cells. These diverse effects on cellular membranes, along with the effects of certain growth factors, may explain why cells grown under anchorage-independent conditions are more sensitive to retinoids than cells grown in anchorage-dependent conditions.[52]

c. Growth Factors

Retinoids modulate the effects of many mitogens and transforming growth factors which affect the cell membrane, such as epidermal growth factor (EGF), platelet-derived growth factor (PDGF), colony-stimulating factor (CSF), sarcoma growth factor, other tumor promoters (Teleocidin), and hormones (insulin).[53] EGF, one of the most important growth factors, regulates growth and differentiation of epithelial and mesenchymal cells and plays a role in embryogenesis and neoplastic transformation. EGF interacts with many enzymes. Most notably, it increases the activity of ODC, and it is integrally involved in the PK-C cascade.[54] The activated PK-C then phosphorylates the EGF receptor which inhibits binding to EGF. This feedback mechanism controls EGF activity. Loss of EGF requirement for growth *in vitro* has been associated with malignant transformation. It has been shown in several cell lines that retinoids enhance EGF binding by producing an increase in EGF receptor sites without affecting receptor activity.[55] The precise influence of these mitogens and growth factors on carcinogenesis, cell differentiation, and proliferation remains to be defined. Initially, retinoids were thought to act in a way very similar to steroid hormones by altering gene expression, but the experimental work in the last few years has not verified this concept.[56]

d. Binding Proteins

There is evidence that the retinoids combine with a cellular retinol-binding protein (CRBP) or cellular retinoic acid-binding protein (CRABP) which is delivered to the appropriate target tissue. Both retinol and its derivatives and retinoic acid and its synthetic analogs show a high specificity for their intracellular binding proteins.[26] These different binding proteins are independently controlled, which suggests that retinol and retinoic acid affect the regulation of growth and differentiation in different ways.

Although there are an estimated 100,000 to 300,000 binding sites per nucleus for CRBP and slightly fewer for CRABP, most binding is to nuclear membranes, not to DNA.[57] In contrast to the steroid receptor protein, the specific DNA sequences have not yet been identified. Possibly, some tumors express higher numbers of the cellular binding proteins, which may enhance their susceptibility to the differentiating or antiproliferating effects of retinoids. Higher concentrations of CRBP in tumors compared to normal tissue have been found in many human and experimental tumors and in many cancer cell lines. Furthermore, recent findings suggest that CRABP mediates the increase in cAMP-dependent protein kinases which are associated with retinoic acid-induced differentiation of embryonal carcinoma cell lines. In contrast, some retinoid responsive cell lines (e.g., HL-60) do not express CRABP.[58] Also, it has been found that some melanoma cell lines which were resistant to the effects of retinoids contained levels of binding proteins higher than levels in sensitive cell lines.[3] These data suggest that retinoid-binding proteins alone may not confer antiproliferative activity.

e. Genomic and Postgenomic Expression

Genomic and postgenomic expression is the hypothesis compatible with the multitude of *in vitro* and *in vivo* effects; the retinoids modify the genomic expression. Recently, by using hybridization selection and *in vitro* translation to identify several independent retinoid-inducible gene sequences in F_9 cells, it has been demonstrated that retinoids regulate the transcription of specific genes.[59] Retinoids may also antagonize the action of oncogenes, which are normally genetically repressed polypeptides that change the regulated growth pattern of normal cells to a more malignant pattern. Thus, it was found that retinoic acid modifies C-myc gene transcription. The C-myc oncogene plays an important role in the cell differentiation process. Retinoic acid turns off the expression of the myc gene. The lack of expression is not due to resting differentiated cells. Recently, it has been shown that retinoic acid-induced C-myc transcriptional down regulation in HL-60 cells occurs at the level of elongation, not initiation.[60] Declined C-myb expression after retinoic acid treatment is also associated with loss of cell proliferation. N-myc, a gene which shares limited homology with C-myc, is amplified in neuroblastoma cell lines.

A recent study showed that during retinoic acid-induced differentiation of neuroblastoma cells, a decreased level of N-myc expression preceded cell cycle changes and morphologic differentiation. These findings suggest that the mediation of transformation at the molecular level by retinoids may be heterogenous depending on the cell type and/or the tranasforming agent.[39,61] It has also been shown that the activation of specific oncogenes in transformed Syrian hamster embryo cells can influence their response *in vitro* to retinoids.

Although the mechanism by which retinoic acid interferes with the expression of oncogene products is not known, it is postulated that retinoic acid may influence V-src and V-Ha-ras activities by playing a critical role in the synthesis and response to endogenous growth factors, which are regulated by the oncogenes.[62] Retinoids might also control protein synthesis by post-transcriptional control of RNA processing. These proteins may include α-tubulin and glycoprotein synthesis through the formation of glycosyl phosphoryl retinoid intermediates.[63]

f. Extracellular Effects

Retinoids also have major biologic effects which are expressed extracellularly, including modifying the synthesis of plasminogen activator and collagenase, and certain prostaglandins. Plasminogen activator (PA), which is described in Chapter 1, is thought to be a specific biologic marker for differentiation in early embryogenesis for some tumor cells and for retinoid-dependent differentiation. Retinoids inhibit synovial and skin collagenase synthesis, a process that is synergistic with steroids. The beneficial activity those retinoids have shown in certain proliferative disorders, such as experimental arthritis, may be due to this inhibition of collagenase synthesis.[64] These results have clinical implications for the treatment of other proliferative diseases characterized by excessive synovial and skin collagenase synthesis, such as psoriatic and rheumatoid arthritis and epidermolysis bullosa dystrophica. Skin carcinogenesis is enhanced by certain prostaglandins and inhibited by retinoids and/or prostaglandin inhibitors. An important mechanism of action of retinoids may be the inhibition of prostaglandin synthesis.

g. Retinoids and the Immune System

Recent studies indicate that retinoids play an important role in immune-host defense systems. Thus, Vitamin A deficiency is associated with loss of lymphoid tissue and with impaired immune function; these abnormalities improve after replacement of Vitamin A. Administration of pharmacologic doses of retinoids is associated with enhanced ability to resist bacterial infections and increased cell-mediated immunity. Vitamin A and retinoids can act as adjuvants for the development of both humoral immunity and antigen-specific,

T-lymphocyte-mediated cytotoxicity. Retinoids in pharmacologic doses also inhibit the NK activity and interferon production, but they stimulate production of interleukin-2 (IL-2) by T-helper cells, which results in T-killer cell proliferation. Mice injected with retinoids display an enhanced capacity to produce IL-2.[65] Retinoids inhibit proliferation of several B-lymphocyte leukemia cell lines, but lower concentrations of retinoids enhance thymocyte proliferation. Vitamin A potentiates antibody formation, increases the phagocytic and tumoricidal activity of macrophages, and activates polymorphonuclear leukocytes.[66] Aromatic retinoic acid analogs inhibit *in vivo* the growth and metastases of transplantable syngeneic tumors. In all cases, the tumor inhibitory effect was T-cell dependent. This phenomenon was abolished in congenital athymic nude mice and also in thymectomized mice by irradiation along with cytarabine which interferes with IL-2 response.[67] Retinoid pretreatment of rodents improves their survival after implantation of certain tumors. Retinoids promote the delayed cutaneous hypersensitivity. Retinyl palmitate apparently potentiates the antitumor effect of the immune-enhancer BCG (bacille Calmette-Guérin). These immune properties of retinoids may be responsible, in part, for their antitumor effects seen *in vivo*. Thus retinoids exert a biphasic effect on the immune system; low doses stimulate, while high doses inhibit immune functions.

h. The Protein Kinase-C (PK-C) Cascade System

This system could be a unifying concept to explain the complex anticarcinogenic action of retinoids. The PK-C/phosphoinositol cascade system could explain the myriad of reported actions of retinoids, and provides a unifying mechanism which can play a central role in retinoid anticarcinogenic effect.

PK-C, the phorbol ester receptor, is a Ca^{2+}-activated, phospholipid-dependent enzyme, which is a major cell surface signal transduction pathway, and plays a critical role in the carcinogenic process.[54,68] Recent work supports the theory that retinoids modulate the PK-C activity. Although the molecular mechanisms of action which cause various cellular changes by retinoids are not precisely understood, it is possible that the PK-C system alters phosphorylation of cellular retinoid-binding proteins, which could affect the regulation of enzyme synthesis, membrane structure, growth factors, binding proteins, gene transcription, postgenomic effects, and extracellular actions. PK-C modulation may also be involved in retinoid antagonism with phorbol esters (TPA), and synergistic activity with other agents (tamoxifen and selenium), as well as the ability to reverse cytotoxic drug resistance.

Interaction with the PK-C cascade system may explain the synergistic anticarcinogenic activity of retinoids with other agents, such as antiestrogens (tamoxifen) and selenium, but it cannot explain the biphasic effects of retinoids on the immune system. Despite the fact that Vitamin A and retinoids have shown a potential therapeutic effect in several premalignant and malignant *in vivo* and *in vitro* models, their clinical therapeutic use lags behind the *in vitro* work, which unequivocally established their therapeutic value in many cancer cell lines, as well as in several animal tumor models. A major advance would be to develop new screening tests to detect the "retinoid-sensitive" tumors and cancer cells in earlier stages and to find new retinoids equal in efficacy to existing ones, but significantly less toxic at the therapeutic level. Some of the new synthesized retinoids lack the systemic toxic effects, such as liver dysfunction, teratogenicity, and bone toxicity.[69] Combining retinoids at lower doses with other agents, including cytotoxic drugs, hormones, growth factor, irradiation, micronutrients, and other biologic modifiers, will enhance their therapeutic potential since *in vitro* studies showed that they have additive and synergistic effects.

At present, there is enough experimental and epidemiologic evidence to indicate that Vitamin A and many retinoids have a potential anticancer activity and are able to suppress or retard the tumor growth in animal tumor models as well as in human cancers. Studies in animals indicate that Vitamin A deficiency generally increases susceptibility to chemically

TABLE 3
Chemopreventive Action of Retinoids in Human Cancer

Malignancy	Ref.
Dermatologic	
Actinic keratosis	72—74
Keratoacanthoma (Multiple keratoacanthomas—Ferguson-Smith syndrome)	75
Basal cell carcinoma	76
Dysplastic nevi	77, 78
Epidermodysplasia verruciformis	79
Xeroderma pigmentosum	100
Nondermatologic	
Oral leukoplakia	80—83
Bronchial metaplasia	4, 28, 31, 84, 85
Laryngeal papillomatosis	86
Cervical dysplasia	87—89
Carcinoma *in situ* (Bowen's disease)	
Myelodysplastic syndromes (MDS)	40, 90—92, 93
Superficial bladder carcinoma	94—99,
Colon Cancer	70

induced tumors and that the supplementation or addition of the vitamin or retinoids prevents or delays the incidence and development of most, but not all, cancers. Retinoids have been shown to inhibit chemically induced tumors of the breast, urinary bladder, skin, and lung. Epidemiologic studies indicate that there is an inverse relationship between the risk of cancer and the consumption of foods containing Vitamin A (e.g., liver), or its precursors (some β-carotenoids in dark green and deep yellow vegetables). It has been found that there is an inverse relationship between Vitamin A and β-carotene intake and a reduced risk of cancer of the lung, urinary bladder, larynx, and colon/rectum.[70]

In this section, we will focus on the role of Vitamin A and retinoids as chemopreventive agents in human cancers and as therapeutic agents in human cancers. The usefulness of the retinoids in the treatment of non-neoplastic dermatologic diseases (acne, psoriasis, and Darier's disease) will not be discussed in this section.

3. Chemopreventive Agents in Human Cancers

Although the cause and effect relationship between Vitamin A and cancer is far from being established, the action of retinoids on tumor initiation and promotion is complex and appears to be carcinogen- and cocarcinogen-specific. Initially, retinoids were mainly used in chemoprevention of cancer. Many clinical studies, however, demonstrated a substantial preventive as well as therapeutic activity in several types of dermatologic and nondermatologic premalignant and malignant conditions (See Table 3).

Since retinoids accumulate preferentially in the skin, their widest application has been in the management of skin diseases.[2,25,38,71] Most cancers, almost 90%, are of epithelial origin, and retinoids are mostly effective on epithelial carcinogenesis, especially in the postinitiation phase of carcinogenesis. Thus, retenoids delay the transformation of premalignant cells into malignant cells, and consequently the expression of premalignant cells.[6]

Actinic keratosis — This is a common skin disease that occurs following a long exposure to high levels of ultraviolet light. About 5% of these premalignant lesions undergo malignant transformation and lead to nonmelanomatous skin cancer. Impressive prophylactic and therapeutic results have been achieved by treatment with topically applied and oral retinoids. Previous clinical studies revealed that when 93 patients with actinic keratosis were treated with topical retinoic acid cream, a complete regression occurred in 46 (49.4%) and partial response occurred in 47 patients (50.5%).[72] Another study using topically applied retinoic acid cream (0.1 to 0.3%) noted a complete regression in 24 (40%) and partial regression in 27 (45%) from 60 patients.[73] The arotinoid RO 13-6298 was studied in 16 patients, who were given a dose of 1 μg/kg/d orally for 28 d, and improvement was seen in 10 patients. Side effects, including cheilitis, pruritus, palmar-plantar exfoliation, and eczema were seen in 11 patients.[74] These studies demonstrate the efficacy of retinoids in the treatment of actinic keratosis and indicate that a maintenance retinoid therapy is required to prevent relapses and disease progression.

Keratoacanthoma — This is a hyperkeratotic lesion which is morphologically similar to squamous cell carcinoma of the skin (SCC). These tumors undergo either spontaneous regression, or where multiple lesions are present (Ferguson-Smith syndrome), frank malignant changes. Preliminary findings showed impressive sustained responses to isotretinoin (2 mg/kg/d) in five of eleven patients with multiple keratoacanthomas.[75] Also, patients showed complete regression after 2 to 3 months of taking oral etretinate (1 mg/kg/d). One year after discontinuing therapy some patients remained in complete remission.

Basal cell carcinoma (BCC) — In addition to their therapeutic role in BCC, retinoids also have a role in preventing the development of this type of skin cancer. It has been reported that patients who had basal cell carcinomas for 6 to 16 years before treatment had a 100% statistical chance of developing new lesions within one year; however, no new lesions had developed following treatment with isotretinoin at an average dose of 1.5 mg/kg/d. Similar chemoprophylactic results have been reported in other high-risk patients with both isotretinoin and etretinate.[76] Several large prevention studies are now under way, using β-carotene, retinol, and isotretinoin in the secondary prevention of skin cancer.

Dysplastic nevi — These are melanocytic nevi characterized by the presence of several pigmented macules which are composed of dysplastic melanocytes. These nevi may occur either familially or sporadically and frequently undergo malignant transformation to melanoma. Thus, they are markers for an increased risk for the development of cutaneous melanoma. Previously a small number of patients (only three) were treated with topical tretinoin (0.05% applied daily) and after 10 to 12 weeks, dysplastic histologic features underwent marked reduction to benign nevocellular nevi.[77] However, a more recent study on eleven patients with dysplastic nevi treated with oral isotretinoin in doses of 40 mg twice a day for 4 months, showed no clinical or histologic changes in these patients. Thus, oral isotretinoin does not appear to have a significant biologic effect on the clinical or histologic appearance of dysplastic nevi in the treatment schedule employed.[78] However, it is possible that higher doses or a longer course of isotretinoin would affect some changes in dysplastic nevi syndrome.

Epidermodysplasia verruciformis — This is a familial skin disease, characterized by multiple squamous cell carcinomas and flat wart-like lesions beginning in childhood. The lesions contain human papillomavirus Type V(HPV-5), which is oncogenic. Administration of etretinate, in doses of 1 mg/kg/d given orally for 2 months, produced a regression of lesions in a few cases. Clinical improvement occurred in some cases despite persistence of the virus. The improvement may be due to changes in cell-mediated immunity following retinoid treatment.[79] Xeroderma pigmentosum prevention was obtained in some cases after the use of etretinate. However, the findings in these studies are preliminary, and further trials are needed for confirmation.

Chemoprevention of nondermatologic cancers recently has received more attention than that of dermatologic cancers. Thus, in a variety of premalignant lesions, such as oral leukoplakia, bronchial metaplasia, laryngeal papillomatosis, cervical dysplasia, myelodysplastic syndromes, superficial bladder cancer, and colorectal carcinoma, some evidence of improvement following retinoid therapy was reported.

Oral leukoplakia — Retinoids may reduce the chance of this developing into an overt malignancy and thus are considered standard therapy for this premalignant lesion. In Syrian hamsters, retinyl acetate delayed the development of leukoplakia and oral cancer.[80] In humans, treatment with retinoids may be associated with a decreased incidence of leukoplakia and possibly of oral cancer. This treatment with isotretinoin etretinate or tretinoin at a dose of 70 mg/d for 8 weeks in 90 patients with advanced leukoplakia showed positive responses after 3 weeks in a majority of these patients. Responses were controlled by histologic grading and followup biopsies. Followup examinations revealed that treatment with etretinate produced higher response rates (91%), more sustained remissions (50%), reduced relapses (46%), and fewer progressions (4%) as compared to patients treated with isotretinoin (87, 44, 47, and 9%) or tretinoin (59, 43, 40, and 17%). Relapses occurred within 1 or 2 months, indicating the need for maintenance or periodic therapy. Etretinate is more active and less toxic, and causes no discontinuation of therapy, whereas, tretinoin and isotretinoin did so in 11 and 4%, respectively.[81] Based on these initial results, a second study was conducted in 48 patients receiving only oral etretinate for 6 weeks, with 50% also treated with local application of 0.1% etretinate paste and oral etretinate. Both groups had a high response rate after 2 weeks (CR + PR = 83.5% in the combined, and 71% in the oral etretinate-alone group). Relapse occurred after 2 months of stopping therapy. Repeated courses of retinoid therapy are recommended to reduce relapses.[82] In a recent prospective randomized double-blind trial, it has been found that isotretinoin was effective in suppressing leukoplakia. Thus, 44 patients were treated with 2 mg/kg/d for 3 months for leukoplakia. A complete or partial objective response was seen in 67% of the patients receiving retinoid as compared to only 10% of the patients receiving placebo.

Despite the significant therapeutic response, however, relapse with progression of lesions usually occurred within 2 to 3 months after treatment was stopped. Thus, retinoids appear to have significant therapeutic effect in the treatment of leukoplakia.[83] Further studies regarding the efficacy of retinoids in oral "hairy" leukoplakia in AIDS patients, in patients with head and neck squamous cell carcinoma, as well as in those with Barrett's esophagus (chronic peptic ulcer and metaplasia of the lower esophagus), are needed. Although retinoids exert beneficial therapeutic effects, further studies are required to determine which compound is most active and least toxic and to establish the guidelines for maintenance therapy.

Bronchial metaplasia — It is well documented that Vitamin A deficiency induces bronchial squamous metaplasia, a precancer lesion which often leads to lung cancer, and administration of Vitamin A reverses these changes.[4,28,31] These observations led to several studies to determine the effects of Vitamin A and its derivatives in patients with high risk of developing lung cancer. Experience with oral etretinate at a dose of 25 mg/d for 6 months has been reported in heavy smokers with bronchial metaplasia, and reduction in metaplasia occurred in 23 of the 30 evaluable patients.[84] Complete resolution of metaplastic changes was noted also in patients who had stopped smoking; a more recent study including blinded pathologic review of biopsies showed significant results in heavy smokers. Thus, 40 heavy smoker subjects with a >15% index of metaplasia received 25 mg/d of etretinate for 6 months. When a second bronchoscopy was performed on 36 evaluable patients, a significant decrease of metaplasia (from 34.57 to 26.96%) was observed. These results are significant and suggest that retinoids may play an active role in reversing this precancerous lesion. Confirmation of these findings in more randomized trials would be an important step in order to accept this approach as a standard therapy for heavy smokers.[85]

Laryngeal papillomatosis — This is a benign proliferation of polypoid lesions on the vocal cords which may lead to squamous cell carcinoma (SCC). Retinoids have been tried because of their antiproliferative activity on the transforming epithelial tissues and also because of their lack of toxicity. Both isotretinoin and etretinate were used in patients with recurrent progressive papillomatosis of the larynx and produced similar results. Thus, from 42 patients with laryngeal papillomatosis treated with 1 mg/kg/d of etretinate, 28 patients (67%) achieved a complete resolution and 11 patients (26%) had a partial remission.[86]

Cervical dysplasia and carcinoma *in situ* — These were treated with retinoids based on the retinoid activity in reversing preneoplastic epithelial proliferation in the other tissues and on the epidemiologic association of cervical dysplasia with decreased intake of dietary Vitamin A.[87] Several studies using retinoin or retinyl acetate gel were conducted in patients with cervical dysplasia and carcinoma *in situ*. In one Phase I study, 36 patients were treated topically with retinoid for 4 d. Doses were escalated from 0.05 to 0.48% tretinoin cream, and a complete response was seen in 33% of the patients. Response was clearly dose-related since 45% of the complete responders were on high doses (0.15 to 0.48%) compared to only 14% who received low doses (0.05 to 0.11%).[88] Similar results were obtained with tretinoin concentration of 0.37% in 20 patients, and a complete response was achieved in 50%. In another study conducted in 50 patients with histopathologic diagnosis of mild or moderate dysplasia, placebo and varying doses of retinyl acetate gel were self-administered using a vaginal application for 7 d beginning on the fifth day of the menstrual cycle. Doses ranged from 3 to 18 mg, and several patients had a decrease in erythema and a general improvement in the transformation zones; no patient had a progression of her dysplasia.[89] Although the results of using retinoids in treatment of cervical dysplasia, vulvar leukoplakia, and carcinoma *in situ* are promising for chemoprevention and for the long-term management of cervical preneoplasia, the embryotoxic potential of tretinoin may limit the clinical use at present and must wait for extensive followup and the development of new, less toxic drugs.

Myelodysplastic syndromes (MDS) — These are a heterogenous group of diseases and represent a preleukemic state in which progressive clonal abnormalities of hemopoietic stem cells give rise to a variety of hematologic aberrations, including single or multiple cytopenias.[90] Clinical manifestations range from chronic refractory anemia to overt leukemia in approximately 40% of patients, and for this reason MDS is considered as a preleukemia state. Since Vitamin A deficiency is associated with anemia in humans and with reduced bone marrow precursors in animals, and since Vitamin A replacement corrects these abnormalities, these findings have opened the door for evaluating retinoids in MDS.[40] Several *in vitro* studies have shown that retinoids, especially those with a free terminal carboxyl group, such as 13-*cis* and β-all *trans*retinoic acid, have potent hematopoietic activity. These reports also have demonstrated that retinoic acid induced terminal differentiation and cessation of growth in several human leukemic cell lines from certain patients with MDS and acute myelocytic leukemia.[40,91] However, cells from less mature leukemic cell lines are often resistant to retinoid-induced differentiation. These *in vitro* studies have demonstrated a differential effect of retinoic acid on normal and neoplastic hematopoietic cells, leading to the use of isotretinoin in patients with MDS. However, some of these studies used a small number of patients (4 to 5 patients) and a wide range of doses. Thus, it would be difficult to draw a definite conclusion regarding the therapeutic effects. In two more recent studies, one reported the results of 15 MDS patients treated with isotretinoin at a dose of 1.5 to 4 mg/kg/d for 8 weeks; eight patients (53%) had a >20% increase in peripheral blood neutrophils and five of these had an absolute increase of >500. Abnormalities recurred after cessation of the drug but responded again to its readministration.[92] A more recent randomized therapeutic trial with 13-*cis*-retinoic acid was carried out in 70 patients with MDS having 5% or fewer marrow blast cells. Among nonsideroblastic patients the 1-year survival in the treated group was 77%, compared with 36% in the control group.[93] The results also suggest a significant increase in survival in patients with refractory nonsideroblastic anemia taking 13-*cis*-retinoic acid (13-CRA) at the relatively low dose of 20 mg/d. In conclusion, an overall response rate in MDS of 38% (26 of 69 patients), with four well-documented complete responses, indicates that isotretinoin is active in treatment of this disease. Clinical trials using retinoids with more potent *in vitro* hematopoietic activity, such as the retinoidal benzoic acid derivative TTNPB, should be of interest.[40] Combination therapy with other cytotoxic agents or vitamins (vitamin D_3) should also be evaluated.

Superficial bladder carcinoma — This has been treated with retinoids (tretinoin, etretinate, fenretinide) before or following resection of superficial bladder tumors. Experimental and epidemiologic studies showed that isotretinoin and etretinate inhibited carcinogen-induced transitional and squamous cell carcinoma of the urinary bladder in rats and mice.[94] Other studies have correlated low levels of dietary Vitamin A with an increased incidence of bladder cancer in humans.[95] Retinoic acid receptors have also been identified in transurethral resected specimens from human bladder cancer.[94] A controlled study has compared placebo and etretinate 50 mg/d in 73 patients with recurrent, noninvasive bladder tumor and showed inconclusive results. A recent randomized, placebo-controlled, multicenter trial lasting 24 months, conducted in 86 patients with propensity for bladder tumor recurrence, showed a lower tumor recurrence for the oral etretinate-treated group than for the placebo-treated patients at 3 months (29 vs. 40%), 12 months (35 vs. 55%), and 24 months (29 vs. 56%). Multifocal recurrences were also lower in the etretinate group, 17 vs. 48%.[97] Compared to therapy with intravesical cytotoxic therapy in randomized, double-blind trials, prolonged (>1 year) low-dose etretinate 25 mg/d appears to be similarly effective with cytotoxic agents.[98] Also, the local instillation of Vitamin A alone or in conjunction with oral retinoids showed encouraging results following resection of urinary bladder tumors.[99]

Colon cancer — Recently a total of 112 subjects were evaluated, including 41 with colorectal cancer with distal metastases, 40 patients with benign colorectal disease (polyps, gastric ulcers, diverticulosis), and 31 healthy subjects. All patients with colon cancer had lower values of Vitamin A as compared to healthy controls. The differences between the cancer cases and the patients with benign GI disease were not found to be significant. It appears, therefore, that the biochemical evidence of Vitamin A deficiency is a common factor for both benign and malignant GI disease.[70] Also, β-carotene has been found to exert protective effects in rats, mice, and hamsters against tumors at various sites. It was found that β-carotene at 20 mg/kg diet exerts a significant inhibitory effect against colon tumors in mice, induced by 1,2-dimethyl hydrazine (DMH). Both the incidence and multiplicity of tumors were reduced by about half; adenomas, the predominant type of tumors were reduced by 40%, and adenocarcinomas were largely absent.[70]

Xeroderma pigmentosum — This is a rare, disfiguring skin disease, inherited as an autosomal recessive trait, and characterized by hyperpigmentation and telangiectasia. Frequently it develops into squamous cell carcinomas. Prevention of tumors with etretinate has been recently reported.[100] Thus, Vitamin A (retinol), retinoids, and carotenoids exert important preventive effects of cancer development, inhibiting the transformation of premalignant lesions into malignant tumors. They are potential inhibitors of human cancer. β-Carotene therapy is an effective treatment for erythropoietic protoporphyria (EPP) in high doses of Solatene (15 to 180 mg/d).

4. Retinoids as Therapeutic Agents in Human Cancers

Although retinoids have been investigated primarily for cancer prevention, considerable laboratory and clinical evidence now supports the use of retinoids as anticancer drugs as well.[2,6,15,25,27,43,71,73,101] The parent compound Vitamin A (retinol) appears to have only limited antitumor activity in humans at clinically tolerable doses.[102] Thus, the immediate future for retinoids in human cancer clearly lies with the far more effective and less toxic synthetic retinoids, such as isotretinoin, etretinate, and the retinoidal benzoic acid derivatives, or arotinoids.[2,22,25,40,43,71,102.]

Although the precise mechanism of retinoid action remains unclear, the recent discovery that the retinoic acid receptor is homologous to the steroid and thyroid hormone receptors suggests that the retinoid mechanism of action may be analogous to that of steroid hormones.[103] Retinoids have shown impressive activity against premalignant skin lesions and other epithelial precancers (oral leukoplakia, bronchial metaplasia, cervical dysplasia). In

TABLE 4
Therapeutic Action of Retinoids in Human Cancer

Neoplasia	Drug	Total response (%) (CR + PR)	Ref.
Basal cell carcinoma (BCC)	Topical tretinoin	98.43 (38.22 + 60.21)	72, 73, 105
	Isotretintoin	53.02 (7.86 + 45.16)	71, 76, 102
	Etretinate	42.50 (7.50 + 35%)	106
Squamous cell carcinoma (SCC)	Etretinate	50.00 (25 + 25)	106
	Arotinoid	100 (0 + 100)	74
	Isotretinoin	77.77 (22.22 + 55.55)	109, 120
Malignant melanoma	Retinoic acid	100 (50 + 50)	104, 113
	Isotretinoin	15	
Mycosis fungoides (cutaneous T-cell lymphoma)	Isotretinoin	61 (14 + 47)	114
	Etretinate	50 (50 + 0)	115
	Arotinoid	84 (67 + 17)	115, 116
Myeloid leukemia	Isotretinoin	57.92	117, 118
Squamous cell cancer of the head and neck	Isotretinoin	15.78	120

established basal cell skin cancers, topical retinoid treatment has produced a complete response rate of 33%, and systemic retinoids have produced an objective response rate of 51%. In advanced squamous cell skin cancers, systemic retinoids have produced a response rate of over 70%. Combined treatment of retinoids and α-interferon enhances the therapeutic effects in advanced skin cancers.[104] Therefore, retinoids show promise as a relatively nontoxic preventive and adjuvant cancer therapy. Further investigations should be focused on combination of retinoids with other biologic response modifiers (BRM), such as interleukin-2 (IL-2), CSF, hormones, cytotoxic drugs, radiation, or other vitamins, which will potentiate their therapeutic effects and will offer exciting prospects for primary and neoadjuvant therapy for advanced malignancy. The therapeutic anticancer activity of various retinoids will be examined in the treatment of established malignancies such as basal cell carcinoma (BCC), squamous cell carcinoma (SCC), malignant eccrine poroma, malignant melanoma, mycosis fungoides, leukemia, squamous cell cancer of the head and neck, lung cancer, and Kaposi's sarcoma (See Table 4).

Basal cell carcinoma (BCC) — Basal cell carcinoma and squamous cell carcinoma (SCC) of the skin are the two most common malignancies in the U.S. accounting for over 300,000 cases per year.[104] Although BCC is the most common type of skin cancer, accounting for over 75% of cases in the U.S., its metastatic potential is lower than that of cutaneous SCC. Early studies used topical retinoic acid in 49 BCC patients and achieved a 33% complete response (CR) and 65.30% partial response (PR), an overall of 98.50% (CR + PR) response rate.[72,73,105,106] Systemic retinoid therapy has produced an overall response rate (CR + PR) of 51% in 57 BCC patients.[76] One of these patients had xeroderma pigmentosum with actinic keratoses in addition to BCC and had a CR to etretinate.[107] Although retinoids have been used mainly to treat local disease, patients with bone metastases from BCC can also be treated; one patient avoided decompressive laminectomy.[106] Discontinuing therapy and reducing drug doses, generally are associated with recurrence, especially in patients with multiple lesions. Another study used oral etretinate to treat 40 patients, 20 with isolated and 20 with multiple BCC skin lesions. Despite the fact that the response rates were equivalent in both groups (CR + PR = 40 to 50%), the relapse pattern is different. Thus, at followup after 1 year, 86% of the patients with multiple lesions relapsed, compared to relapses in only 10% with isolated lesions.[106] As with isotretinoin, maintenance therapy with etretinate appears necessary, especially in patients with multiple lesions. Another study of 15 patients treated with retinoic acid was done; 2 patients developed a complete response (CR =

13.40%), 13 experienced a partial response (PR = 86.66%) with a decrease in tumor area, and histologic examination showed cancer cell necrosis after treatment.[105] In three other studies using oral retinoids, namely, high-dose isotretinoin (4.5 mg/kg/d), complete clinical and histologic regression was achieved in 10% of 248 tumors in 11 patients. Maintenance retinoid therapy was necessary for preventing relapses. Small tumors (<10 mm diameter) responded completely more often than did larger tumors (21% vs. 3%). An improvement in two thirds of all the lesions, and also a partial response (PR) lasting over 16 months in one of three study patients with multiple BCC was observed. Several of these tumors resolved completely. Patients who discontinued treatment had relapses in 8 to 18 months.[76]

Squamous cell carcinoma (SCC) — This is a more malignant tumor and has a higher tendency to metastasis than BCC. The preclinical evidence for using retinoids in SCC is based on data from *in vitro* and *in vivo* studies which showed retinoid activity against SCC cell lines as well as in chemically induced SCC in mice and rats. *In vitro* studies have shown that in the 1483 SCC line, retinoic acid significantly suppressed cell growth by decreasing EGF receptors, EGF kinase activity, and EGF binding. The suppression of EGF receptor gene expression appeared to be selective since retinoids did not affect other genes.[108] A marked inhibition of chemically induced (by 3-methyl-cholanthrene) SCC in mice and BCC in rats by a topical application of Vitamin A (retinol) has been recently reported.[30] The antitumor activity of retinol is accompanied by a significant decrease of DNA synthesis studied by [³H]-thymidine, also advanced ultrastructural (cytolytic, mitochondrial, and lysosomal) changes and cell surface disorganization. These findings suggest that Vitamin A exerts its anticarcinogenic action by inhibiting DNA synthesis, cytolysis, and disorganization of cell membranes of neoplastic cells. However, despite this demonstrable antitumor activity in cell lines and in animal models, the retinoid therapy for SCC in humans has been limited. Thus, in 14 patients with advanced squamous skin cancers, the overall response rate was 71% including three complete sustained remissions.[74,106] Treatment of patients with SCC and Bowen's disease resulted in some partial and a few complete remissions and no relapses at 12 months in patients with either disease.[106,107] In a study including patients with both active keratosis and SCC treated with arotinoid (RO 13-6298) daily at a dose of 1 μg/kg for 28 d, one patient experienced a dramatic reduction in tumor size after 4 weeks of treatment.[107] In a recent study conducted on four patients who received 1 mg/kg/d of isotretinoin, two had complete responses lasting 19 and 3 months, and the other two had partial responses of 2- and 9-month durations. All patients had well-differentiated SCC of the skin.[109] Retinoids are less effective in tumors that: (1) have poor histologic differentiation, (2) are necrotic and often superinfected, and (3) have spread lesions in the head and neck region. This suggests a correlation between retinoid anticancer activity and cell differentiation. Therefore, retinoids are a highly effective and well-tolerated systemic therapy for SCC of the skin.

Malignant eccrine poroma — This is a rare tumor originating in the sweat or eccrine glands. Experience with retinoids is very limited in this type of cancer. In one case in which surgery, irradiation, and chemotherapy had failed, treatment with isotretinoin 3 mg/kg/d produced a dramatic improvement within 1 week; lesions became dry and necrotic. Rebiopsy after 9 d of treatment revealed cell differentiation toward normal tubules and ducts and some degree of cellular necrosis.[110] However, other patients do not respond.

Melanoma and dysplastic nevus syndrome — These are also responsive to retinoid therapy. Early *in vitro* studies showed that retinoids can suppress growth of cells from human melanoma lines and inhibit growth of murine melanoma and colony-forming human melanoma cells from tumors.[3,41,111] A significant inhibition of tumor growth following treatment with Vitamin A of a transplantable murine melanoma in mice has been reported. Immunologic changes have been achieved in melanoma by treating transplanted melanomas with intralesional Vitamin A, and this cured 79% of tumors in histoincompatible donor mice.[112] Partial responses of cutaneous melanoma metastases in a few patients were previously reported. A recent study including patients with dysplastic nevus syndrome and malignant melanoma revealed that topical retinoic acid therapy under tape occlusion produced two complete responses in three treated patients. Oral isotretinoin produced no clinical or histologic improvement in seven patients. Two patients with malignant melanoma have been treated with topical retinoid therapy. One had a prolonged complete response and the other had a short-lived partial response. Systemic isotretinoin therapy produced less dramatic results than those of topical treatment, thus only a 15% response rate in 20 patients treated with isotretinoin.[113] This rate is similar to those of α-interferon and cytotoxic chemotherapy.

Mycosis fungoides or cutaneous T-cell lymphoma (CTCL) — This is an uncommon T-cell lymphoproliferative disorder which primarily involves the skin, and progresses from small to extensive plaques, then to tumors and generalized erythroderma. The broadest experience with retinoids has been in the rare cases of T-cell lymphoma called mycosis fungoides. Since 1983, subsequent retinoid trials with isotretinoin have been performed and produced an impressive response rate of 62% (21% complete responses) in 92 patients treated with CTCL.[114] A completed Phase II study from the same clinical trials reported a 44% response (CP + PR) rate in 25 patients. The median duration of response was over 8 months in this study. The most complete and prolonged responses generally occurred in patients with less advanced disease (early plaque stage or parapsoriasis-en-plaque). Responses were less dramatic in patients with advanced tumor-stage disease. No responses were seen in patients with Sézary's syndrome treated with retinoids. Continued retinoid administration is necessary for maintenance of these responses. Preliminary data in mycosis fungoides suggest that the arotinoid RO 13-6298 may be more effective and non-cross-resistant with earlier generation retinoids. In a study using RO 13-6298 in four patients with advanced plaque and tumor-stage disease, three complete responses and one partial response were achieved.[115] A recent CTCL report documented a complete response to RO 13-6298, given as salvage therapy after isotretinoin had failed.[116] Whether the beneficial effects are due to immune-mediated events, alterations in target organ response, or a direct effect of retinoids on neoplastic lymphocytes, is unclear. Further investigations of the interaction of retinoids and mycosis fungoides are needed.

Myeloid leukemia — Although there are extensive studies of *in vitro* human leukemic cell lines and animal *in vivo* data indicating that retinoids have potent antiproliferative and differentiation activity (encouraging the use of retinoids in leukemia), the clinical trials are limited).[39,40,61,91] In many patients, retinoids are combined with cytotoxic drugs, biologic modifiers (α-interferon), or other vitamins (Vitamin D_3). This situation makes it difficult to evaluate the therapeutic value of retinoids per se in different types of leukemias. The most promising clinical results are achieved in acute promyelocytic leukemia (APL), despite the fact that cases are limited. Remarkable responses were achieved in four of seven previously refractory patients, including two patients with prolonged ($\geq$ 1 year) complete responses.[117] A recent study reported a heavily pretreated patient with acute promyelocytic leukemia and residual malignant cells in his bone marrow after multiple courses of chemotherapy (cytosine arabinoside) was given 13-*cis*-retinoic acid orally, in a dose of 100 mg/m² in two doses. The patient achieved a complete remission for 1 year with retinoid maintenance therapy; then he relapsed with a population of cells resistant to retinoic acid-induced differentiation.[118] Despite *in vitro* studies, clinical results in other types of leukemias, such as acute nonlymphocytic leukemia (ANLL) and lymphoid leukemias, are less impressive. In bone marrow cells from chronic myeloid leukemia (CML), tretinoin produced a dose-dependent decrease in colony and cluster growth and retinoid-induced myeloid differentiation. However, uncontrolled studies involving 28 chronic phase CML patients achieved no obvious improvement or complete remission with isotretinoin.[119] Thus, there is a discrepancy between *in vitro* and *in vivo* responses, which may be due to structure-function specificities of different retinoids.[40]

Squamous cell cancer of the head and neck — Isotretinoin has been used to treat patients with various types of advanced head and neck cancers. A study of 29 patients from whom 19 were evaluable patients, only three partial responses were observed.[120] A limited number of studies evaluated a combined retinoid therapy with either chemotherapy or radiation therapy in patients with cancer of the head and neck. However, impressive results were reported by a Japanese group in 48 patients who received Vitamin A and 5-FU administered before each daily radiotherapy. Thirty-three of these patients had laryngeal cancer and an overall 4-year survival rate of 78% as compared to controls of approximately 55%. Fifteen patients were treated for hypopharyngeal cancer and had an overall 3-year rate of 60%, as compared to an overall 3-year rate of <50% in patients treated with surgery or radiation.[121] Although these combination studies are promising, their therapeutic design makes the exact contribution of Vitamin A unclear. Further evaluation of a single-agent retinoid and the overall response (CR + PR) rate in patients with advanced head and neck cancer is needed

Lung cancer — There are no conclusive studies regarding the role of retinoids in patients with squamous cell carcinoma (SCC) of the lung. Thus, in a small number of patients, nine male patients with unresectable SCC were treated with Vitamin A palmitate or isotretinoin; only one objective response was demonstrated in a patient with histologically proven cancer.[122] In a Phase II trial involving 33 lung cancer patients, 22 of whom were evaluable, only two minor responses and six disease stabilizations were reported. These results indicate that retinoids are not effective in the treatment of advanced nonsmall cell lung cancer.[102]

Ovarian cancer — One partial response occurred in an ovarian cancer patient with a 50% decrease in a pelvic mass and resolution of ascites. Two complete responses (CR) were achieved in five patients with minimal disease choriocarcinoma. One of these has been sustained for $3^1/_2$ years. This is a high rate of response.[102] No objective responses occurred in other types of cancers, such as breast, prostate, colon, bladder, cervical, and brain cancer, and carcinoid, testicular, or Kaposi's sarcoma associated with AIDS.

5. Side Effects and Toxicity

The adverse and toxic effects of excessive intake of retinoid, or hypervitaminosis A, in humans have been known for years. First reports of acute hypervitaminosis A involved Eskimos and arctic explorers who ingested excessive amounts of Vitamin A (retinol) from polar bear or seal liver (5 to 8 mg of retinol/g of liver) and then acutely developed severe headache, drowsiness, irritability, nausea, and vomiting. Later (12 to 24 h) after ingestion, erythema and desquamation of skin developed. All symptoms resolved within 7 to 10 d. Hypervitaminosis A occurs when the intake of retinol exceeds the liver capacity to remove and store. Since there are differences in storage, distribution, and metabolism of Vitamin A (retinol) and its esters, isotretinoin, etretinate, and tretinoin, the toxic effects of Vitamin A and its esters may differ significantly in both type and degree, and seem to be related to the specific analog. In this section, we will discuss separately the side effects of the prototype molecule, Vitamin A (retinol), as well as the toxic effects of the widely used derivatives of Vitamin A, including isotretinoin, etretinate, and tretinoin.

Vitamin A (retinol) — This given in excessive amounts (at least 350,000 IU of Vitamin A by infants and 1,000,000 IU by adults) will produce major acute toxic effects in 12 to 24 h after ingestion. Later minor acute side effects which are more frequent will occur. Chronic toxic effects result from the ingestion of lower daily amounts of retinoids over months or years. Most side effects are reversible after Vitamin A intake is stopped. Compared to Vitamin A the synthetic retinoids tend to have less severe and fewer central nervous system and liver side effects (Table 5).[22,26,38,40,69,102-126]

Isotretinoin — Isotretinoin is the 13-*cis* retinoic-acid, and was synthesized in 1955. A lag of 30 min to 2 h is observed between ingestion and the appearance of the drug in the

TABLE 5
Side Effects of Vitamin A (Retinol) in Humans

Major acute effects	%	Minor acute effects	%
CNS symptoms		Mucocutaneous symptoms	
Severe headache	28	Cheilitis	>90
Increased CSF pressure	17	Xerosis	30—50
Papilledema, exophthalmos	26	Pruritus	10—20
		Alopecia	0—5
Irritability	19	Epistaxis	25—35
Dizziness	17	Conjunctivitis	38—75
Nausea, vomiting, fatigue, lethargy	5—15	Skin and nail fragility	30
		Bone pain	16
		Hepatomegaly	16
		Splenomegaly	5
		Edema	10
		Menstrual disorders	3
		Laboratory abnormalities, elevated SGOT	10—20
		SGPT, alk. phos., elevated sed rate (ESR)	40
		Increased cholesterol	7

Major chronic effects		Minor chronic effects	
Embryologic defects, teratogenic effects	1—3	Cheilitis	40
		Xerosis	50
Bone and joint pain	10—20	Musculoskelatal abnormalities	50—60
Periosteal calcification,			
Cranial hyperostosis	10	Pruritus	35
Hypertriglyceridemia, cholesterolemia	<10	Hair loss	40
		Visual disorders	30
		Headache	40

systemic circulation, with maximum blood concentrations occurring between 1 and 4 h after ingestion.[123] Approximately 99% of the drug is bound to serum albumin. Isotretinoin undergoes oxidation and glucoronidation by the liver. The major metabolite of isotretinoin is 4-oxy-isotretinoin, while 20 to 30% of the parent drug isomerizes *in vivo* to tretinoin. Enterohepatic recycling and biliary secretion are characteristic. The drug and its major metabolites are excreted in the urine and the feces. The mean elimination half-life is 20 h, reaching a steady state in 5 to 7 d.[127] The side effects of isotretinoin are generally mucocutaneous, dose-dependent, and reversible with discontinuation of the drug (See Table 6).[123,124,128,129] Isotretinoin has a higher teratogenic effect in animals, including defects such as cleft palate, craniofacial malformations, and abnormalities of the eye. Also, birth defects occur (48 congenital malformations reported to the FDA by 1986) in those born to patients taking isotretinoin during the first trimester of pregnancy.[129] Birth defects, including small or absent ears, severe central nervous system defects (hydrocephalus, microcephalus, cardiovascular defects, facial dysmorphia, cleft palate, and spontaneous abortions) have occurred at rates as high as 100% when patients are taking the drug into the second month of gestation. Therefore, the drug must not be recommended for pregnant women or those women who may become pregnant while undergoing treatment. More than 60 mg/kg/d of isotretinoin was found to produce severe headache, vertigo, ataxia, and desquamative dermatitis. The side effects are resolved without residua when the drug is discontinued.

Etretinate — This is widely used in Europe and has only recently been approved in the U.S. It produces fewer skeletal and lipid abnormalities, but severe hepatotoxicity and marked teratogenesis due to its long half-life (80 to 100 d), as compared to isotretinoin.

TABLE 6
Side Effects of Isotretinoin in Humans

Central nervous system
Headache   6—25
Insomnia   5
Psychological changes   1
Musculoskeletal
Bone, joint, muscle pain   12—15
Mucocutaneous
Cheilitis   90—100
Xerosis   30—60
Pruritus   15—25
Hair loss   10—15
Palmoplantar desquamation   0—5
Conjunctivitis   36—77
Epistaxis, petechiae   25—35
Skin fragility   31
Gastrointestinal
Nausea/vomiting   20
Anorexia   4
Laboratory abnormalities
Elevated cholesterol level   7
Hypertriglyceridemia   25—50
Elevated transaminase   10—15
Elevated platelet count   10—14
Elevated ESR   40—50
Decreased RBC indices   10—15
Decreased WBC   10

Note: Values are expressed as percentages.

The common clinical findings include mucocutaneous symptoms, such as cheilitis (78%), palmar plantar exfoliations (31%), xerosis (21%), and pruritus (15%).[126,127] Reports of hepatotoxicity with abnormal liver function are increasing and now occur in 8 to 40% of etretinate-treated patients.

Topical tretinoin — This commonly causes skin irritation (erythema, desquamation) and reversible hypopigmentation. Toxic effects accompanying oral tretinoin are similar to those with Vitamin A, except severe hepatotoxicity, because tretinoin is not stored in the liver. These various side effects are described in Table 7. Most of the adverse effects are reversible after discontinuation of treatment.[130]

B. B VITAMINS (B_1, B_2, B_6, B_{12}, NIACIN) AND CARCINOGENESIS

These are large, water-soluble vitamins which play a crucial, coenzymatic role in nucleic acid synthesis, protein metabolism, cell proliferation, and host immunocompetence. However, their role in carcinogenesis is not yet clearly established. In many instances, the roles of Vitamin B in carcinogenesis are largely extensions of, and linked to, their role in normal metabolism.

1. Vitamin B_1 (Thiamin)

Early studies carried out in animal tumor models are conflicting, due to the relationship among the B vitamins and their relationship with other major dietary components; it is difficult to explain specifically their role in different stages of carcinogenesis as initiation or promotion. There are no epidemiologic studies relating the dietary B vitamins to the occurrence of cancers. Early laboratory investigations indicated no significant differences

TABLE 7
Side Effects of Tretinoin in Humans

Mucocutaneous	
Erythema/desquamation	80
Reversible hypopigmentation	
Xerosis, epistaxis	25—50
Cheilitis	80
Pruritus	23
Hair loss	10
Central nervous system	
Headache, dizziness	80
Lethargy, failure	43
Anorexia	30
Increased intraocular pressure	11
Mental status changes	10
Nausea/vomiting	30

Note: Values are expressed as percentages.

in the incidence of tumors among groups of animals fed minimal, moderate, or high levels of the B vitamins. In three of four experiments, however, the rate of tumor development was faster in mice ingesting moderate amounts of vitamins than in mice ingesting either high or low amounts.[131]

It has also been reported that when intake of all B vitamins was low, the incidence of tumors in mice was decreased.[132] In these early experiments, dietary thiamin, riboflavin, pyridoxine, panthotenate, niacin, and choline, were varied, from levels just adequate for growth to three, and five, or nine times these amounts. Four experiments on the influence of B vitamins in carcinogenesis were performed: two with spontaneous mammary carcinoma and two with carcinogen-induced skin tumors. In each experiment, there were no significant differences in the incidence of tumors among the groups fed the minimal, moderate, or high levels of B vitamins.

However, in three of the four experiments, the carcinomas developed at a faster rate in the mice ingesting moderate amounts of vitamins than in those on either low or high intake.[132] Since the tumor derives its energy mainly from glucose, and this increases the demand for thiamin (B_1), it is interesting that Vitamin B_1 therapy is beneficial in a neurologic paraneoplastic syndrome (opsoclonic cerebellopathy). It is possible that thiamin may have some beneficial therapeutic effects in Wernicke's encephalopathy.

2. Vitamin B_2 (Riboflavin)

It may influence the rates of growth of spontaneous tumors as well as those induced by specific carcinogens. Thus, riboflavin deficiency decreases the rate of growth of spontaneous tumors in laboratory animals but enhances the carcinogenicity of specific drugs, such as the azo dyes, which are degraded by a microsomal hydroxylase system requiring riboflavin.[133] The relationship of riboflavin to cancer was first reported in 1941, namely, its role in liver cancer.[134] It has been demonstrated that riboflavin provided partial protection against hepatic cancer caused by orally administered dimethyl aminoazobenzene in rats by enhancing the detoxification of that carcinogen by a flavin-dependent enzyme system. Since then, antitumor effects of riboflavin deficiency have been extended in a number of animal species and with a wide variety of tumor types.[133] Thus, in C3H mice fed a riboflavin-deficient diet, the development of spontaneous mammary tumors was markedly depressed. Manipulations of dietary riboflavin content were followed by predictable changes of tumor growth rate. In mice fed a diet containing no riboflavin for 3 weeks, the average tumor size was half that of mice fed a riboflavin-supplemented diet.[135] When riboflavin was reintroduced into the deficient diet, tumor size rapidly returned to normal. If riboflavin was again removed from the diet, tumor size decreased in response to dietary change. Also, growth rates of lymphosarcoma in mice, Walker carcinoma, and Novikoff hepatoma in rats are inhibited by dietary riboflavin deficiency.[133,136,137] It is of interest that structural analogs of riboflavin that have appreciable biologic activity, such as 7-methyl-8-ethyl flavin, do not inhibit the growth of tumors. The reason that dietary riboflavin deficiency inhibits the growth of spontaneous tumors in laboratory animals is not known.

Interestingly, riboflavin deficiency is not confirmed to reduce the tumor growth rate, but also tends to enhance the carcinogenicity of certain drugs such as the azo dyes. Azo dye reductase activity is markedly decreased in livers of riboflavin-deficient rats. This microsomal enzyme is important for degradation of carcinogens (azodye). For example, when a small number of mice were treated with dimethyl nitrosamine, those receiving a riboflavin-deficient diet had more lung adenomas and liver carcinomas than riboflavin-fed controls. Thus, with riboflavin deficiency, in which drug degradative capacity is diminished, the dose of carcinogen delivered to susceptible tissues is likely to be greater and the half time of disappearance more prolonged than in normally replete animals.[138]

It has also been reported that local application of riboflavin in the form of tetrabutyrate to the skin of mice treated topically with 3-methylcholanthrene markedly delayed the appearance of skin tumors and reduced their overall incidence. The incidence of papillomas in riboflavin-treated mice was less than one third that of controls, and that of squamous cell carcinomas was two thirds that of controls.[139] Thus, riboflavin deficiency either decreases or increases the tumor development rate in experimental animals with certain carcinogens, and depends on the metabolic degradation of the carcinogen and the species sensitivity.

At present, little is known of the possible role of riboflavin in the etiology of human cancer. Because the microsomal drug hydroxylation system requires flavin coenzymes, it can be stipulated that dietary riboflavin deficiency might retard the degradation and inactivation of carcinogens and thereby enhance their delivery to susceptible tissues. However, direct evidence to support this hypothesis is difficult to obtain, particularly in humans. The antitumor activity in experimental animals prompted some investigators to explore the riboflavin analogs in the treatment of neoplastic and myeloproliferative diseases in humans. A decrease in tumor size occurred in six patients with advanced cancer, such as colon cancer, lymphosarcoma, and lymphadenopathy. Two patients with Hodgkin's disease and several with polycythemia also showed improvement. These patients were treated by a combination therapy using galactoflavin, a potent riboflavin antagonist in rats, together with a riboflavin deficiency.[140] These preliminary findings raise the possibility that riboflavin deficiency was characterized by weight loss, glossitis, cheilosis, seborrheic dermatitis, normocytic anemia, and particularly neuropathy. The preventive or therapeutic potential of this approach is limited, however, by the toxic side effects. Abnormalities in riboflavin metabolism have also been reported in certain patients with multiple myeloma, namely, high specific binding and marked delay in riboflavin excretion, which should prompt investigations for possible metabolic disorders of riboflavin in other tumors.[133,140] Recent epidemiological studies revealed a high riboflavin deficiency in patients with esophageal cancer in different countries (Iran, China, U.S.). Thus, an increased incidence of esophageal cancer was found to be associated with a high riboflavin deficiency associated with deficiencies of other B vitamins, and Vitamins A and C in Iran, China (Linxian Province), among black men in Washington, D.C., and different African populations at risk for esophageal cancer.[141,142]

Although riboflavin deficiency has been detected in several population groups around the world that are at high risk for esophageal cancer, the etiological role of riboflavin deficiency in human esophageal cancer remains to be defined since B_2 vitamin deficiency has been associated with deficiencies of other vitamins or key nutrients. Possible mechanisms of riboflavin in carcinogenesis were suspected long ago, particularly in riboflavin-deficient patients with the Plummer-Vinson syndrome, which is often associated with esophageal cancer. Observations on animal tumor models revealed that early manifestations in riboflavin-deficient mice occurred in the esophagus and squamous epithelial lining of the stomach, and these oxidative damages render the tissue more vulnerable to carcinogens.[141] Riboflavin deficiency may damage other epithelial tissues, but tumor tissue is generally more resistant to dietary deprivation of riboflavin. Previous studies have shown that the progressive development of riboflavin deficiency resulted in a much slower rate in mouse mammary tumor than in muscle or liver from tumor-bearing animals.[135] Thus, the concentration of Vitamin B_2 in tumors from deficient animals is greatly reduced, or in many samples, not detected. Riboflavin affects carcinogenesis, and cancer affects riboflavin metabolism, too.[133]

Recent studies have also shown that riboflavin deficiency greatly increases the rate of prostaglandin biosynthesis, specifically PGE_2 and $PGF_{2\alpha}$, in the rat kidney *in vitro*. Prostaglandins are thought to be mediators of paraneoplastic syndromes such as fever and hypercalcemia. It is possible that control of prostaglandin synthesis may relate to tumor survival and metabolism.[143] Riboflavin deficiency also decreases the glutathione concentration in the erythrocytes and glutathione reductase in the hepatic cells. Both are required for PGE_2 synthesis. Riboflavin deficiency also increased lipid peroxidation of cellular and microsomal membranes. Other investigators have shown that a riboflavin-deficient diet lowers the hepatic activity of ligandin, an enzyme which reacts with chemical carcinogens and reduces the susceptibility of the liver to azodye and aromatic amine-induced carcinogens.[144]

However, it is still difficult to relate all these various activities of riboflavin to carcinogenesis, and further investigations are needed in order to define a direct role of riboflavin in carcinogenesis.

3. Vitamin B 6 (Pyridoxine)

The term "Vitamin B_6" refers to a group of interconvertable compounds that act as an enzyme cofactor for many amino acid interconversions. The predominant dietary forms are pyridoxine, pyridoxal, pyridoxamine, pyridoxal 5′-phosphate (PLP) and pyridoxamine 5′-phosphate (PMP). They cross the intestinal mucosa by a passive transfer after being dephosphorylated; then they are transported to the liver, muscle, and other organs and are converted to the biologically active forms, PLP and PMP. These forms, predominantly PLP, are then used as coenzymes for over 100 known enzymatic reactions. Due to the high chemical reactivity of these forms of the vitamin, they may react and modulate many regulatory compounds, including certain carcinogens.

Vitamin B_6 deficiency involves an essential nutrient, and an abnormal metabolism of tryptophan, which results in the production of tumors. The interaction of Vitamin B_6 and tryptophan involves, instead, normal and abnormal metabolism of compounds essential to life.

Thus, Vitamin B_6 deficiency has been implicated in the production of bladder tumors and kidney hyperplastic nodules, as a result of the excess exposure to tryptophan metabolites, and in the production of breast tumors, possibly by suppression of the immune system or alteration in the regulation of polyamine synthesis.[145] PLP, which is the biologically active form of Vitamin B_6, plays a crucial coenzymatic role in nucleic acid synthesis, protein metabolism, and cell proliferation. A deficiency of this vitamin in animals and humans has been correlated with atrophy of lymphoid organs and impairment of both humoral and cell-mediated immunity.[146] Several investigators have reported that pyridoxine deficiency can inhibit the development of epithelial tumors and sarcomas in mice.[147] An early study found that spontaneous mammary carcinoma and chemically induced skin tumors grew more rapidly in mice that ingested moderate amounts of six B vitamins (including B_6) than those in animals consuming the same vitamins at either low or high levels.[131] Additionally, high levels of pyridoxine or pyridoxal either suppress growth or exhibit cytotoxicity against animal or human cancer cells *in vitro*.[148]

A recent study showed suppression of tumor growth and enhancement of immune status with high levels of dietary Vitamin B_6 in BALB/c mice. Thus, high dietary intake of Vitamin B_6 (megadoses) decreased significantly the volume of primary tumor as well as the number of metastases in mice with tumors induced by herpes simplex virus Type 2-transformed (H238) cells. There is a dose relationship between Vitamin B_6 and tumor growth. Mice fed lower doses (2 mg) had the largest primary tumor volume, the highest incidence of lung metastases, and the greatest number of metastatic nodules per animal at 7 weeks post-injection, as compared to animals fed with high doses (7.7 and 74.3 mg), which had lower tumor volumes and metastases. These data suggest that high doses of Vitamin B_6 have suppressed tumor development by either immune enhancement or PLP growth regulation of this tumor.[149] Also, mice with Vitamin B_6 deficiency developed significantly larger tumors (Moloney sarcoma virus-induced tumors) than those fed with adequate Vitamin B_6 diet.[150] Several studies reported alterations in Vitamin B_6 levels and clinical manifestations of certain cancers (breast and bladder cancer, Hodgkin's disease, and melanoma).[151-153] Breast cancer patients who excreted subnormal amounts of 4-pyridoxic acid had a significantly high probability of breast cancer recurrence after mastectomy. PLP was normal in early breast cancer, but was significantly lower in cases of local recurrence and systemic metastases. Abnormal tryptophan metabolism, after a tryptophan load, occurred in patients with bladder cancer, breast cancer, and Hodgkin's disease. Abnormal tryptophan metabolism and low Vitamin B_6 metabolic levels are of great concern for cancer patients since metabolic disturbances are of importance in view of the immunosuppressive effects of pyridoxine deficiency. Additionally, it was found that Vitamin B_6 exerts cytotoxic effects to several cancer cells, including melanoma cell line.[148] A topical cream of pyridoxal was applied to patients with recurrent malignant melanomas, and it was found to produce a significant reduction in the size of subcutaneous nodules and a complete regression of cutaneous papules.[154] However, these results are preliminary and require confirmation. Also, pyridoxine megatherapy in certain psychiatric disorders needs to be confirmed.

4. Vitamin B_{12} (Cyanocobalamin) and Folate

The roles of Vitamin B_{12} and folate in carcinogenesis are large extensions of, and linked to, their roles in normal metabolism, particularly 1-carbon unit metabolism. A possible key area may be hypomethylation to "switch on" genes and methylation to "switch them off". Some vitamin analogs may act as antivitamins in these reactions, as may some vitamin-binding proteins. Others may act as specific delivery proteins. Using appropriate radioactive substrates and suspensions of vitamin-dependent normal and malignant cells, it is possible to work out their positive and negative control of DNA synthesis.[155] A significant body of experimental evidence supports the notion that a deficiency of either Vitamin B_{12} or folic acid enhances the activity of various carcinogens. Vitamin B_{12} is not vitamin active in its stable pharmaceutical form, cyanocobalamin. The cyanide must be removed for vitamin function to occur.

Although the cocarcinogenic effect of methionine deficiency is well recognized, the consensus of opinion has been that B_{12} and folate deficiencies should decrease the risk of cancer development. As early as 1950, a marked procarcinogenic effect of Vitamin B_{12} on p-dimethyl aminoazobenzene (DAB)-fed rats had been reported.[156] Thus, the addition of 50 μg Vitamin B_{12} to the diet increased the incidence of hepatomas to 78%. On the other hand, adding 0.6% DL-methionine to the basal diet with or without a Vitamin B_{12} supplement, decreased the hepatoma incidence to 11 and 33%, respectively. The control group of rats receiving Vitamin B_{12}-supplemented diet without DAB had no hepatic tumors. This study clearly demonstrated that Vitamin B_{12} is not a carcinogen by itself, but markedly enhanced the carcinogenic effect of a chemical carcinogen. The procarcinogenic effect of Vitamin B_{12} has since been repeatedly demonstrated. Thus, in experiments with a larger number of animals involving the addition of 50 μg of Vitamin B_{12}/kg to female rats fed with DAB (200 mg/kg), after 6 months only 37% of the surviving deficient rats had liver tumors, whereas 78% on the diet supplemented with B_{12} had developed liver tumors. The potentiating effect of Vitamin B_{12} has also been demonstrated with 2-acetylamino-fluorene and diethylnitrosamine in rat liver, azoxymethane in rat colon, and methylcholanthrene in skin tumors and sarcoma induction in mice.[157-159]

In humans, vitamin B_{12} deficiency appears to slow down the course of hematopoietic malignancy associated with pernicious anemia. Administration of B_{12} accelerates the progression of the already established malignant disease. Numerous reports support the notion that patients with Vitamin B_{12} deficiency are at increased risk of developing hematopoietic malignancy and several isolated cases of pernicious anemia and leukemia have been reported. Thus, in 1625 patients with pernicious anemia, the incidence of death secondary to leukemia was in excess of three times the expected rate. A total of ten patients developed leukemia, predominantly of the myeloid type, and a high incidence of stomach cancer.[160] An antitumor effect of Vitamin B_{12} has also been reported in human cancers. Massive doses (1 mg injected i.m. daily or every other day) of Vitamin B_{12} have been used to treat neuroblastoma in children and retinoblastoma, and it has been claimed to obtain tumor regression or arrest in 55 of 101 patients.[161] However, subsequent studies have failed to confirm these reports.[162]

In summary, the data from literature suggest that Vitamin B_{12} may act as cocarcinogen, anticarcinogen, or procarcinogen, depending on its level in nutrition. A cocarcinogenic effect can be demonstrated when body stores of the vitamins are depleted, a condition that may experimentally induce, or that may develop secondary to, B_{12} malabsorption in humans. This Vitamin B_{12} deficiency markedly enhances the activity of chemical carcinogenesis in hepatocarcinogenesis, or in humans, deficiency increases the risk of hematopoietic malignancy in pernicious anemia. At slightly higher levels, the cocarcinogenic effect disappears, and an anticarcinogenic effect takes place. At higher levels, Vitamin B_{12} exerts a carcinotrophic effect, directly stimulating the growth of each tumor.[163]

A recent study showed a significant improvement in bronchial squamous metaplasia in heavy smokers treated with folate and Vitamin B_{12}. Seventy-three men with a history of heavy smoking who had metaplasia on one or more sputum samples were divided in two groups and were treated for 4 months with either placebo or 10 mg of folate plus 500 μg of hydroxocobalamin. Direct cytological comparison of the two groups after 4 months showed significantly greater reduction of atypia in the Vitamin B_{12} supplemented group. This provides preliminary evidence that atypical bronchial squamous metaplasia may be reduced by supplementation with folate and Vitamin B_{12}. However, this procedure should not be used for preventing lung cancer in individuals who continue to smoke.[164]

5. Niacin and Nicotinamide

Niacin is pyridine-3-carboxylic acid (See Figure 2). Niacin is present in foods and is available in drug form. Niacin is easily bioconverted to the metabolically active form nicotinamide. Dietary deficiencies and excesses of these vitamins by themselves do not appear to exert any influence on *in vivo* carcinogenesis in animals. Administration of nicotinamide at pharmacologic doses concurrently with, or following, carcinogen administration to mice or rats has produced different results; in some studies tumor formation increased,[165] whereas carcinogenesis was significantly inhibited,[166] or no effects were observed in other investigations.[167] The lung and kidney were affected in mice, whereas pancreas, intestine, and urinary bladder were affected in rats. Nicotinamide was reported to promote the development of kidney tumors induced by DEN in rats.[165]

The mechanisms by which nicotinamide influences carcinogenesis are not known.[168] Epidemiological studies have not determined the relationship between niacin deficiency or excess and carcinogenesis in humans. It has been suggested that diets relatively deficient in niacin, zinc, magnesium, and possibly riboflavin, may play a role in the etiology of esophageal cancer.[169] The modulation of carcinogenesis by the B vitamins under conditions of normal dietary intake is probably minimal. However, these vitamins may also modulate other processes, such as immunosurveillance, which may affect the ultimate outcome of carcinogenesis. Thus, impairment of the immune function has been demonstrated in pyridoxine-deficient animals, and it seems likely that major disruption of energy or carbohydrate metabolism by riboflavin or thiamin deficiencies, as well as disruption of normal cell replication by Vitamin B_{12} deficiency, would affect immunosurveillance and carcinogenesis. However, due to the inter-relationship among the B vitamins and their relationship with other major dietary components, it is difficult to evaluate specifically the role of each vitamin on different stages of carcinogenesis.

C. VITAMIN C (ASCORBIC ACID) IN CARCINOGENESIS

Vitamin C is an essential nutrient whose protective role in carcinogenesis has been discussed for more than 50 years. Epidemiological studies suggest that the consumption of Vitamin C-rich foods is associated with a lower risk of cancers of the esophagus and stomach. The observation that cancer patients have low leukocyte Vitamin C levels, led to therapeutic trials with controversial results.[170] Experimental studies in animal tumor models, or *in vitro* using cell cultures, showed that Vitamin C can effectively inhibit the formation of carcinogenic nitrosamines and thus prevent tumor development.[171] Vitamin C supplementation has been reported to inhibit skin, nerve, lung, and kidney carcinogenesis. The addition of Vitamin C to the diet resulted in a marked inhibition of pulmonary tumors in mice induced by nitroso compounds.[172] Ascorbic acid also inhibits urinary bladder tumors induced by 3-hydroxyanthranilic acid in mice and reduces the frequency of diethylstilbestrol (DES)-induced kidney clear cell carcinoma in male Syrian hamsters.[173]

Furthermore, the survival rate of mice with leukemia and Ehrlich carcinoma was increased after daily treatment with 4 mg Vitamin C, plus 2 mg Vitamin B_{12} i.p. The decreased mortality of ascorbate-treated mice might result from the reduced density of microvilli on the surface of the cancer cells.[174] Growth of 3-methylcholanthrene-induced tumors in guinea pigs increased when the animals were put on high ascorbic acid diet after the tumors became palpable. Tumors tended to have a shorter latent period in the group of guinea pigs receiving Vitamin C.[175] The guinea pig is the only laboratory animal that, like primates, does not synthesize Vitamin C. Inhibition of colon carcinogenesis induced by 1.2-dimethylhydrazine (DMH)-initiated in rats has also been reported following ascorbic acid treatment. Others found no effect of ascorbic acid on DMH-induced colon carcinogenesis. Thus, ascorbic acid had no effect on colon carcinoma or lymphosarcoma in mice, mammary tumors in rats, or urinary bladder tumors induced by nitrosamine and FANFT in rats.[176,177] However, Vitamin C or sodium ascorbate supplementation has been reported to inhibit skin cancer (mouse skin papillomas induced by DMBA-croton oil), neurogenic cancer (ethylurea-induced peripheral nervous system tumors in the offspring of pregnant hamsters), lung (pulmonary adenomas), and kidney cancer (induced by DES in male hamsters). It also has been reported to inhibit, not to affect, or enhance mammary gland and colon carcinogenesis, and to enhance urinary bladder carcinogenesis (when given as sodium ascorbate, but not as ascorbic acid).

Thus, the effects of Vitamin C on animal carcinogenesis are still conflicting. The picture has become complex because various types of cancer have been studied using different carcinogens at various doses, with different routes of administration and with different animal species. Sufficient evidence suggests that Vitamin C can inhibit tumors produced by nitrosamine in animals through inhibition of nitrosamine formation.[171]

Ascorbic acid is reported to have various effects on the metabolism of tumor cells and to change cellular manifestations of malignancy. When C3H10T^1/$_2$ mouse embryo cells are exposed to 3-methylcholanthrene, morphological transformation occurs. However, the transformation is prevented if ascorbic acid is added to the culture medium. Addition of the ascorbic acid as late as 23 d after the treatment with 3-methylcholanthrene still completely inhibits transformation and causes reversion of chemically transformed cells to normal-appearing morphological phenotypes by adding ascorbic acid to the culture medium.[178] The effects of ascorbic acid on human leukemia cells in culture have also been studied. Low concentrations of ascorbic acid were found to suppress growth of human leukemia cells from patients with acute nonlymphocytic leukemia under conditions in which growth of normal myeloid colonies was not suppressed.[179]

Vitamin C has been shown to reduce the *in vitro* mutagenic actions of several carcinogens which are nitroso compounds. Sodium ascorbate causes chromosomal damage in Chinese hamster ovary cells in culture and this damage is further enhanced by some metals (Cu, Mn, Fe).[180] The intrinsic mechanism of action of Vitamin C on tumor cells is still unknown. It has been postulated that in order to produce selective cell death in tumor tissue, it is necessary that the tumor cells generate enough intracellular H_2O_2 to cause cell deaths. Tumor cells can also accomplish this by an accumulation of large amounts of intracellular Vitamin C and/or by an inhibition of catalase activity. Normal cells have both catalase and peroxidase activities, whereas tumor cells have predominantly catalase activity with little or no peroxidase due to a mutational event. Therefore, the efficacy of Vitamin C treatment may vary depending upon the number of cells having predominantly catalase activity with little or no peroxidase in a tumor mass at the time of Vitamin C treatment.[181]

Interestingly, from a therapeutic point of view, *in vitro* data reveal that Vitamin C at a nontoxic concentration with certain pharmacologic agents and ionizing radiation produced a synergistic or an additive effect on the growth inhibition of mouse neuroblastoma (NBP_2) cells in culture; it did not produce such an effect on rat glioma (C-6) cells in culture. For example, sodium ascorbate at a nontoxic concentration potentiates the growth inhibitory effect of 5-FU, bleomycin sulfate, and sodium butyrate on neuroblastoma cells in culture, but it does not produce such effect on glioma cells in culture. Sodium ascorbate (Vitamin C) did not enhance the growth inhibitory effect of vincristine, or 6-thioguanine; however, at higher drug concentrations, it potentiated the effect of these drugs in a synergistic manner. The potentiating effect of Vitamin C in combination with certain tumor therapeutic agents is not prevented by the addition of catalase in the growth medium, and suggests that this effect of the combined treatment is not mediated by H_2O_2. Sodium ascorbate can also reduce the cytotoxic effect of certain pharmacologic agents, such as reducing the cytotoxic effect of methotrexate on neuroblastoma cells in culture. The modification of the effect of ionizing radiation is dependent upon the type of tumor cell. Sodium ascorbate increased the effect of ionizing radiation on neuroblastoma cells in culture, but it did not modify the effect of irradiation on survival of glioma cells.[181] *In vivo* studies showed that Vitamin C, when combined with ionizing radiation, also increased the survival of mice with ascites tumor cells in comparison to those treated with X-irradiation alone.[181] These studies indicate that Vitamin C may modify the effect of pharmacologic agents in a variety of ways.

1. Possible Mechanisms of Action

Vitamin C intervenes in the regulation of the oxidation-reduction potential of the cell. It acts as a reducing compound in the aqueous medium of the cell. Vitamin C may act synergistically with Vitamin E, exerting a stronger antioxidant effect than either vitamin alone. As an antioxidant, Vitamin C may also have potential anticancer activity. It is established that Vitamin C can inhibit the formation of nitrosamines from precursors.

Several possible mechanisms of action are suggested, such as modifying the metabolic pattern of polycylic hydrocarbons by shifting the equilibrium between metabolic activation and inactivation of carcinogenic compounds. Thus, most carcinogens require activation by enzymes present in the cells in order to react with cell nucleophiles such as DNA.

Antioxidants may act in several ways to modify the activation of chemical carcinogens by affecting the activity of enzymes. They may modify the activity of enzymes involved in oxidative xenobiotic metabolism. These are microsomal enzymes which catalyze Phase I reactions to increase the activities of enzymes in liver and peripheral tissues, which can inactivate reactive electrophilic metabolites of many xenobiotics. There are also enzymes catalyzing Phase-II reactions. Thus, microsomal hydroxylation and demethylating systems and the associated electron transport protein, such as cytochrome P-450, are decreased in animals under conditions of ascorbic acid depletion. Hepatic microsomal hydroxylation and demethylation systems were depressed by 50% in ascorbic acid-deficient guinea pigs.[182] Antioxidants may act to reduce mutagenic activity by blocking the formation of mutagenic and carcinogenic nitrosamines, mutagenesis by nitroso compounds, and DMBA, a colon and breast carcinogen.[183] As with the activation and inactivation of carcinogens, antioxidants may modify the metabolism of premutagens and mutagens, shifting metabolic pattern toward the production of inactive metabolites. Antioxidants may also react with genotoxic free radicals. These free radicals can interact with a variety of cellular molecules resulting in inhibition or alteration of lipid peroxidation, DNA damage, and enzyme inactivation. Certain promoters of carcinogenesis act by generation of oxygen radicals. Furthermore, many complete carcinogens also cause the production of oxygen radicals. Examples are nitroso compounds, hydrazines, quinones, polycyclic hydrocarbons, cadmium and lead salts, nitro compounds, and radiation. Some of these free radicals, like those initiated by ionizing radiation, may serve as a continuous source of tumor initiators and promoters, and subsequently result in tumor formation.[184] Vitamin C inhibits the cell growth of several cell lines (neuroblastoma, glioma, and melanoma) in culture. From these studies, it appears that Vitamin C action is dependent upon the cell type. Generally, cells require a very large concentration of Vitamin C to produce a growth inhibitory effect. The effect of high doses of Vitamin C on cell growth inhibition is mediated by hydrogen peroxide (H_2O_2) which is formed at the cell surface because the addition of exogenous catalase to the growth medium prevents Vitamin C-induced growth inhibition.[185] Vitamin C enhances cellular immunity acting as a biologic redox agent and stimulates functions of leukocytes and macrophages, such as chemotaxis and phagocytosis.[170] The cellular immune response is compromised when the leukocyte Vitamin C is low, and it has been suggested that lung cancer patients with or without resection, have a better prognosis if they have higher lymphocyte counts.[186]

Hence, there is no single cellular or biochemical mechanism which can explain the effects of Vitamin C on cancer development. Vitamin C acts by complex mechanisms and has multiple functions. Thus, Vitamin C is a potent redox agent as well as a prooxidant, depending on the dose used, and may act as a chelating agent for copper and iron. It is also involved in mutagenesis, collagen biosynthesis, enzyme activity (cytochromic P-450), maintenance of polysomes, stimulation of chemotaxis and phagocytosis, protection against infection, detoxification processes, enhancement of the immune system, wound healing, prevention of thiol group oxidation, biosynthesis of norepinephrine, and metabolism of histamine, cyclic nucleotides, and prostaglandins.[187]

2. Epidemiological Studies

These studies revealed an inverse relationship between concentration of Vitamin C and risk of cancer. In general, the data suggest that Vitamin C may lower the risk of cancer, particularly in the esophagus and stomach. However, the association of Vitamin C with cancer in epidemiological studies is mostly indirect since it is based on the consumption of foods known to contain high concentrations of the vitamin, and not on actual intake of Vitamin C. Thus, an inverse association of both Vitamin A and Vitamin C consumption with esophageal cancer has been observed. The relationship was statistically significant for Vitamin C, but not for Vitamin A after controlling for smoking and alcohol use.[188] Based on correlational and case-control studies, an inverse relationship between esophageal cancer and consumption of fresh fruits and calculated intake of Vitamin C in human populations in the Caspian litoral of Iran has been found.[189]

Similar inverse associations between fresh fruit, i.e., citrus fruit consumption, and gastric cancer have been reported by several investigators.[190-192] These observations are consistent with the hypothesis that Vitamin C protects against gastric cancer by blocking the reaction of secondary and higher amines with nitrite to form nitrosamines. Recently, a hospital-based case-control study of gastric cancer precursor lesions in the U.S. showed a two-fold increased risk in patients with nitrite at pH > 5.0 in stomach juice. The case control comparison showed a protective effect associated with fruit, vegetable, and dietary Vitamin C. The formation of *N*-nitroso compound is increased when less Vitamin C-containing fruits and vegetables are consumed.[193] This was confirmed recently in patients with cancer of the uterus, cervix, and ovary, and in patients with leukemia and lymphoma.[194] A decrease of Vitamin C plasma levels due to irradiation treatment has been reported. Combined administration of Vitamin C reduced the side-effects of radiotherapy.[195] A protective role for Vitamin C in laryngeal cancer was also reported in a case-control study. An inverse relationship between cancer risk and indices of both Vitamins C and A, after controlling for smoking and alcohol consumption, has been found. There was a similar relationship for vegetable consumption in general, but not for cruciferous vegetables in particular.[196]

A similar inverse association between Vitamin C consumption and uterine dysplasia in a case-control study of women in New York, has been recently reported. These findings persisted after the investigators controlled for age and sexual activity in the analysis.[197] However, no association between Vitamin C consumption and colon cancer in a case-control study based on quantitative data obtained from dietary history has been found.[198] Thus, the epidemiologic data regarding the effect of Vitamin C on the occurrence of cancer are not extensive. Furthermore, they provide mostly indirect evidence since they are based mainly on the consumption of foods, especially fresh fruits and vegetables, known to contain high concentrations of vitamin, rather than on actual measurements of Vitamin C intake. The results of several case-control studies and a few correlation studies suggest that the consumption of Vitamin C-containing foods is associated with a lower risk of certain cancers, particularly gastric and esophageal cancers.

3. Clinical Trials

These are based on certain *in vitro* and *in vivo* data which showed that Vitamin C exerts some antitumor effects on animal models as well as in various neoplastic cell lines in culture. Also, epidemiological studies revealed that consumption of a low Vitamin C diet increases the risk of cancer, particularly esophageal and gastric cancers. In fact, the finding of low ascorbate levels in leukocytes of cancer patients provided the impetus for clinical studies using high doses of Vitamin C or megadoses (megavitamin therapy or orthomolecular therapy).[199,200] It has also been postulated that increased amounts of ascorbic acid are reduced in collagen synthesis for the protective encapsulation of tumors; that it provides feedback inhibition of lysosomal glycosidases, which are responsible for malignant invasiveness; and that it functions by stimulating the immune system of host resistance, including immunocompetence.[201]

Vitamin C was postulated to increase host resistance against cancer by a variety of mechanisms, including enhancing lymphocyte function, increasing the resistance of the intercellular ground substance to hydrolysis by hyaluronidase elaborated by tumor cells, and protecting the pituitary-adrenal axis from the effects of stress. Also, ascorbic acid is cytotoxic to mammalian cells from a variety of species. It potentiates the *in vitro* cytotoxicity of several chemotherapeutic agents.[181,182,186]

The first large-scale trial of Vitamin C in human cancer therapy started in the early

1970s. One hundred terminal cancer patients were given large doses of ascorbate (10 g/d) as part of their routine management; 1000 similar patients who were treated identically, but received no ascorbate, served as controls. This study, conducted at the Vale of Leven Hospital in Scotland, suggested that ascorbate had a remarkably positive effect on survival; the mean survival time of those receiving ascorbate was more than 4.2 times (210 d) greater than survival time for the controls (50 d).[202] In addition, regression of grossly measurable tumors occurred in several cases.[203]

A similar study at the Mayo Clinic involved 150 patients with advanced cancer in a controlled double-blind study in which 10 g of ascorbic acid was given daily; the other group received a comparably flavored lactose placebo. The results were clear-cut: Vitamin C was no better than placebo with respect to either amelioration or survival time and median survival for all patients was about 7 weeks.[204] However, this study was criticized in that the cytotoxic chemotherapy given to a large majority of patients before the study entry might have compromised the ability of Vitamin C to stimulate the host defense. Thus, this study has been repeated in a controlled double-blind clinical trial in 100 patients with colorectal cancer who had not received chemotherapy or irradiation. The results showed that administering 10 g of Vitamin C by mouth each day did not improve survival of control symptoms, as compared with placebo. In addition, none of the 19 patients with measurable tumor masses had shrinkage of tumors.[205] The use of antioxidants to control large bowel adenomas was tested in a randomized, double-blind study of 49 patients with polyposis coli. Of 36 patients who were evaluated at completion, 19 had received 3 g/d of ascorbic acid and 17 had received placebo. A significant reduction of polyposis coli was found and it was suggested that ascorbic acid may play a role in chemoprevention.[206]

D. ROLE OF VITAMIN D (CALCIFEROL) IN CARCINOGENESIS

Vitamin D has long been studied in relation to bone and calcium homeostasis only. Recently, it has been shown that Vitamin D is progressively metabolized by the liver and then the kidney by hydroxylation to an active hormonal form, $1\alpha,25$-dihydroxyvitamin D_3 ($1\alpha,25(OH)_2D_3$), which is the active form of Vitamin D responsible for calcium and phosphorus homeostasis in the blood.[207] Recent evidence, however, suggested a wider biologic role of $1\alpha,25(OH)_2D_3$ in tissues or cells not primarily related to mineral metabolism. It has been found that $1\alpha,25(OH)_2D_3$ binds to a specific cytosol receptor and exerts its biologic action by a mechanism analogous to that proposed for other steroid hormones (estrogens, progesterone, glucocorticoids). Thus, the receptor-ligand complex acts on the chromatin to induce transcription of specific genes. Intracellular receptors that bind $1\alpha,25(OH)_2D_3$ with high affinity have been found in a large number of normal mammalian cell types (intestine, kidney, bone-osteoblasts, parathyroid glands, epidermal cells, fibroblasts, myocardium, mammary tissue, uterus, ovary, testes, pituitary gland, colon, thymus, circulating monocytes, and lymphocytes) as well as in a large number of cancer cells (osteosarcoma, melanoma, breast carcinoma, colon carcinoma, medullary thyroid carcinoma, myeloid and lymphocytic leukemia, pancreatic adenocarcinoma, bladder carcinoma, cervical carcinoma, and fibrosarcoma).[208-210] The $1\alpha,25(OH)_2D_3$ receptor in these cells has similar characteristics to the receptors in bone and intestine, the known target tissues of the hormone. In fact, $1\alpha,25(OH)_2D_3$ inhibits the proliferation of melanoma, osteosarcoma, and breast carcinoma cells.

More recently, $1\alpha,25(OH)_2D_3$ has been shown to suppress the growth and induce monocytic differentiation of murine and human myeloid leukemia cells *in vitro*. A recent study also showed clear-cut, time- and dose-dependent, yet reversible, effects of $1\alpha,25(OH)_2D_3$ on the replication of human cancer cells *in vitro* and *in vivo*, which are possibly mediated through changes in growth factor receptor levels. These results suggest a significant involvement of Vitamin D in cell differentiation and replication in human cancers. Hence, analogs of the Vitamin D hormone may be of interest as possible therapeutic agents in cancer treatment.

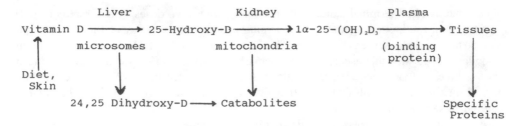

FIGURE 3.   Metabolic pathways of Vitamin D_3 and its metabolites.

Thus, Vitamin D plays an important role in cancer biology. To date, as many as 20 metabolites of Vitamin D have been identified and characterized chemically.[211] Whether any of these products has a unique biologic acitivity, however, is not known.

In addition to the kidney, synthesis of $1\alpha,25(OH)_2D_3$ has been found in other tissues, including cells which are targets for the actions of $1\alpha,25(OH)_2D_3$, and might prove to be important for an autocrine role of this vitamin in the regulation of its target tissues.

Vitamin D and its metabolites are transported in blood bound to the plasma D-binding protein (DBP). This is an α-globulin identical to the human group specific component (GC), and is synthesized in the liver and is structurally homologous to two other blood proteins, albumin and α-fetoprotein at both the protein level and the genomic DNA level.[212] It has an estimated molecular weight of between 50 and 60 kDa, and has one binding site for the Vitamin D secosteroids. At present, there is no evidence that DBP enters the cells. The relatively low affinity of DBP for $1\alpha,25(OH)_2D_3$, in combination with the high affinity of the intracellular receptor, allows this hormonal metabolite to enter its target cells readily.[210] The preferential entry of $1\alpha,25(OH)_2D_3$ is of paramount importance in the function of the Vitamin D endocrine system. Thus, Vitamin D from the diet and the skin is converted in the liver at the level of microsomes to 25-hydroxy-D and then in the kidney at the level of the mitochondria to $1\alpha,25$-dihydroxy-D_3 ($1\alpha,25(OH)_2D_3$), which binds to plasma proteins, enters the cells, and acts on specific proteins. Schematically, these metabolic pathways can be seen in Figure 3.

These metabolic pathways can be significantly influenced by hormones, such as thyroid hormones, and low concentrations of $1\alpha,25(OH)_2D_3$ were found in hypothyroidism, whereas estrogens, calcitonin, growth hormone, prolactin, insulin, and glucocorticoids can increase serum levels of $1\alpha,25(OH)_2D_3$, particularly estrogens. Testosterone does not change the serum levels of Vitamin D metabolites.

Understanding of metabolic regulation of Vitamin D_3, particularly of its active metabolic product, $1\alpha,25(OH)_2D_3$, is of paramount importance for its therapeutic use. The concentration of DBP in normal adult human plasma is approximately 500 mg/l, but 3 to 5% of DBP is normally saturated. This huge binding capacity provides a large storage, and DBP serves as a reservoir during periods of inadequate light exposure and dietary deprivation. However, from a physiologic point of view, only the free fraction of $1\alpha,25(OH)_2D_3$ (which is not bound to DBP), is biologically active.[213] Changes in DBP have no physiologic significance for the function of Vitamin D hormone.

Intensive research during the last 15 years has disclosed that $1\alpha,25(OH)_2D_3$ exerts its actions via specific intracellular receptors in a manner similar to that of steroid (estrogens) and thyroid hormones. The discovery of its receptors in normal as well as in cancer cells has contributed greatly to our understanding of the Vitamin D endocrine system and its role in pathophysiology and cancer biology. It has now been established that the $1\alpha,25(OH)_2D_3$ receptor is a protein with a molecular weight of 50 to 60 kDa and with a sedimentation coefficient of 3.1 to 3.75. The receptor represents less than 0.001% of the soluble cellular protein (10,000 to 20,000 receptor sites/cell). The isolated receptor protein binds $1\alpha,25(OH)_2D_3$

TABLE 9

Normal Cells Possessing $1\alpha,25(OH)_2D_3$

Receptor

TABLE 8

Cancer Cells Possessing

$1\alpha,25(OH)_2D_3$ Receptor

Cancer Cells (Table 8)	Normal Cells (Table 9)
	Kidney
	Intestine
	Bone (osteoblasts)
	Mammary tissue
	Skin (keratinocytes, fibroblasts)
Melanoma	Hair follicle
Breast carcinoma	Testes
Osteosarcoma	Ovary
Lymphoma	Uterus
Colon carcinoma	Placenta
Lung carcinoma	Pancreas
Medullary thyroid carcinoma	Colon
Myeloma	Pituitary gland
Pancreatic adenocarcinoma	Myocardium
Cervical carcinoma	Thymus (thymocytes)
Fibrosarcoma	Parathyroid gland
Pituitary adenoma	Tonsils
Transitional cell bladder carcinoma	Circulating monocytes and activated lymphocytes
Myeloid and lymphocytic leukemia	B-lymphocytes (activated)
Mouse myeloblastic leukemia	Myoblasts
Papillomas	Brain

with high affinity. The 1-hydroxyl and the 25-hydroxyl groups are the most critical for receptor recognition. The biology potency of the various Vitamin D analogs correlates well with the binding activity of these substances for the receptor protein. The receptor interacts with nuclei, chromatin, and DNA. Using limited trypsin cleavage, it has been found that the DNA-binding domain is located at one end of the molecule; the ligand-binding domain is distinct and distal to that end. This steroid-receptor complex is translocated to the DNA in the nucleus of target cells to initiate the synthesis of specific RNA encoding proteins. Strong homologies occur in the putative DNA-binding region of the receptor with the DNA-binding domains of other steroid hormone receptors and with the v-erb A oncogene.[214] This suggests that the $1\alpha,25(OH)_2D_3$ receptor belongs to the same super gene family as all other steroid hormone receptors.

The $1\alpha,25(OH)_2D_3$ receptor is found in several cancer cells (see Table 8) and normal cells (see Table 9). Some investigators have reported that $1\alpha,25(OH)_2D_3$ has very rapid effects (within 1 to 15 min). Clear evidence exists that the very rapid effect of this $1\alpha,25(OH)_2D_3$ on fibroblasts is receptor mediated since fibroblasts from patients with defective $1\alpha,25(OH)_2D_3$-receptor proteins did not respond to the hormone.[215] Because 60% of all cancer cells examined contained the Vitamin D receptor, it is logical to examine what influence this vitamin might have on malignant cells in culture. Vitamin D deficiency has not been related to an increased incidence of malignancy. Epidemiological studies are very difficult because Vitamin D deficiency is rare in human populations (at least in advanced civilizations), and in most cases, there is a borderline or marginal Vitamin D_3 deficiency. However, men who consume little Vitamin D and calcium are about $2^1/_2$ times as likely to develop colorectal cancer as compared to individuals who consume higher amounts of these nutrients. Thus, there is a great risk as well as great mortality for colorectal cancer among humans who consume little or deficient Vitamin D and calcium diets.[216]

Recently, it has been found that the $1\alpha,25(OH)_2D_3$ receptor-expressing cell line also expressed C-myc mRNA. In contrast, the cell line in which the $1\alpha,25(OH)_2D_3$ receptor was not found, did not express c-myc mRNA. The association between the myc gene and the $1\alpha,25(OH)_2D_3$ receptor protein might help to explain the ubiquity of this receptor and thus its widespread role in the regulation of cell growth and differentiation of normal and neoplastic cells.

During the last few years, it has been suggested that Vitamin D_3, in addition to regulating a variety of normal cells (see Table 9), plays a role in controlling cancer cells. Many cancer and other malignant cells have now been found to possess receptors for $1\alpha,25(OH)_2D_3$ that are indistinguishable from the receptors found in the normal cells (see Table 8). *In vitro* as well as *in vivo* evidence suggests that $1\alpha,25(OH)_2D_3$ can influence the growth and differentiation of cancer cells. Specifically, $1\alpha,25(OH)_2D_3$ was found to inhibit the replication of breast cancer cells, melanoma, osteosarcoma, colon cancer, hematopoietic cells, and epidermal cells.[217,218] The replication of several of these cell types has also been shown to be regulated by this hormone, both *in vitro* and *in vivo*. Thus, studies on human breast cancer cells (T47-D) treated with 10^{-9} to $10^{-6} M$ $1\alpha,25(OH)_2D_3$ for 6 d found a significant reduction of cell numbers to approximately one half of those found in control cultures at 6 days. This decline was also associated with a doubling of the proportion of cells in the $G_2 + M$-phase of the cell cycle and was accompanied by a significant decline in the proportion of G_0/G_1 cells. At higher concentrations there was a significant decline in S-phase cells, with accumulation of cells in both G_0/G_1- and $G_2 + M$-phases. The antiestrogen, tamoxifen, at a concentration which caused similar effects on cell number, produced a proportional decrease in both the S- and $G_2 + M$-phase cells and accumulation of G_0/G_1 cells. The effects of $1\alpha,25(OH)_2D_3$ were associated with reduction in epidermal growth factor receptor levels; the *in vivo* experiments demonstrated marked inhibition of the growth of human cancer xenografts in immunosuppressed mice by $1\alpha,25(OH)_2D_3$, which were inhibited with $1\alpha,25(OH)_2D_3$ (0.1 μg i.p. three times per week), but growth was rapidly restored when the vitamin was withdrawn. Thus, the effects of $1\alpha,25(OH)_2D_3$ were time- and dose-dependent, yet reversible, on the replication of human cancer cells, which are possibly mediated by changes in growth factor receptor levels.[217]

Recent studies on the proliferation of a human colon cancer cell line *in vitro* called LoVo, which possesses a receptor for $1\alpha,25(OH)_2D_3$ with a low capacity, showed a significant inhibition of the proliferation in the presence of 10 nM to 1 μM of $1\alpha,25(OH)_2D_3$. After 8 d of treatment, the cell morphology was also changed from cuboidal cells to spindle-like cells. The growth inhibitory effect was modulated by verapamil (a calcium channel blocker), hydrocortisone, and moxestrol (1 mM), an estrogen analog. The LoVo cells also possess estrogen and glucocorticoid receptors. Therefore, a modulation of human colon cancer cells is possible through a vitamin hormone, $1\alpha,25(OH)_2D_3$, (hydrocortisone, estrogen analog) and a calcium channel blocker.[219] Other investigators reported biphasic effects on the replication of two distinct human cell lines, i.e., the breast cancer T-47D and the malignant melanoma MM96, thus, to stimulate cancer cell replication at low "physiologic" concentrations and to inhibit it at higher concentrations. The inhibitory effects were accompanied by marked morphological changes. The stimulatory, but not the inhibitory effect of $1\alpha,25(OH)_2D_3$, was abolished by cortisone. These $1\alpha,25$-dihydroxy Vitamin D_3 metabolites show promise for the inhibition of cancer growth, analogous to the effect of estrogens and antiestrogens in breast cancer, but with a wider potential application in a much wider range of human cancers.[218] Inhibitory effects of the vitamin on tumor growth were also found in *in vivo* conditions. The administration of $1\alpha,25(OH)_2D_3$ reduced the size of transplanted sarcoma cells in mice and reduced the number of Lewis lung carcinoma cells in mice. In contrast, tumor growth was enhanced by the administration of $1\alpha,25(OH)_2D_3$ to mice that had been inoculated with rat osteosarcoma cells. Also, antitumor activity of $1\alpha,25(OH)_2D_3$ at doses of 1 μg/d was found in patients with low-grade non-Hodgkin's lymphoma.[220] Moreover, the $1\alpha,25(OH)_2D_3$-induced stimulation of fibronectin production by a variety of human cancer cells was putatively implicated as a possible antimetastatic effect of the hormone. Although the majority of findings show an inhibitory effect of $1\alpha,25(OH)_2D_3$ on tumor growth, they suggest that the effects of the hormone may vary with the cell type. Also, topical application of $1\alpha,25(OH)_2D_3$ inhibited phorbol-ester-dependent chemical carcinogenesis in mouse skin. However, 20 to 80% of primary breast carcinoma cases have been shown to have Vitamin D receptors (VDR) or $1\alpha,25(OH)_2D_3$ receptor, which suggests involvement of $1\alpha,25(OH)_2D_3$ in growth modulation of human breast cancer. Typical VDR have been demonstrated in chemically induced rat mammary tumors, and this animal tumor can serve as a good model for evaluating the effect of $1\alpha,25(OH)_2D_3$ on tumor growth. Administration of $1\alpha,25(OH)_2D_3$ (1 or 2 μg twice a week for 16 weeks) in rats with DMBA-induced mammary tumors does not decrease the incidence nor the size of the tumors, but decreases the estrogen and progesterone receptor contacts of the tumor.[221]

Recently, receptor proteins specific for $1\alpha,25(OH)_2D_3$ were found in a number of tissues, including skin, which suggests that skin is also a target for this hormone.[222] Studies regarding the effect of $1\alpha,25$-dihydroxy Vitamin D_3 on the morphologic and biochemical differentiation of human epidermal keratinocytes *in vitro* showed that $1\alpha,25(OH)_2D_3$ caused a dose-dependent decrease in proliferation and an increase in the morphologic differentiation of human keratinocytes. Therefore, it appears that $1\alpha,25(OH)_2D_3$ is a potent inhibitor of keratinocyte proliferation as well as a stimulator of epidermal terminal differentiation.[223] It also inhibits DNA synthesis. In psoriasis, a hyperproliferative skin disease, the therapeutic use of calcitriol, $1\alpha,25(OH)_2$ Vitamin D_3 or calcipotriol (less active on calcium metabolism) orally or topically, in doses of 0.5 to 2 μg/d orally or 0.5 to 3 μg of vitamin per gram of petrolatum/topically for approximately 6 months, showed a significant improvement at the end of treatment. Fibroblasts are found to be more resistant than keratinocytes to calcitriol administration.[224] Vitamin D_3 should be taken at bedtime (to metabolize overnight), and dietary calcium intake should be less than 800 mg/d. Vitamin D_3 also plays an important role in hematopoietic cell differentiation. Since 1981, it has been clearly demonstrated that $1\alpha,25(OH)_2D_3$ suppressed growth and induced differentiation of mouse myeloid leukemia cells as well as human promyelocytic leukemia cells and human histiocytic monoblast-like lymphoma cells.[225,226] Using HL-60, a very useful cell line in determining the direction of differentiation, it was found that $1\alpha,25(OH)_2D_3$ is a potent, natural inducer in monocyte-macrophage differentiation. It was also demonstrated that $1\alpha,25(OH)_2D_3$ strikingly increases the proportion of cells accumulating in the G_0/G_1-phase and decreased that in the S-phase. Vitamin D_3 also decreases the interleukin-3 (IL-3) production.

Using both vitamins, $1\alpha,25(OH)_2D_3$ and retinoic acid, on human promyelocytic leukemia cells (HL-60), it was demonstrated that both vitamins suppressed proliferation and induced differentiation of HL-60 cells, but $1\alpha,25(OH)_2D_3$ was 70 to 100-fold more potent than was retinoic acid on a molar basis. Thus, both vitamins exhibit additive effects in suppressing growth and inducing differentiation of the cells, but monocyte-macrophage differentiation by $1\alpha,25(OH)_2D_3$ occurs much more readily than does granulocyte differentiation by retinoic acid.[227] Although studies *in vivo* and *in vitro* on human preleukemic and leukemic cells showed that high concentrations (10^{-6} M) of $1\alpha,25(OH)_2D_3$ can induce differentiation of leukemic blast cells *in vitro*, the administration of vitamin to patients with myelodysplastic syndrome (preleukemia) does not have an enduring therapeutic effect. These studies are hampered by the occurrence of hypercalcemia, and development of new Vitamin D_3 analogs with less hypercalcemic effect will be medically useful for treatment of preleukemic and leukemic patients. Also, there are cooperative effects of recombinant human gamma-interferon (γ-IFN) and $1\alpha,25(OH)_2D_3$ in inducing monocytoid differentiation of the leukemic blast cells. Thus, it is now well established that $1\alpha,25(OH)_2D_3$ promotes the differentiation of leukemic and preleukemic as well as normal myeloid stem cells toward the macrophage phenotype. The effect of Vitamin D_3 and its analogs seems to be synergistic or cooperative with other agents, such as γ-interferon, other lymphokines, glucocorticoids, and retinoic acid. A recent study estimating by immunocytochemical method the $1\alpha,25(OH)_2D_3$ receptor status of tumors from 136 patients with primary carcinoma of the breast, showed that patients with receptor-positive tumors had significantly longer disease-free survival than those with receptor-negative tumors. Effects of $1\alpha,25(OH)_2D_3$ studied *in vitro* revealed that this vitamin inhibits the proliferation of several established human breast cancer lines. Also, a study using a nitrosomethylurea (NMU)-induced rat mammary tumor model, which is biologically similar to hormone-responsive human breast cancer because these tumors contain substantial amounts of estrogen receptor (ER) and regress on ovariectomy, showed that treatment of tumor-bearing animals with 0.1 μg of the synthetic analog, 1α-hydroxy Vitamin D_3 given three times weekly, produced significant inhibition of tumor progression. These studies suggest that the levels of $1\alpha25(OH)_2D_3$ occurring *in vivo* may exert an inhibitory effect on receptor positive tumors.[228]

The recent discovery of receptors for $1\alpha,25(OH)_2D_3$ in several cells of the immune system and the multifaceted influence of this vitamin on humans are less impressive. At present, little is known regarding the therapeutic usefulness of Vitamin D metabolites in human cancer. This can be due, in part, to the hypercalcemic effects of Vitamin D and its derivatives which hamper their antiproliferative effects. This situation would be overcome with the development of newer analogs with greater specificity in their anticancer effects and lesser hypercalcemic potency. Recently fluorinated analogs of Vitamin D at C-26 and C-27 were five- to tenfold more potent and less hypercalcemic. Although many anticancer effects *in vitro* are clear-cut and time- and dose-dependent, the clinical results are conflicting and seem to suggest that pharmacologic doses are required in order to achieve sustained therapeutic effects. Thus, the reason for the discrepancy between *in vitro* and *in vivo* antitumor effects of $1\alpha,25(OH)_2D_3$ on certain cancers is still unclear. Although the treatment of NMU-induced rat mammary cancer, which is a hormone-responsive tumor similar to human breast cancer, with a synthetic analog 1α-hydroxy Vitamin D_3 three times weekly, produced a significant inhibition of tumor progression, further studies are required to evaluate the role of Vitamin D_3 metabolites in the treatment of human breast cancer.[228] Several new Vitamin D analogs, including $1\alpha,25S$, 26-trihydroxy Δ-22 Vitamin D_3, have been recently developed that induced differentiation of HL-60 cells, but with less ability than $1\alpha,25(OH)_2D_3$ to cause hypercalcemia. The *in vitro* studies suggest that $1\alpha,25(OH)_2D_3$ may be useful in the treatment of myelodysplastic syndrome (MDS) and, possibly, acute myeloid leukemia since the vitamin may induce the abnormal hematopoietic cells to differentiate into more mature monocytes and lymphocytes. These findings have raised the possibility that $1\alpha,25(OH)_2D_3$ is an immunoregulatory agent. The expression of the $1\alpha,25(OH)_2D_3$ receptor in lymphocytes coincides with the cell entry into the G_1-phase of the cell cycle, and the concentration of the receptor protein reaches a peak at the end of the G_1-phase and declines during the S-phase. It has also been shown that $1\alpha,25(OH)_2D_3$ inhibits IL-1 production and, consequently, IL-2 production and T-cell proliferation. These effects are mediated via IL-1. Both γ-interferon (γ-IFN) and granulocyte/monocyte-colony stimulating factor (GM-CSF) are decreased in the presence of $1\alpha,25(OH)_2D_3$.[229] Peritoneal macrophages from Vitamin D-deficient mice, in contrast to macrophages from normal mice, had impaired phagocytosis and chemotaxis; repletion with $1\alpha,25(OH)_2D_3$ restored these functions. Recent studies showed that $1\alpha,25(OH)_2D_3$ exerted a biphasic effect on α-IFN. Significant stimulation of α-IFN occurred at lower concentrations of the hormone (10^{-12} to 10^{-10} M), and inhibition was evident only at supraphysiologic concentrations (10^{-8} M).[230] Systemic levels of the vitamin may aid in maintaining tonic immunosuppression and thus prevent trivial antigenic stimuli from initiating an immune response.[223]

At present, it is becoming increasingly apparent that $1\alpha,25(OH)_2D_3$ may be capable of both stimulating responses in certain circumstances and suppressing them in others. However, the available clinical information and the *in vivo* experiments are consistent with an immunostimulating role of $1\alpha,25(OH)_2D_3$. Thus, Vitamin D deficiency states are associated with defective, rather than enhanced, immunity, and cellular immunity is impaired in the end stage of renal disease where the production of $1\alpha,25(OH)_2D_3$ has virtually ceased.[230] Whether the role of Vitamin D_3 in immunobiology is exerted through systemic or localized actions, remains unclear at this stage. Instead of being a systemic immunomodulator, $1\alpha,25(OH)_2D_3$ may be a local mediator of macrophage-lymphocyte interactions. Evidence has been presented that macrophages and transformed lymphocytes as well as granulomata and giant cells synthesize $1\alpha,25(OH)_2D_3$ locally; thus, the vitamin may act in a paracrine fashion as a local modulator of interactions between cells of the immune system.[231] Calcitriol is a potent inhibitor of T-cell activity as well as of IL-2 and IFN-r. Thus, there is experimental evidence as well as clinical information which supports a role of $1\alpha,25(OH)_2D_3$ in immunobiology. However, the physiologic, pathophysiologic, and pharmacologic implications of the immunomodulating activity of $1\alpha,25(OH)_2D_3$ have not been well established.

1. Possible Mechanism of Action of Vitamin D

Recently, the discovery of $1\alpha,25(OH)_2D_3$ receptors in a variety of previously unexpected normal as well as cancer cells (see Tables 8 and 9) suggests that this hormone-like vitamin might have a much wider biologic role than that related to calcium and phosphorus metabolism. It has also been associated with the function of other tissues not primarily related to calcium metabolism, such as stimulation of insulin secretion, modulation of prolactin synthesis, skeletal and cardiac muscle, and thyroid gland and the gonads.[232] Substantial evidence has accumulated that the mechanism of action of $1\alpha,25(OH)_2D_3$ is similar to that of other steroid and thyroid hormones, and Vitamin D should be more appropriately classified as an exohormone.[233] $1\alpha,25(OH)_2D_3$ is known to interact noncovalently, but stereospecifically with a nuclear receptor protein. This steroid receptor complex is then associated with DNA in the nucleus of target cells, either to initiate the synthesis of specific RNA encoding proteins that mediate the biologic responses or to mediate a selective repression of gene transcription. The $1\alpha,25(OH)_2D_3$ receptors from several species, including man, have been biochemically characterized as DNA-binding proteins of 50 to 60 kDa that bind $1\alpha,25(OH)_2D_3$ with a high affinity. The ligand affinity of the intracellular receptor proteins for Vitamin D_3 metabolites is usually correlated with their biologic activity. Strong homologies occur in the putative DNA-binding region of the receptor with the DNA-binding domains of all the other steroid hormone receptors and with the v-erb A oncogene.[214]

Some investigators have reported that $1\alpha,25(OH)_2D_3$ has very rapid effects (within 1 to 15 min), which therefore cannot be explained by genomic actions. Perhaps the most intriguing evidence is that $1\alpha,25(OH)_2D_3$ has a role in controlling cellular proliferation and differentiation of several cancer cell lines, including human cancer cells (melanoma, breast, colon, osteosarcoma, and leukemia).[208,217-219,225,226] A unifying hypothesis for the generalized mechanism of action of $1\alpha,25(OH)_2D_3$ in such a diversity of cell types has yet to be proposed, but the fundamental role of vitamin in regulating intracellular calcium has appeal; $1\alpha,25(OH)_2D_3$ may regulate its various cellular processes by altering intracellular calcium. Recent reports showed that increased extracellular calcium can block the growth inhibitory effect of $1\alpha,25(OH)_2D_3$ and also can modulate the hormone's effect in promoting cellular differentiation.[234] Finally, Vitamin D_3 interacts with specific areas of chromatin to modify gene expression, which can raise the possibility that it may modify or enhance expression of oncogenes (v-erb A, C-myc) involved in neoplastic transformation.

Therefore, Vitamin D_3 may exert its antitumor effects on various malignant cells: (1) by binding to its specific intracellular receptor proteins and transferring to certain areas of DNA, where by a transcription process it synthesizes a new m-RNA that in turn elicits by a translation process the synthesis of new proteins and, consequently, exerts its biological effects; (2) by controlling the homeostasis of intracellular calcium, which plays an important role in cell growth and differentiation; (3) by modifying the oncogene expression, which exerts a significant role in the carcinogenic process; and (4) by association with growth factors, through paracrine and autocrine mechanisms. These findings suggest that some Vitamin D_3 analogs may provide a tool for treatment of cancer.[235]

2. Clinical and Therapeutic Implications

The clinical and therapeutic implications of Vitamin D_3 and its active form $1\alpha,25(OH)_2D_3$ reveal that it acts as a hormone or hormone-like substance, particularly similar to other steroid hormones (estrogens, progesterone, or glucocorticoids) and has a potential therapeutic effect in certain malignancies, or proliferative diseases, such as, psoriasis, leukemia, and lymphoma. Despite the initial observations that $1\alpha,25(OH)_2D_3$ inhibits cancer cell proliferation and replication in a variety of cancer cells (breast, melanoma, colon, osteosarcoma, leukemia) *in vitro* as well as the animal tumor models (mammary rat carcinoma, leukemia, Lewis lung adenoma, papilloma) and human cancer cell xenografts, its anticancer therapeutic effects in humans are less impressive. Also, *in vivo* the administration of $1\alpha,25(OH)_2D_3$ in mice with myeloid leukemia cells significantly prolonged survival. Similar results were obtained with $1\alpha(OH)D_3$. However, the administration of $1\alpha,25(OH)_2D_3$ (2 µg/d) did not result in an improvement of hematopoiesis in patients with MDS, following 12 weeks of treatment.[236] Some mild therapeutic effects were reported in a few cases with lymphoma treated with alfacalcidol. More encouraging results were obtained recently in a clinical trial where $1\alpha,25(OH)_2D_3$ was administered orally in combination with retinoic acid, α-interferon (α-IFN), and low doses of cytosine arabinoside. From eight patients with acute myeloid leukemia, two complete remissions (CR) and three partial remissions (PR) were achieved.[237] Favorable therapeutic results were reported in 40 patients with psoriasis vulgaris treated with calcitriol ($1\alpha,25(OH)_2D_3$) at doses starting with 0.5 to 1.0 µg/d orally or 0.5 µg/g of petrolatum topically for 6 months. The mechanism of action of $1\alpha,25(OH)_2D_3$ on psoriatic lesions may be due to suppression of growth and induction of differentiation of keratinocytes.[224] Patients with hypercalcemia and hypercalciuria should not be placed on Vitamin D_3 therapy. Treatment should be started with 0.25 µg at bedtime and increased every 2 weeks by 0.25 µg to a maximum dosage of 2 µg/d.

3. Side Effects of Hypervitaminosis with Vitamin D

The side effects of hypervitaminosis with Vitamin D therapy can result from hypercalcemia. This is mainly due to an excessive production of 25-hydroxy-D in the liver. This accumulated 25-hydroxy-D is likely to be the cause of intoxication with Vitamin D_3. The first symptoms are fatigue, anorexia, headache, nausea, and vomiting, followed by polyuria, polydipsia, weakness, irritability, and pruritus. Renal function is impaired (proteinuria, casts, azotemia), and in most severe cases, metastatic calcification, particularly in the kidney, osteoporosis, and coma can occur. In these cases, discontinuation of treatment, large amounts of fluids, and glucocorticoids are recommended. Therefore, dietary calcium intake should be limited to less than 800 mg/d, and frequent serum and urine calcium determinations should be made every 2 weeks in all patients receiving large doses of Vitamin D.

E. VITAMIN E (α-TOCOPHEROL) AND ITS ROLE IN CANCER BIOLOGY AND THERAPY

The term Vitamin E includes at least eight compounds, called tocopherols (α, β, γ and δ) and tocotrienols. The most biologically active tocopherol is d-α-tocopherol. Since 1980, Vitamin E activity in the RDA has been expressed in milligrams of tocopherol equivalent and has replaced the international unit (IU). Usually, 1 mg of tocopherol is equal to 1 IU of α-tocopherol. The daily requirements for adults are approximately 20 mg, and for children and adolescents, 8 mg.

During the last 30 years, several articles have been published concerning the effects of

Vitamin E on dietary procarcinogens and carcinogens, and in patients with cancer.[238,239] Recent studies indicate that Vitamin E and its derivatives play an important role in regulation of growth, differentiation, and transformation of normal, as well as neoplastic cells; thus it exerts a potent antitumor activity *in vitro* and *in vivo* in animal tumor models and cancer cell lines. Thus, Vitamin E has been shown to inhibit skin, liver, oral, ear duct and forestomach carcinogenesis; and to enhance, to have no effect on, or to inhibit mammary gland or colon carcinogenesis, depending upon the method of administration, the level of dietary selenium or fat, and the species and strain of animals used. Vitamin E can inhibit mutagenesis and carcinogenesis *in vitro* and also can inhibit tumor cell growth and carcinogen-induced DNA damage.[171] Epidemiologic studies are few and inconclusive. No definite links between dietary Vitamin E and human cancer have been demonstrated.

Epidemiologic data may prove difficult to obtain for several reasons. First, Vitamin E is present in a wide variety of foods, which makes it difficult to identify groups of people with different levels of intake. Also, a clear-cut deficiency has not been established in humans. Since Vitamin E is relatively unstable during storage, its concentration can vary greatly in individual foods. However, a recent 10-year longitudinal study among men in Finland established a strong inverse relationship between serum Vitamin E and risk of cancer. The strongest inverse association was observed for cancers of stomach, pancreas, and urinary tract organs, and for all cancers unrelated to smoking. The strongest association between α-tocopherol and cancer risk was observed in the youngest group. These findings support the hypothesis that high Vitamin E intake protects against cancer and demonstrates a relationship between serum Vitamin E and the risk of cancer.[240]

Studies regarding the effects of Vitamin E on mammalian tumor cells in culture revealed that inhibitory effects depend upon the form of Vitamin E and state of cell proliferation. For example, α-tocopheryl succinate (Vitamin E succinate) induces growth inhibition in murine neuroblastoma, human neuroblastomas, rat glioma, and human prostate cancer *in vitro*.[5,238,241] Also, Vitamin E acid succinate induces dramatic morphological changes and reduction by 50%. Most round melanoma cells exhibit a fibroblastic morphology. This cell differentiation is induced after 4 d of treatment and remains irreversible after Vitamin E is removed. However, there are Vitamin E acid succinate-resistant cells in culture. In addition, Vitamin E succinate induces growth inhibition and differentiation in mouse melanoma (B-16) cells in culture. Other forms of Vitamin E, such as α-tocopherol, α-tocopheryl acetate, and α-tocopheryl nicotinate, were ineffective.[5] These findings show that Vitamin E acid succinate is the most potent form of Vitamin E in causing morphological changes and growth inhibition in melanoma cells in culture.

The exact reason for these differences is unknown. It is possible that: (1) Vitamin E acid succinate may be relatively more soluble and stable in growth medium, (2) it may easily cross the cell membrane, and (3) it may be converted to α-tocopherol more slowly so that the intracellular level of α-tocopherol remains high for a longer period of time. Also, Vitamin E succinate inhibited the growth of human neuroblastoma cells in culture and in nude mice.[242] An evaluation of the modulation by Vitamin E of antitumor effects due to radiation of a murine tumor revealed that low doses of Vitamin E augmented them while high doses were inhibitors.[243] It has been reported that α-tocopheryl acetate (Aquasol E) had both growth inhibitory and differentiative effects on murine neuroblastoma, while Vitamin E acid succinate was a most potent form of Vitamin E for inducing irreversible growth inhibition in some melanoma cells in culture.[241] Experiments with radiolabeled Vitamin E (D-α{5-methyl-^{3}H} tocopherol) in tumored mice showed differences between i.p. and i.v. routes. The spleen, liver, and lungs appeared to be preferred sites of radioactive Vitamin E accumulation while preferential accumulation in tumor tissue was not observed. Oral administration of Vitamin E was ineffective in treating heterotransplanted subcutaneous neuroblastoma tumors in nude mice. However, when Aquasol E was administered to the drinking water of tumored mice in adequate amounts, an antitumor effect was observed which strongly suggests that the vitamin itself has antitumor activity.[242] Studies regarding the effects of Vitamin E acid succinate showed that Vitamin E had specific effects which depend on cell type; thus, administration of 5 μg/ml on mouse fibroblast (L-cells), rat glioma (C-6), and mouse neuroblastoma (NBP₂) cells in culture did not affect the morphology or growth of mouse fibroblasts in culture; however, it inhibited the growth of mouse NB cells and rat glioma cells in culture.[242]

DL-α-tocopherol induces morphological differentiation in mouse myeloid leukemia cells in culture without affecting the growth rate. The reason for the occurrence of resistant cells to Vitamin E in melanoma cells in culture is unknown. Thus, Vitamin E exhibits anticancer activities by increasing the expression of morphological differentiation in neuroblastoma cells and by enhancing the growth inhibition and morphological differentiation produced by ionizing radiation on these cells. It has also been reported that α-tocopherol significantly inhibits the differentiation of the mouse myeloid leukemia cells induced by dexamethasone.[244]

It has been reported that Vitamin E is more potent than other antioxidants at decreasing carcinogen-induced chromosomal breakage in leukocyte cultures. Others reported that Vitamin E protected against chromosomal damage of cultured Chinese hamster lung and ovary cells induced by benzo(a)pyrene.[245] It has been demonstrated that covalent binding of aflatoxin B to liver DNA and RNA of chicks fed a diet deficient in Vitamin E and selenium was greater than that of chicks supplemented with Vitamin E or selenium, or both.[246] Hence, Vitamin C can inhibit mutagenesis and inhibit *in vitro* carcinogenesis. Vitamin E also inhibits tumor cell growth, binding of the active carcinogen metabolite to cellular DNA, and chromosomal breakage induced by carcinogens.[171] It has also been reported that Vitamin E inhibited bacterial mutagenesis induced by DMBA.[183] α-Tocopheryl, a Vitamin E analog, is effective in decreasing X-ray-induced transformation in mouse C3H10 T½ cells in culture. It was effective when present throughout the entire treatment period or when treatments began after confluence was reacehd at day 12 post-irradiation. It was ineffective if present only for the early portion of the radiation transformation assay period, suggesting that its effect may be reversible.[247] The effects of Vitamin E on the transformation of C3H10 T½ cells in culture, induced by X-ray, benzo(a)pyrene, or tryptophan pyrolysate, have also been studied. Incubation of the cells with α-tocopheryl succinate for 24 h prior to exposure to X-rays or to chemical carcinogens resulted in an inhibition of transformation.[248]

1. The Mechanisms of Action of Vitamin E

The mechanisms of action of Vitamin E on neoplastic cell growth inhibition and differentiation are poorly understood. Butylated hydroxyanisole (BHA), a lipid soluble antioxidant, also inhibits the growth of NB cells and melanoma cells.[241] This suggests that part of the mechanism of action of Vitamin E succinate on cell growth may be mediated by an antioxidation mechanism.

A recent study showed that Vitamin E exhibited a protective role by inducing alveolar macrophage cytotoxicity for lung parenchymal cells. Thus, the cytotoxicity induced on normal rat lung parenchymal cells by smoker alveolar macrophages removed from alveolar fluid, was inversely related to the Vitamin E content of the parenchymal cells. Alveolar fluid in young asymptomatic smokers at baseline was relatively deficient in Vitamin E, compared to nonsmoker fluid (3.1 μg/ml vs. 20.7 ng/ml). After supplementation with a 3-week course of oral Vitamin E (2400 IU/d), the smoker alveolar fluid Vitamin E levels increased, but they still remained significantly lower than nonsmoker baseline levels. These findings suggest that Vitamin E is an important alveolar fluid antioxidant; the deficiency seen in young smokers may predispose them to an enhanced oxidant attack on their lung parenchymal cells and may contribute to the pathogenesis of emphysema. Vitamin E in the alveolar fluid may neutralize the oxidants and free radicals present in cigarette smoke and those released by lung inflammatory cells. The cytotoxicity experiments revealed the potentially important protective role of Vitamin E.[249]

Recently, it has been shown that Vitamin E (α-tocopherol) is an effective inhibitor of platelet adhesion. The platelet adhesiveness was tested *ex vivo* in a group of six normal individuals receiving varying doses of α-tocopherol. The average decrease in adhesion after 2 weeks of 200 IU Vitamin E was 75%. After 2 weeks of 400 IU Vitamin E, platelet adhesion was reduced by 82%. The inhibitory effect of α-tocopherol was dose-dependent. Scanning electron microscopy revealed a striking decrease of pseudopodia formation, and suggested that Vitamin E may also be an effective antiadhesive agent *in vivo*.[250]

2. Experimental Studies

These revealed that Vitamin E may inhibit skin, liver, oral, ear duct, and forestomach cancers, but have no effect on, enhance, or inhibit mammary and colon carcinomas. The antitumor activity depends upon the route of administration, the level of dietary selenium or fat, and the species of animals used. Efforts to inhibit cancer development by increased amounts of Vitamin E have a long history and started more than 40 years ago. The vast majority of studies on experimental carcinomas have been conducted with α-tocopherol. In one of the earliest studies (1946), it was reported that the number of mixed tumors resulting from intraperitoneal injection of 3-methylcholanthrene (3-MCA) was lower in rats receiving a diet with added wheat germ oil than in rats on a control diet.[251] Subsequent studies also showed that α-tocopherol inhibited the occurrence of subcutaneous sarcomas induced in mice by injecting 3-MCA.[252] Recently, Vitamin E (α-tocopheryl acetate) has been found to significantly reduce the incidence of skin papillomas by 54%, induced by DMBA in the Egyptian toad. The exact mechanism by which this tumor regression occurs is not known. However, it is possible that Vitamin E may act as antioxidant and stimulates the host's immune system.[253]

Several investigators have studied the effects of α-tocopherol on DMBA-induced formation of mammary tumors. Thus, ingestion of high levels of α-tocopherol only before DMBA was administered did not inhibit the occurrence of mammary tumors. Also, an increased intake of Vitamin A was reported to have no inhibitory effect on epidermal neoplasia in mice.[252] In comparative experiments using high and low doses of Vitamin E on dimethylhydrazine-induced carcinomas in the large intestine of mice, it has been shown that even though the tumor incidence was similar in both groups, the average number of tumors per animal was less in the high Vitamin E group than in the low Vitamin E group.[254]

In a recent study, a prevention by Vitamin E of experimental oral carcinogenesis has been reported. Thus, hamster buccal pouch carcinogenesis, induced by topical application of a 0.5% solution of DMBA (7,12-dimethylbenz(a)anthracene) in oil, has been shown to be significantly inhibited by Vitamin E administered systemically by mouth (10 mg of α-tocopherol twice a week). With a less potent carcinogen (0.1% DMBA), Vitamin E was shown to prevent tumor development in Syrian hamsters. In hamsters painted only with DMBA, but that had received no Vitamin E, the presence of epidermoid carcinoma was demonstrated grossly and microscopically.[255] Vitamin E combined with adriamycin has been shown to enhance the growth-inhibitory effects of adriamycin on human prostatic carcinoma cells *in vitro*. Also, adriamycin-Vitamin E (tocopherol) combination therapy reduced the tumor volume in N_b rat prostate adenocarcinoma by 80%, but the mortality rate was 57%. No animals showed complete tumor regression, but the group treated with an early large dose of Vitamin E had no mortality and a high rate of tumor regression.[256]

Our own investigations, started more than 15 years ago, on the study of preventive and therapeutic effects of various vitamins, hormones, and prostaglandins on cancer development and regression revealed interesting data regarding their role in tumor biology and neoplastic cell physiology. We used epidermal neoplasia, squamous cell carcinomas in mice, and basal

TABLE 10
Influence of Hormones, Vitamins, and Prostaglandin on Squamous Cell Carcinomas
in Mice

Group	Treatment[a]	Dose	Administration
1	Controls + diluent	0.2 ml	Locally (once)
2	MCA[b] + diluent	0.2 ml (= 800 μg)	Locally (once)
3	MCA + estradiol (E)	0.2 ml MCA + 200 μg E	Locally (once) 2 × weekly, i.m.
4	MCA + thyroxine (T$_4$)	0.2 ml MCA + 2 μg T$_4$	Locally (once) 2 × weekly, i.m.
5	MCA + calcitonin (C)	0.2 ml MCA + 2 MRCU[c]C	Locally (once) 2 × weekly, i.m.
6	MCA + progesterone (P)	0.2 ml MCA + 2 mg P	Locally (once) 2 × weekly, i.m.
7	MCA + hydrocortisone (HC)	0.2 ml MCA + 1 mg HC	Locally (once) 2 × weekly, i.m.
8	MCA + PGE$_2$	0.2 ml MCA + 10 μg PGE$_2$	Locally (once) 2 × weekly, i.m.
9	MCA + Vitamin A (retinol)	0.2 ml MCA + 8 mg A	Locally (once) 2 × weekly, i.m.
10	MCA + Vitamin E	0.2 ml MCA + 50 IU E	Locally (once) 2 × weekly, locally
11	MCA + Vitamin C (ascorbic acid)	0.2 ml MCA + 50 mg C	Locally (once) 2 × weekly, orally
12	MCA + hypophysectomy	0.2 ml MCA + total hypophysectomy	Locally (once)

[a]   All experiments in mice were carried out for 9 months.
[b]   MCA (3-methylcholanthrene).
[c]   MRCU (Medical Research Council Units).

cell carcinomas in rats, chemically induced by topical application and initiation of a dose of 800 μg of a strong chemical carcinogen, 3-methylcholanthrene (3-MCA), on their dorsal skin (young male albino Swiss mice), and followed up for a period of 9 months. After initiation by 3-MCA, animals were treated by continuous i.m. injections of certain hormones (estradiol, thyroxine, calcitonin, progesterone, and hydrocortisone) twice a week. With hormone deprivation (hypophysectomy), prostaglandin E$_2$ (PGE$_2$), in i.m. injections of Vitamin A, topical application (E), and oral administration (C) were given at various doses (See Table 10). Since epidermal carcinomas are the only visible tumors, their incidence, development, and regression under the treatment of vitamins, hormones, and prostaglandins can be easily monitored by the naked eye, without the sacrifice of animals; thus, the mouse skin became an ideal model for the study of vitamins and hormones on cancer development and regression.

In order to study the multifaceted and complex mechanism of action of vitamins and hormones on cancer cells, we used modern techniques, such as light and electron microscopic (high resolution) autoradiography using [³H]-thymidine for DNA synthesis, [³H]-uridine for RNA synthesis, and [³H]-leucine for protein synthesis. At the end of the experiments (9 months) and 2 h prior to sacrifice, each mouse received i.m. 8 μCi/g/bwt from each nucleotide. Some mice received 8 μCi/g/bwt of [³H]-thymidine for DNA synthesis; others received 8 μCi/g/bwt [³H]-uridine for RNA synthesis; and others received i.m. 8 μCi/g/bwt [³H]-leucine for protein synthesis. At the end of the experiments, tumor specimens and control skin were fixed in Bouin's solution, dehydrated, and embedded in paraffin. Sections (5 μm thick) were covered with Kodak Nuclear Emulsion NTB$_2$ or Ilford K$_5$ and exposed

TABLE 11
Autoradiograms: Percentage of Mouse Epidermal Cells Labeled with [³H]-Thymidine, [³H]-Uridine, and [³H]-Leucine Following MCA-Initiation and Hormone, Prostaglandin, and Vitamin Treatments

Group	Treatment	[³H]-thymidine no. of labeled cells/total no. of cells	%	[³H]-uridine no. of labeled cells/ total no. of cells	%	[³H]-leucine no. of labeled cells/ total no. of cells	%
1	Controls + diluent	82/1000	8.2[a]	75/1000	7.5	88/1000	8.8
2	MCA + diluent	180/1000	18.0[a]	160/1000	16.0	175/1000	17.5
3	MCA + estradiol	250/1000	25.0[a]	220/1000	22.0	240/1000	24.0
4	MCA + thyroxine	375/1000	37.5[a]	350/1000	35.0	370/1000	37.0
5	MCA + calcitonin	320/1000	32.0[a]	305/1000	30.5	310/1000	31.0
6	MCA + progesterone	140/1000	14.0[a]	130/1000	13.0	142/1000	14.2
7	MCA + cortisol	52/1000	5.2[a]	48/1000	4.8	55/1000	5.5
8	MCA + PGE₂	352/1000	35.2[a]	341/1000	34.1	350/1000	35.0
9	MCA + Vitamin A	50/1000	5.0[a]	55/1000	5.5	51/1000	5.1
10	MCA + Vitamin E	125/1000	12.5[b]	110/1000	11.0	128/1000	12.8
11	MCA + Vitamin C	127/1000	12.7[b]	105/1000	10.5	130/1000	13.0
12	MCA + hypophysectomy	49/1000	4.9[a]	47/1000	4.7	50/1000	5.0

[a] Statistically significant ($p < 0.001$) from the respective controls.
[b] Statistically significant ($p < 0.002$) from the respective controls.

for 14 d at 4°C in dark boxes. The filmed sections were processed in D_{19} Kodak developer, then stained with Hematoxylin-Eosin (H & E), and examined under light microscope. Quantitative estimation was made by counting the labeled cells from 1000 consecutive epithelial cells in the basal layers of epidermal neoplasms or control mice. The ratio between labeled cells with [³H]-thymidine, [³H]-uridine, and [³H]-leucine, and 1000 counted cells, as well as the percentage of labeled neoplastic cells, were recorded in each experimental group (see Table 11). Tumors were counted in each group at 3, 6, and 9 months and expressed as tumorigenetic curves for each group (see Figure 4).

For ultrastructural studies and intracellular organelle distribution, small specimens were removed, diced and fixed in cold 3% cacodylate buffered glutaraldehyde (GTA), postfixed in 1% phosphate osmium tetroxide (O_4O_s), dehydrated and embedded in a mixture of Epon-Araldite. Ultrathin sections were cut using an ultrotome equipped with a diamond knife, then stained with a solution of uranyl acetate and lead citrate, and examined under a transmission electron microscope. For cell surface studies, larger specimens were removed and fixed in the same 3% cacodylate buffered GTA, dehydrated, and embedded using critical point method with Freon-13; then they were coated with gold (200 Å) and examined under a scanning electron microscope.

Both squamous cell and basal cell carcinomas are histologically almost identical to those found in humans. From these multidisciplinary studies, it appears clearly that vitamins and hormones exert a profound effect on cancer development, tumor cell biology, and physiology, including DNA, RNA, and protein synthesis, ultrastructural pathology, and cell surface changes. Thus, Vitamin A (retinol) markedly reduced the incidence and development of epidermal neoplasms, at a level comparable to those of cortisol and hypophysectomy, followed by Vitamin E (α-tocopherol) which is close to progesterone, and a slight decrease in vitamin C (ascorbic acid) treated animals. On the contrary, hormones (estradiol, thyroxine, calcitonin) and PGE_2 increased the tumor growth (see Figure 4).

Autoradiographic studies also revealed a significant decrease in DNA, RNA, and protein synthesis in epidermal cancer cells (nuclei, nucleoli, ribosomes) in Vitamin A-treated animals; followed by a moderate, but significant reduction in Vitamin E-treated animals and a

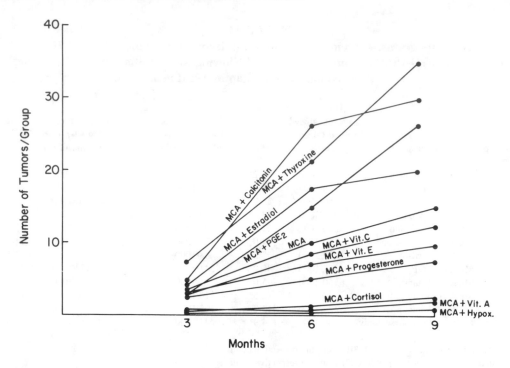

FIGURE 4.   Influence of certain hormones, vitamins, and prostaglandins on tumor (squamous cell carcinoma) growth and regression in mice.

mild decrease after Vitamin C treatment. These effects are similar to those observed in cortisol-treated, progesterone-treated, or hypophysectomized animals. Hormones, such as thyroxine, estradiol, calcitonin, and PGE_2, increased DNA, RNA, and protein synthesis in epidermal cancer cells (see Table 11).

Ultrastructural pathology of neoplastic cells revealed significant changes, such as advanced cytolysis, membrane alterations, shrunken nuclei and nucleoli, and mitochondrial, lysosomal and polysome reduction, after vitamin treatment. Most advanced ultrastructural changes occurred in epithelial cancer cells of Vitamin A-treated animals.[30] Also, significant cytotoxic cellular changes are observed in epidermal tumor cells following Vitamin E treatment. Thus, polygonal or elongated cells with enlarged nuclei and nucleoli, an increased number of mitochondria with membrane disruption and condensation and tonofilaments, can be frequently seen in neoplastic cells following 3-methylcholanthrene administration (see Plate 1 *). Advanced cytotoxic changes, such as cytolysis, membrane disruption, reduction of mitochondria and polysomes, increase in dense granules or lysosomes, nuclear abnormalities, and chromatolysis are frequently seen in epidermal cancer cells following Vitamin E treatment (see Plate 2 *). Scanning electron microscopic observations revealed interesting cell surface changes of epidermal cancer cells following vitamin administration. Thus, round and polyhedral cells covered by several blebs and microvilli, separated by enlarged, and interconnected by a vast network of microfibrils, are visible in neoplastic cells in 3-methylcholanthrene-treated animals (see Plate 3 *). Interesting cell surface changes with predominance of enlarged polygonal cells devoid of blebs and microvilli and advanced cytolysis and marked reduction of microfibrils are seen in cancer cells following Vitamin E administration. Thus, an advanced cytotoxicity and cell differentiation occurs in neoplastic cells of Vitamin E-treated neoplasms (see Plate 4 *). These cell surface changes are similar to those previously reported in Vitamin A and some in Vitamin E-treated cancer cells.[30,257] Both mild ultrastructural and cell surface alterations are seen in epidermal cancer cells

---

* Plates 1, 2, 3 and 4 appear following page 198.

following Vitamin C administration. Therefore, these studies *in vivo* strongly suggest a therapeutic role of vitamins in cancer therapy. Some of these findings are similar to those of hormones and prostaglandin-treated neoplasms.[258]

3. Effect of Vitamin E on Immunity and Drug Resistance

This is an important component of the host's immune system defense mechanism or immune surveillance mechanisms which may allow the transformed cells to escape and thereby allow the development of detectable cancer. An enhancement or augmentation of the host's immune system may also be important for the success of cancer treatment. Vitamin E, supplemented to diets in pharmacologic doses, four to six times above the currently used levels, stimulates humoral antibody production by increasing proliferation of B-lymphocytes (antibody producing cells), and consequently promoting a rapid transition from less efficient IgM antibody production to more efficient IgG antibody production. No direct enhancement of T-cell activity or cell-mediated immunity can be attributed to Vitamin E. Thus, the role of Vitamin E as a potent immunoenhancer or immunoaugmentator is more important in humoral immunity than in cell-mediated immunity.

There is strong evidence that prostaglandins (PG) play a regulatory role in this process and that Vitamin E modulates PG biosynthesis. It has also been shown that DL-α-tocopherol free alcohol at high doses stimulates the immune system in humans. Also, Vitamin E is a most potent immunoenhancer when administered as a water-in-oil type adjuvant mixed with the antigen.[259] It has also been reported that Vitamin E enhances the effect of tumor therapeutic agents on tumor cells in culture, such as: (1) ionizing radiation; (2) synthetic cytotoxic agents (vincristine, adriamycin, 5-fluorouracil); (3) naturally occurring nontoxic agents (Vitamins A, C); and (4) hyperthermia. If this concept is applicable to *in vivo* conditions, the effectiveness of pharmacologic agents can be greatly enhanced by vitamin manipulation.[260]

4. Mechanisms of Vitamin E Action on Cancer Cells

The exact mechanisms of the antitumor effects of Vitamin E are still unknown. However, there are several possible mechanisms by which Vitamin E may act on cancer cells: (1) cytotoxicity (advanced cytolysis); (2) antioxidation; (3) cell differentiation; (4) cell membrane stabilizer; (5) inhibiting DNA, RNA, and protein synthesis; (6) mitochondrial metabolism; (7) heme synthesis; (8) immunoenhancement; (9) inhibiting prostaglandin biosynthesis; (10) reducing mutagenic activity; (11) preventing platelet adhesion; (12) modifying the metabolic pattern of polycyclic hydrocarbons; (13) enhancing the effects of ionizing radiation, hyperthermia, and chemotherapeutic drugs; (14) changing the enzyme activity involved in oxidative xenobiotic metabolism (cytochrome P-450); and (15) reacting with genotoxic free radicals. Some of these free radicals may result in tumor formation by serving as a continuous source of tumor initiators and promoters.[184] Thus, Vitamins E and C may act as quenching molecules to remove hydroxy radicals (OH). Hence, these multiple inhibitory effects of Vitamin E on cancer cells indicate that it has a potential usefulness in the prevention and treatment of cancer.

Vitamin E in cancer therapy can have a promising role. Since several experimental *in vitro* and *in vivo* studies demonstrate a potential therapeutic effect, is is likely that Vitamin E at high doses may exhibit antitumor activity on human cancers. Because of poor absorption of orally ingested Vitamin E (ester or free alcohol), it is thought that oral administration of Vitamin E may not increase the plasma Vitamin E level enough, and thus its intracellular concentration (at high levels), to suppress or kill the growth of cancer cells. Therefore, it is postulated that intravenous infusion of Vitamin E would be most suitable for treatment of human cancers.

Clinical trials using DL-α-tocopherol free alcohol in a Phase I trial infused 2300 mg/m^2 daily for 2 to 3 d in patients with metastatic neuroblastomas, primitive neuroectodermal tumor, and retinoblastoma, after patients had become unresponsive to other known thera-peutic modalities for 9 d, and some antitumor and analgesic effects were observed. The major adverse side effect of high doses of Vitamin E is an increased bleeding tendency, which is corrected with Vitamin K infusions. It should be pointed out that DL-α-tocopherol, which has been used in the treatment of human tumors, is much less potent than DL-α-tocopheryl succinate; however, the pharmacology and toxicology of the latter has not been defined. These data suggested Phase II trials with Vitamin E (Ephynal at 2300 mg/m^2/d preceded by 10 mg Vitamin K$_3$ for 5 d which led to minor objective and subjective responses in patients with neuroblastoma, primitive neuroectodermal tumor, and retinoblastoma. The most important aspect of this clinical study was the virtual lack of toxicity at high doses.[261] The lack of major responses and their brief duration may be due to the heterogeneity of tumors.

Conflicting reports have also been published regarding the role of Vitamin E in patients with chronic cystic mastitis.[262] Thus, Vitamin E may be useful in the treatment of human tumors by inhibiting growth or inducing differentiated cell phenotypes in several types of tumors. It can also kill newly transformed cells directly or indirectly by stimulating the host's immune system and reverse the malignant phenotype to a normal cell phenotype in certain tumors. However, there are Vitamin E-resistant cells in culture and *in vivo*.

Vitamin E will be more effective in combination with Vitamins A and C, β-carotene, and selenium, since together they act synergistically in some ways. They will exert additive effects on tumors. Also, Vitamin E may enhance the effects of chemotherapeutic drugs, radiation therapy, and hyperthermia and may reduce their toxic effects. All these studies suggest that Vitamin E may be one of the important anticancer agents which could play a significant role in cancer treatment and prevention.

5. Toxicity and Side-Effects

A minimum daily requirement is estimated to be about 15 to 30 IU, an amount that is likely to be present in almost every type of diet consumed by human populations. Vitamin E appears to be nontoxic in moderate doses; intake of 800 IU daily for 3 years caused no adverse effects in man. However, very high doses (3000 IU/d) for several years (up to 11 years) may produce gastrointestinal problems in a few patients (8%). A higher incidence of necrotizing colitis has been found in premature infants after high doses of Vitamin E.

F. VITAMIN K IN CANCER TREATMENT

Vitamin K is a generic term for a homologous group of fat soluble vitamins which promote clotting of the blood by increasing prothrombin synthesis in the liver. There are at least three such vitamins: (1) Vitamin K$_1$ (phytonadione); (2) Vitamin K$_2$ (menaquinone), and (3) Vitamin K$_3$ (menadione). Despite the fact that all Vitamin K naphtokinones share certain biochemical properties and can serve as electron acceptors for mammalian redox enzymes, there are differences in prosthetic group substitution which impart important bio-chemical and physiologic differences among the Vitamin K congeners. From all Vitamins K, only Vitamin K$_3$ (menadione) is assumed to play a role in cancer development and treatment. Although Vitamins A, C, and E have received the most intensive scrutiny, considerable evidence is accumulating that the Vitamin K group is also worthy of clinical and experimental investigation.[263]

Thus, experimental investigations have revealed the antineoplastic potential of Vitamin K compounds, such as Vitamin K$_1$ (phylloquinone) and warfarin, on L1210 murine leukemia cell growth and Vitamin K$_3$ on various human tumor explants. A complete inhibition of L1210 growth in culture was obtained at concentrations of 200 μg/ml of warfarin, 75 μg/ml of Vitamin K$_1$, and 4 μg/ml of Vitamin K$_3$. Combined use of Vitamin K$_3$ and warfarin enhanced cytotoxicity since a concentration of 1 μg/ml of Vitamin K$_3$ together with 70 μg/

ml of warfarin resulted in early complete inhibition of L1210 growth. Comparable inhibition of malignant cell growth with Vitamin K_3 at concentrations of 6.4 μg/ml for L1210 leukemia and 1 μg/ml for Hll$_4$E hepatoma lines, where a >70% decrease in colony formation in both experiments, was seen. The cytotoxic activity of Vitamin K_3 was also tested *in vitro* against 34 human tumor explants, including adenocarcinoma of the breast, ovary cancer, colon carcinoma, stomach and kidney tumors, melanoma, squamous cell carcinoma of the lung, bladder transitional cell carcinoma, and hepatocellular carcinoma. A >50% decrease in colony formation occurred in 91% of human tumors tested at 10 μg/ml and in 86% tested at 1 μg/ml; a >70% inhibition in control colony formation occurred in 65% tested at 10 μg/ml and in 25% tested at 1 μg/ml. Therefore, the antineoplastic activity of Vitamins K_1 and K_3 is enhanced by combination with warfarin; Vitamin K_3 also exerts cytotoxic activity against human tumor explants *in vitro*.[264]

Vitamin K_3 was found to be approximately 25 times more cytotoxic than Vitamin K_1 in human neuroblastoma cell line. Vitamin K_3 also increases the thermosensitivity of Ehrlich ascites carcinoma cells, and enhances *in vitro* the antineoplastic activity of 5-fluorouracil in Friend murine erythroleukemia cells. Recent studies showed that combined i.p. administration of Vitamins K_3 and C before or after a single i.p. dose of six different cytotoxic drugs, all commonly used in human cancer therapy, produced a distinct chemotherapy-potentiating effect for all drugs, especially when injected before chemotherapy, on the survival of ascitic liver tumor (TLT)-bearing mice. Thus, Vitamins K_3 and C are cancer chemotherapy-potentiating agents.[265] With respect to Vitamin K_3 pharmacology, only soluble derivative menadiol sodium diphosphate (synkavite) has been studied. Using ^{3}H-K_1 suggests a biexponential decay which is between 20 and 25 min, and 2 to 2.8 h with a total clearance of 115 ml/min.

2. Clinical Trials

Vitamin K_3 as menadiol sodium diphosphate has been used as a radiation sensitizer. Some improvements were noted in radiation therapy plus synkavite in patients with bronchogenic carcinoma and buccal carcinoma. Thus, 39% of patients treated with radiation plus synkavite were alive and disease-free at 5 years, as opposed to 20% (from 70 patients) treated with radiation alone.[266] It has also been shown that injection of Vitamin K_3 (menadione) delays the occurrence of tumors in rats injected with DMBA or benzo(a)pyrene. Vitamin K_1, however, does not reduce the rate of tumor appearance.[267]

The anticoagulant warfarin has a similar quinone-based structure and has been used in different clinical trials in small cell lung cancer, breast cancer, prostate cancer, osteogenic sarcoma, and adenocarcinoma of the colon, showing some beneficial effects.[268] Rationale for the use of warfarin anticoagulation was originally based on animal studies which demonstrated that coagulation inhibition reduced the incidence of metastases. Other investigators noted tumor necrosis in patients receiving synkavite, which is metabolized to its active form of menadione (Vitamin K_3), and subsequently it was used as a radiation sensitizer as well as a targeting agent for the delivery of radioisotopes.[269] Combination of Vitamin K with antimetabolites was also used. This combination of Vitamin K_3, warfarin, and 5-FU was given to 15 patients with metastatic adenocarcinoma of the colon, and objective responses have lasted more than 12 months in four responding patients.[269]

3. Possible Mechanism(s) of Action of Vitamin K in Cancer Cells

The exact mechanism by which Vitamin K acts as an antineoplastic agent is currently unknown. Vitamins K_1 and K_3, as well as warfarin, are inhibitors of DNA synthesis in malignant cells as measured by incorporation of [^{14}C]-thymidine and [^{3}H]-deoxyuridine, mainly [^{14}C]-thymidine incorporation, which suggests a preferential inhibition of the salvage rather than *de novo* pathway of DNA synthesis. Thus, the K vitamins induce their cytotoxicity by inhibiting DNA synthesis in neoplastic cells; by possible generation of peroxides followed by membrane lipid alterations, especially electron transfer producing semiquinone free radical intermediates; and by inducing changes in transmembrane ionized calcium flux, observed in hepatocytes, pancreatic islet cells, and leukocytes.[270] In addition to producing cytotoxicity, menadione may act by noncytotoxic mechanisms. An inhibition of binding the epidermal growth factor to its receptor by Vitamin K_3 has been reported. In contrast, Vitamin K_1, K_2, and anthracyclic antitumor agents, such as doxorubicin, had no effect on EGF binding.[271] Menadione affects the secretion and activity of other growth modifiers, such as insulin and prostaglandin. It is likely that menadione (K_3) may prevent activation of polycyclic hydrocarbon carcinogens *in vivo* and may exhibit antimetastatic activity by affecting coagulation.

Therefore, the data, mostly *in vitro*, suggest that Vitamin K, especially Vitamin K_3 (menadione), exerts a cytotoxic and antitumor activity comparable to the toxic anthracycline quinones in current use. This antitumor activity may be further improved by using Vitamin K_3 in combination with radiation therapy, chemotherapeutic drugs (5-FU and methotrexate), radioisotopes as carriers, or other vitamins, such as Vitamins E and C. These vitamins act in certain ways synergistically and can provide additive therapeutic effects. Use of Vitamin K, either alone or in combination, represents a significant addition to cancer therapy.

II. COMMENTS AND CONCLUSIONS

The role of vitamins in the prevention and treatment of cancers has become increasingly evident in the last 10 to 15 years. In this regard, the biologic and biochemical activities associated with a variety of vitamins have stimulated investigations regarding their direct antitumor potential as well as their potential as adjuvants into antineoplastic therapies, such as radiation therapy, chemotherapy, or immunotherapy. Several investigations *in vitro*, as well as *in vivo,* revealed that certain vitamins exert strong antitumor and cytotoxic activities on tumor cells (Vitamins A, E, C, and K). Further studies will be required to more precisely define these mechanisms, especially to know how vitamins act on cancer cells at cellular and macromolecular levels. This cytotoxic mechanism of vitamins to kill or suppress only the tumor cells and protect the normal cells is of great significance because it is completely different from other antineoplastic agents (radiation and cytotoxic drugs), which destroy normal and neoplastic cells in the same way.

Thus, vitamins are much less toxic than radiation and cytotoxic drugs on cancer cells and also decrease the toxicity of chemotherapeutic drugs and ionizing radiation, thereby enhancing their therapeutic effects. Vitamins act mainly as hormones (hormone-like action) or as growth factors using autocrine and paracrine mechanisms. Although there is no direct evidence that vitamin deficiency plays a role in human carcinogenesis, as it did in animal tumors, it has been suggested that tumors of the esophagus, lung, bladder, stomach, colon, and possibly prostate are caused by carcinogens and precarcinogens in foods; thus, Vitamins A, C, and E are useful in preventing these types of cancers.[102,171,189,239,272] Hence, in recent years, there has been considerable interest in the role of Vitamins A, C, and E in the genesis, prevention, and treatment of cancer.

In contrast, little attention has been paid to Vitamins B, D, and K. No studies at all have been carried out on the effect of other vitamins, such as Vitamin H (biotin); Vitamin M (folic acid); Vitamin L (a new factor necessary for lactation in rats), as L_1 (found in beef-liver extract) and L_2 (found in yeast); Vitamin U (ulcer-preventing found in fresh cabbage juice); and Vitamin P complex (bioflavonoids), regarding their role in cancer prevention and treatment. From the entire collection of vitamins, the compounds classified under the general term ''Vitamin A'' are of the greatest current interest because of their possible association with carcinogenesis and cancer therapy and because of their important role in cell differentiation and proliferation.

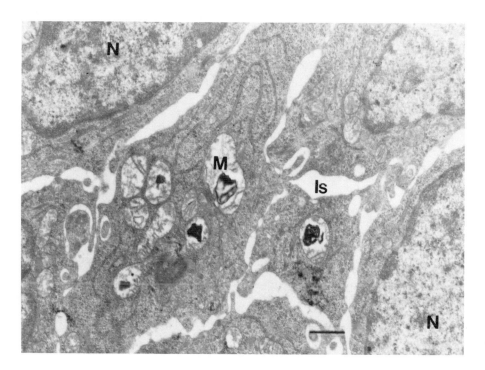

PLATE 1. Electron micrograph showing characteristic neoplastic cells with enlarged nuclei (N), mitochondrial alterations (M), and separated by intercellular spaces (Is) in a mouse with squamous cell carcinoma following 3-MCA. Bar = 1 μm. (Uranyl acetate and lead citrate × 8000.)

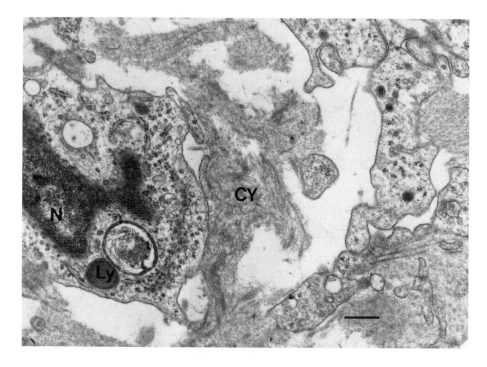

PLATE 2. Electron micrograph showing an advanced cytolysis (CY) cell disorganization with shrunken nucleu (N), and lysosomes (Ly) following 3-MCA and Vitamin E. Bar = 1 μm. (Uranyl acetate and lead citrate × 8000.)

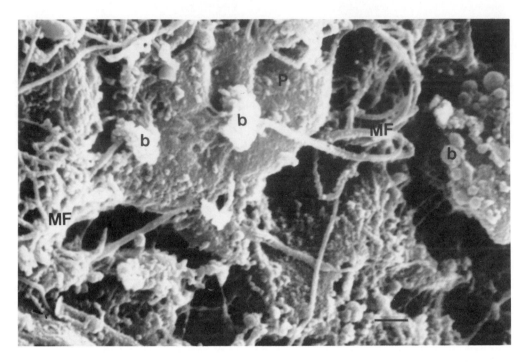

PLATE 3. Scanning electron micrograph showing rounded or polygonal cancer cells (P) covered with microvilli and blebs (b) and connected by a vast network of microfibrils (MF) in a mouse with squamous cell carcinoma following 3-MCA administration. Bar = 1 μm. (Critical point, gold coated × 5000.)

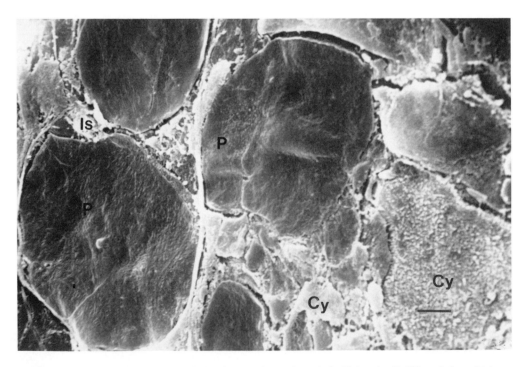

PLATE 4. Scanning electron micrograph showing an advanced cytolysis (Cy) and cell differentiation with large polygonal and flat cells (P) devoid of microvilli and blebs. Cells are connected by narrow intercellular spaces (Is). Mouse treated with 3-MCA and Vitamin E. Bar = 1 μm. (Critical point, gold coated × 5000.)

However, other substances called vitamins or "fake" vitamins, such as laetrile (called Vitamin B_{17}) and pangamic acid (called Vitamin B_{15}), have received great popularity among laymen and have been promoted in "unorthodox" treatment of cancer. At present, there are many "clinics" extensively using these substances for cancer patients who are looking in despair for a cure or improvement in their illness. There is, however, no scientific evidence or clinical controlled trials proving that these substances are vitamins or exert any beneficial effect in cancer treatment. What is needed at present are more studies to clarify the exact mechanisms of action of vitamins at cellular and molecular levels and to define the role of vitamins in cancer biology and neoplastic cell physiology. Unfortunately, the role of most vitamins in cancer cell metabolism is unknown, and they are used primarily on an empirical basis. Also, further studies are needed to develop new synthetic vitamin analogs which should exhibit a more potent antitumor role, less toxicity, and long-lasting activity.[235] Most vitamins, in order to exert their cytotoxic activity and kill cancer cells, should be at higher levels in plasma or within the cells, and consequently toxic effects exceed the therapeutic effects.

Use of vitamins in high doses or megadoses (megavitamin therapy), also called ortho-molecular therapy, is of controversial value. The use of Vitamin C in megadoses in patients with advanced metastatic cancer has provided conflicting results. The therapeutic doses of vitamins should not exceed more than 2 to 10 times the daily vitamin requirement, and undesirable noxious effects ranging from minor to major have been reported in association with the use of high doses of vitamins.

A strong inter-relationship between hormones, vitamins, and growth factors has been demonstrated. Thus, vitamins, hormones, and cytokines may use similar intracellular path-ways. In many cases, therapeutic combinations of hormones, vitamins, and growth factors can act synergistically on neoplastic cells and exert additive therapeutic effects.

An important physiologic phenomenon is the resistance to vitamins (vitamin resistance). The mechanism(s) of vitamin resistance include (1) inherited genetic defect; (2) vitamin-defective receptors; and (3) occurrence by spontaneous mutations of vitamin-resistant clones. The genetic defect occurs in some subjects, especially in absorption, transport, or metab-olism. These patients are nonresponders even to large doses of vitamins. Sometimes, a genetic enzymatic defect, i.e., in the enzyme which converts a provitamin into an active vitamin, is the main reason for the resistance. Some patients are vitamin resistant due to the presence of vitamin-defective receptors. Vitamins, such as A and D, possess several receptor sites for binding and coupling; they form a vitamin-receptor complex that acts on nuclear chromatin (DNA) by a transcriptional process which releases messenger-RNA (m-RNA) in a translation process and ultimately elicits the biologic effect by synthesizing new proteins. The receptors are numerically present, but are nonfunctional; or there is a presence of so-called "wild receptors", which are also defective (Vitamin D-resistant rickets).

Interestingly, the occurrence of vitamin-resistant clones *in vitro* and *in vivo,* is of great significance. For instance, the therapeutic effect of Vitamin C depends on the presence of catalase-containing cells in a certain tumor type. In order to produce a selective cell death in tumor tissue and exert its effects on tumor therapy, it is necessary that tumor cells generate enough H_2O_2 within the cells to cause their death. Normal cells have both catalase and peroxidase activities. Therefore, the inhibition of one of these enzymes may not affect the intracellular H_2O_2, and Vitamin C does not kill these cells. However, some tumor cells, due to a mutational event, contain predominantly catalase activity with little or no peroxidase activity, and consequently, Vitamin C would cause an accumulation of enough H_2O_2 to cause cell death. Also, some tumor cells lose their homeostatic control for the transport of Vitamin C and can accumulate large amounts of Vitamin C by the mechanism involving intracellular H_2O_2. Therefore, the efficacy of high doses of Vitamin C treatment depends upon the number of catalase-active cells, as well as the number of cells having a defective transport for Vitamin C in a tumor mass at the time of Vitamin C treatment. However, the number of these defective transport mechanisms and high catalase activity, may differ from one type of tumor to another, from one patient to another, and in the same individual during treatment.[181] Therefore, the efficacy of Vitamin C therapy in cancer depends mainly on the presence and number of catalase active cells in a tumor mass at the time of Vitamin C treatment.

Vitamins E- and A-resistant cells have also been found in culture, and they exhibit a morphology which is similar to that observed in nontreated cultured cells. It has not been demonstrated whether the mutations of vitamin resistant clones are present at the beginning in a tumor mass, or if they develop during vitamin therapy. It is likely that some mutant cells become more vitamin resistant during vitamin therapy. Because of their particular physiologic mechanism of action and less toxicity as well as very good tolerability, vitamins offer a new approach to cancer treatment, which is different from those of surgery, radiation therapy, chemotherapy, and immunotherapy. Thus, vitamins in contrast to cytostatics, showed no genuine carcinogenicity.[195] Further research is needed to determine if certain tumors are more responsive to a specific vitamin.

Thus, if vitamin responsiveness is a tumor-type specific, this will be an important criteria for selection of cancer patients for vitamin therapy. Most vitamins (Vitamin A and retinoids, Vitamins E, C, and D) are important in the growth and differentiation of epithelial tissues. Thus, vitamins in pharmacologic concentrations exhibit antitumor activity by inducing cell differentiation to normal phenotype and/or by cytotoxic activity causing cell death. Although the exact cellular and molecular mechanisms of Vitamins A, C, E, and D are unknown, there are specific receptors for retinoic acid and one for retinol. There is a statistically significant correlation between ER status and the presence of a cellular regulator for retinoic acid, thus the ER content of the tumor reflects the degree of tumor cell differentiation.[272] Vitamins may influence the management of tumors by inhibiting DNA synthesis and by acting on the cell cycle of tumor cells (see Figure 3A, Chapter 2), i.e., on the S-phase of the cycle.

Certain vitamins (A, E) may change the membrane structure in a way which would alter receptor sites, receptor sensitivity, transport functions, and membrane-bound enzyme activities. These membrane changes could then alter the translation and transcriptional activities of the genome. There are at least three distinct Vitamin E-binding protein receptors (two of these are extranuclear and present in the cytosol, and the third one is associated with the nuclear fraction). The presence of Vitamin E-binding receptors has also been found in tumor cells in culture.[238] Tumor cells resistant to Vitamins A, C, and E are present in tumors. The mechanisms for each of these vitamins on tumor cells appear to be different. Therefore, a combination of more vitamins, such as E and C, or A, E, and C, may act synergistically and thus overcome vitamin resistance. Hence, vitamins can exert additive effects. Further studies are needed to develop a rational strategy for the use of multiple vitamins in pharmacologic doses for the treatment of human cancers.

Vitamins can also modify the effects of tumor therapeutic agents, such as synthetic cytostatic drugs, radiation therapy, immunotherapy, and hyperthermia. Vitamins may enhance their therapeutic potential and render them less toxic; they also may protect normal cells against radiation or cytotoxic agent damages and consequently may markedly improve treatment effectiveness. Thus, it will be possible by using vitamins, vitamin modulation or vitamin manipulation, to enhance the therapeutic effects of conventional therapies, such as chemotherapy, radiation therapy, or immunotherapy, and also to diminish or reduce their toxic effects on normal cells. The combination of vitamins, or vitamins with chemotherapeutic drugs, radiation, or immunological agents, growth factors, and hormones, can better overcome vitamin resistance or drug resistance. Certain vitamins (E, C, D) play an important role in the host's immune system or immune surveillance mechanisms which control the escape of transformed cells to develop a clinically detectable cancer. This system is also important during cancer treatment.

Vitamins A, E, and D exert an enhancement of the immune defense mechanism of the host; they are immunoenhancers or immunoaugmentators, and also increase the resistance to disease. They stimulate humoral immunity and cellular immunity.

Vitamins also may enhance the therapeutic effects of cytotoxic drugs, radiation, and immunotherapy by stimulating the host's immune defense mechanism. Thus, vitamins may increase the effectiveness of current tumor therapeutic agents by increasing their lethal effect on cancer cells and by reducing their noxious effects on normal cells. Each vitamin may act in a different way on tumor cells (cell differentiation, cytotoxicity, antioxidation, DNA synthesis, cell membrane destabilizer, reduction of receptor bindings, paracrine or autocrine mechanism, immunoaugmentation, or prevention of precancer cell transformation into cancer cells), and this depends upon the tumor type, individuals, or cancer cell line. Therefore, vitamins act by a complex and multifactorial mechanism.

However, the exact cellular and molecular mechanisms of vitamins and their analogs on cancer cells still remain unknown. Experiments *in vitro* reveal that vitamins (A, E, D) exert important effects in cell differentiation, cell proliferation, and replication, which strongly suggest that vitamins are significant biologic factors in controlling cancer cell homeostasis. Vitamins, such as Vitamin D_3 and its biologically active form, $1\alpha,25(OH)_2D_3$, act as hormones; they are hormones or hormone-like substances, such as steroid hormones. They bind to specific receptor sites located on the cell membranes. Then they are translocated as vitamin-receptor complexes to the nuclear chromatin, where they trigger at specific regions the transcription process forming m-RNA, and by the translation process synthesize new proteins which elicit the biologic effect on neoplastic cells.

A plethora of experimental and epidemiologic evidence demonstrates that vitamins exert an important antitumor activity in various animal tumor models and in prevention of several human cancers (bronchus, esophagus, colon, skin, prostate, bladder), which indicates that vitamins exert an important chemopreventive and chemotherapeutic effect. There are less impressive studies regarding the therapeutic effects of vitamins in treatment of human cancers. Further investigations should be focused on the development of novel synthetic vitamin analogs which will produce significant antitumor effects without unacceptable toxic or adverse effects. Studies on the role of Vitamins B_1, B_2, B_6, B_{12} and Vitamin K (K_1, K_2, K_3) should be carried out to define their role in cancer prevention and therapy. Recently, it was demonstrated that biotin (vitamin H) is synthesized by microorganisms from biocytin due to enzyme biotinidase. It has many analogs and antagonists, and it was isolated as α-biotin from egg yolk and β-biotin from liver. Biotin is involved in neuromuscular and immune systems and may be involved in the synthesis of growth/transforming factors.[273] Vitamins alone or in combination with other conventional therapy will enhance their therapeutic effects. Clinical oncologists should recommend vitamins or vitamin mixtures more often in cancer treatment. Vitamins, being less toxic and providing the same therapeutic effects, offer new approaches to cancer treatment. In the next decade, research regarding the role of vitamins and their analogs will open an exciting field in cancer treatment and prevention.

REFERENCES

1. **Stähelin, H. B.,** Vitamins and cancer, *Rec. Res. Cancer Res.*, 108, 227, 1988.
2. **Bollag, W.,** Retinoids and cancer, *Cancer Chemother. Pharmacol.*, 3, 207, 1979.
3. **Lotan, R.,** Effects of Vitamin A and its analogues (retinoids) on normal and neoplastic cells, *Biochem. Biophys. Acta*, 605, 33, 1980.

4. **Wolbach, S. B. and Howe, P. R.,** Tissue changes following deprivation of fat-soluble A vitamin, *J. Exp. Med.,* 42, 753, 1925.

5. **Prasad, K. N. and Rama, B. N.,** Modification of the effect of pharmacological agents on tumor cells in cultures by Vitamin C and Vitamin E, in *Modulation and Mediation of Cancer by Vitamins,* Prasad, K. N. and Meyskens, F. L., Eds., S. Karger, Basel, 1983, 244.

6. **Lupulescu, A.,** Control of epithelial precancer cell transformation into cancer cells by vitamins, *J. Cell Biol.,* 103, 29, 1986.

7. Vitamin preparations as dietary supplements and as therapeutic agents, Council Report: *JAMA,* 257, 1929, 1987.

8. **Bässler, K.,** Megavitamin therapy with pyridoxine, *Int. J. Vitam. Nutr. Res.,* 58, 105, 1988.

9. **Pauling, L. and Moertel, C.,** A proposition: megadoses of Vitamin C are valuable in the treatment of cancer, *Nutr. Rev.,* 44, 28, 1986.

10. **Moertel, C. G., Fleming, T. R., Creagan, E. T., Rubin, J., O'Connell, M. J., and Ames, M. M.,** High-dose Vitamin C versus placebo in the treatment of patients with advanced cancer who have had no prior chemotherapy. A randomized double-blind comparison, *N. Engl. J. Med.,* 312, 137, 1985.

11. **Doll, R. and Peto, R.,** The causes of cancer: quantitative estimates of avoidable risks of cancer in the U.S. today, *J. Natl. Cancer Inst.,* 66, 1191, 1981.

12. **Forfar, J. O., Balf, C. L., and Maxwell, J. M.,** Idiopathic hypercalcemia of infancy: clinical and metabolic studies with special reference to the etiological role of Vitamin D, *Lancet,* 1, 981, 1956.

13. **Goodman, D. S.,** Vitamin A and retinoids in health and disease, *N. Engl. J. Med.,* 310, 1023, 1984.

14. **Rosenberg, L.,** Vitamin-responsive inherited metabolic disorders, *Adv. Hum. Genet.,* 6, 1, 1976.

15. **Lippman, S. M., Kessler, J. F., and Meyskens, F. L.,** Retinoids as preventive and therapeutic anticancer agents, *Cancer Treat. Rep.,* 71, 391, 1987.

16. **Israël, L., Hajji, O., Grefft-Alami, A., Desmoulins, D., Succari, M., Cals, M. L., Miocque, M., Bréau, J. L., and Morère, J.F.,** Augmentation par la Vitamine A des effets de la chimiothérapie dans le cancer du sein métastasés après la ménopause, *Ann. Med. Interne (Paris),* 136, 551, 1985.

17. **Bertino, J. R.,** Nutrients, vitamins and minerals as therapy, *Cancer,* 43, 2137, 1979.

18. **Wald, N.,** Retinol, beta-carotene and cancer, *Cancer Surv.,* 6, 635, 1987.

19. **Merriman, R. L. and Bertram, J. S.,** Reversible inhibition by retinoids of 3-methylcholanthrene-induced neoplastic transformation in C3H/10T$^{1}/_2$ clone 8 cells, *Cancer Res.,* 39, 1661, 1979.

20. **Boutwell, R. K.,** Biochemical mechanism of tumor promotion, in *Carcinogenesis, Mechanisms of Tumor Promotion and Carcinogenesis,* Slaga, T. J., Sivak, A., and Boutwell, R. K., Eds., Raven Press, New York, 1978, 49.

21. **Abels, J. C., Gorham, A. T., Pack, G. T., and Rhoads, C. P.,** Metabolic studies in patients with cancer of the gastrointestinal tract. I. Plasma Vitamin A levels in patients with malignant neoplastic disease, particularly of the gastrointestinal tract, *J. Clin. Invest.,* 20, 749, 1941.

22. **Marks, R. and Horton, J. J.,** The oral retinoid agents. Are they the wonder drugs of the 1980s?, *Med. J. Aust.,* 146, 374, 1987.

23. **Brown, M. S., Kovanen, P. T., and Goldstein, J. L.,** Regulation of plasma cholesterol, by lipoprotein receptors, *Science,* 212, 628, 1981.

24. **Wake, K.,** Perisinusoidal stellate cells (fat-storing cells, interstitial cells, lipocytes), their related structure in and around the liver sinusoids, and Vitamin A-storing cells in extrahepatic organs, *Int. Rev. Cytol.,* 66, 303, 1980.

25. **Bollag, W.,** Vitamin A and retinoids: from nutrition to pharmacotherapy in dermatology and oncology, *Lancet,* 1, 860, 1983.

26. **Wolf, G.,** Multiple functions of Vitamin A, *Physiol. Rev.,* 64, 873, 1984.

27. **Sporn, M. B. and Roberts, A. B.,** Suppression of carcinogenesis by retinoids: interaction with peptide growth and their receptors as a key mechanism, in *Diet, Nutrition and Cancer,* Hayashi, Y., Nagao, M., Sugimura, T., Tomatis, L., Wattenberg, L. W., and Wogan, G. N., Eds., Jap. Sci. Soc. Press, Tokyo, 1986, 149.

28. **Nettesheim, P., Snyder, C., and Kim, J. C.,** Vitamin A and susceptibility of respiratory tract tissues to carcinogenic insult, *Environ. Health Perspect.,* 29, 89, 1979.

29. **Shamberger, R. J.,** Inhibitory effect of Vitamin A on carcinogenesis, *J. Natl. Cancer Inst.,* 47, 667, 1971.

30. **Lupulescu, A.,** Inhibition of DNA synthesis and neoplastic cell growth by Vitamin A (retinol), *J. Natl. Cancer Inst.,* 77, 149, 1986.

31. **Moon, R. C., McCormick, D. L., and Mehta, R. G.,** Inhibition of carcinogenesis by retinoids, *Cancer Res.,* 43, (Supp. 5), 2469, 1983.

32. **Marth, C., Mayer, I., and Daxenbichler, G.,** Effect of retinoic acid and 4-hydroxytamoxifen on human breast cancer cell lines, *Biochem. Pharmacol.,* 33, 2217, 1984.

33. **Vitale, C., Rakowski, I., and Raza, A.,** Number of DNA replication cycles completed by HL-60 cells during differentiation induced by 13 *cis*-retinoic acid (RA), *Blood,* 68 (Suppl. 1), 194a, 1986.

34. **Mehta, R. G. and Moon, R. C.,** Inhibition of DNA synthesis by retinyl acetate during chemically-induced mammary carcinogenesis, *Cancer Res.,* 40, 1109, 1980.
35. **Lotan, R. and Nicolson, G. L.,** Inhibitory effects of retinoic acid or retinyl acetate on the growth of untransformed, transformed and tumor cells *in vitro, J. Natl. Cancer Inst.,* 59, 1717, 1977.
36. **Fitzgerald, D. J., Barrett, J. C., and Nettesheim, P.,** Changing responsiveness to all trans retinoic acid of rat tracheal epithelial cells at different stages of neoplastic transformation, *Carcinogenesis,* 7, 1715, 1986.
37. **Lotan, R.,** Mechanism of inhibition of tumor cell proliferation by retinoids, in *Retinoids: New Trends in Research and Therapy,* Saurat, J. H., Ed., S. Karger, Basel, 1985, 97.
38. **Cunningham, W. J. and Ehmann, C. W.,** Clinical aspects of the retinoids, *Semin. Dermatol,* 2, 145, 1983.
39. **Strickland, S., Breitman, T. R., Frickel, F., Hädicke, E., and Sporn, M. B.,** Structure-activity relationships of a new series of retinoidal benzoic acid derivatives as measured by induction of differentiation of murine F_9 teratocarcinoma cells and human HL-60 promyelocytic leukemia cells, *Cancer Res.,* 43, 5268, 1983.
40. **Tobler, A., Dawson, M. T., and Koeffler, H. P.,** Retinoids: structure-function relationship in normal and leukemic hematopoiesis *in vitro, J. Clin. Invest.,* 78, 303, 1986.
41. **Lotan, R., Stolarsky, T., and Lotan, D.,** Relationship between the structure of retinoidal benzoic acid derivatives and their ability to inhibit the proliferation of melanoma cells in culture, *J. Nutr. Growth Cancer,* 1, 71, 1983.
42. **McCormick, D. L., Mehta, R. G., Thompson, C. A., Dinger, N., and Moon, R. C.,** Enhanced inhibition of mammary carcinogenesis by combined treatment with N-(4-hydroxyphenyl) retinamide and ovariectomy, *Cancer Res.,* 42, 508, 1982.
43. **Moon, R. C. and Mehta, R. G.,** Anticarcinogenic effects of retinoids in animals, *Adv. Exp. Med. Biol.,* 206, 399, 1986.
44. **McCormick, D. L., and Moon, R. C.,** Influence of delayed administration of retinyl acetate on mammary carcinogenesis, in *Proc. Int. Cancer Congr ,* 1982, 682.
45. **Russell, D. H. and Haddox, M. K.,** Antiproliferative effects of retinoids related to the cell cycle-specific inhibition of ornithine decarboxylase, *Ann. N.Y. Acad. Sci.,* 359, 281, 1981.
46. **Yuspa, S. H. and Lichti, U.,** Retinoids and skin carcinogenesis: a mechanism of anticarcinogenesis by modulation of epidermal differentiation, in *Retinoids: New Trends in Research and Therapy,* Saurat, J. H., Ed., S. Karger, Basel, 1985, 56.
47. **Martner, J. E. and Bertram, J. S.,** Appearance of tyrosine phosphorylation correlates with time of transformation in $10T^{1/}_2$ cells: inhibition of retinyl acetate, *Proc. Am. Assoc. Cancer Res.,* 25, 146, 1984.
48. **Sidell, N., Lucas, C. A., and Kreutzberg, G. W.,** Regulation of acetylcholinesterase activity by retinoic acid in a human neuroblastoma cell line, *Exp. Cell Res.,* 155, 305, 1984.
49. **Bolmer, S. D. and Wolf, G.,** Stimulation of fibronectin production by retinoic acid in mouse skin tumors, *Cancer Res.,* 42, 4465, 1982.
50. **Grigoriadis, A. E., Petkovich, P. M., Rosenthal, E. E., and Heersche, J. N.,** Modulation by retinoic acid of 1,25-dihydroxy Vitamin D_3 effects on alkaline phosphatase activity and parathyroid hormone responsiveness in an osteoblast-like osteosarcoma cell line, *Endocrinology,* 119, 932, 1986.
51. **Gercel, C. and Schroeder, E. W.,** Relationship between cell surface glycoconjugate and cell-cell interactions of murine and human melanoma cells, *J. Cell Biol.,* 99, 66a, 1984.
52. **Jetten, A. M. and Goldfarb, R. H.,** Action of epidermal growth factor and retinoids on anchorage-dependent and independent growth of nontransformed kidney cells, *Cancer Res.,* 43, 2094, 1983.
53. **Van Zoelen, E. J., Van Oostwaard, T. M., and De Laat, S. W.,** Transforming growth factor-β and retinoic acid modulate phenotypic transformation of normal rat kidney cells induced by epidermal growth factor and platelet-derived growth factor, *J. Biol. Chem.,* 261, 5003, 1986.
54. **Nishizuka, Y.,** Studies and perspectives of protein kinase C, *Science,* 233, 305, 1986.
55. **Jetten, A. M.,** Effects of retinoic acid on the binding and mitogenic activity of epidermal growth factor, *J. Cell Physiol.,* 110, 235, 1982.
56. **Chytil, F. and Ong, D. E.,** Mediation of retinoic acid induced growth and antitumor activity, *Nature (London),* 260, 49, 1976.
57. **Mehta, R. G., Cerny, W. L., and Moon, R. C.,** Nuclear interactions of retinoic acid binding protein in chemically-induced mammary adenocarcinoma, *Biochem. J.,* 208, 731, 1982.
58. **Libby, P. R. and Bertram, J. S.,** Lack of intracellular retinoid-binding protein in a retinol-sensitive cell line, *Carcinogenesis,* 3, 481, 1982.
59. **Wang, S. Y., La Rosa, G. J., and Gudas, L. J.,** Molecular cloning of gene sequences transcriptionally regulated by retinoic acid and dibutyryl cyclic AMP in cultured mouse teratocarcinoma cells, *Dev. Biol.,* 107, 75, 1985.
60. **Bentley, D. L. and Groudine, M. A.,** A block to elongation is largely responsible for decreased transcription of C-myc in differentiated HL-60 cells, *Nature (London),* 321, 702, 1986.

61. **Lawrence, H. J., Hack, F. M., Alhadeft, M., Meyers, F., and Largman, C.,** Effects of retinoic acid on oncogene expression and clonogenic growth of human myeloid leukemia cells, *Clin. Res.,* 34, 40, 1986.
62. **Jetten, A. M., Barrett, J. C., and Gilmer, T. M.,** Differential response to retinoic acid of Syrian hamster embryo fibroblasts expressing V-src or V-Ha-ras oncogenes, *Mol. Cell. Biol.,* 6, 3341, 1986.
63. **Wolf, G., Kiorpes, T. D., Masushige, S., Smith, M., and Anderson, R.,** Recent evidence of the participation of Vitamin A in glycoprotein synthesis, *Fed. Proc.,* 38, 2540, 1979.
64. **Brinckerhoff, C. E., Coffey, J. W., and Sullivan, A. C.,** Inflammation and collagenase production in rats with adjuvant arthritis reduced with 13-*cis*-retinoic acid, *Science,* 221, 756, 1983.
65. **Dennert, G.,** Immunostimulation by retinoic acid, in *Retinoids, Differentiation and Disease,* Nugent, J. and Clark, S., Eds., Pitman, London, 1985, 117.
66. **Tachibana, K., Sone, S., Tsubura, E., and Kishino, Y.,** Stimulatory effect of Vitamin A on tumoricidal activity of rat alveolar macrophages, *Br. J. Cancer,* 49, 343, 1984.
67. **Eccles, S.,** Effects of retinoids on growth and dissemination of malignant tumors: immunological considerations, *Biochem. Pharmacol.,* 34, 1599, 1985.
68. **Cope, F. O., Howard, B. D., and Boutwell, R. K.,** The *in vitro* characterization of the inhibition of mouse brain protein kinase-C by retinoids and their receptors, *Experientia,* 42, 1023, 1986.
69. **Chytil, F.,** Retinoic acid: biochemistry and metabolism, *J. Am. Acad. Dermatol.,* 15, 741, 1986.
70. **Basu, T. K., Temple, N. J., and Hodgson, A. M.,** Vitamin A, beta-carotene and cancer, in *Nutrition, Growth, and Cancer,* Tryfiates, G. P. and Prasad, K. N., Eds., Alan R. Liss, New York, 1988, 217.
71. **Peck, G. L.,** Retinoids in clinical dermatology, in *Progress in Diseases of the Skin,* Fleischmajer, R., Ed., Grune & Stratton, San Francisco, 1981, 227.
72. **Belisario, J. C.,** Recent advances in topical cytotoxic therapy of skin cancer and precancer, in *Melanoma and Skin Cancer,* Proc. Int. Cancer Confer., Sydney, 1972, 349.
73. **Bollag, W. and Ott, F.,** Vitamin A acid in benign and malignant epithelial tumors of the skin, *Acta Derm. Venereol. (Stockh),* Suppl. 74, 163, 1975.
74. **Kingston, T., Gaskell, S., and Marks, R.,** The effects of a novel potent oral retinoid (RO13-6298) in the treatment of multiple solar keratoses and squamous cell epithelioma, *Eur. J. Cancer Clin. Oncol.,* 19, 1201, 1983.
75. **Shaw, J. C. and White, C. R.,** Treatment of multiple keratoacanthomas with oral isotretinoin, *J. Am. Acad. Dermatol.,* 15, 1079, 1986.
76. **Peck, G. L.,** Therapy and prevention of skin cancer, in *Retinoids: New Trends in Research and Therapy,* Saurat, J. H., Ed., S. Karger, Basel, 1985, 345.
77. **Meyskens, F. L., Edwards, L., and Levine, N.,** Role of topical tretinoin in melanoma and dysplastic nevi, *J. Am. Acad. Dermatol.,* 15, 822, 1986.
78. **Edwards, L., Meyskens, F. L., and Levine, N.,** Effect of oral isotretinoin on dysplastic nevi, *J. Am. Acad. Dermatol.,* 20, 257, 1989.
79. **Lutzner, M. A. and Blanchet-Bardon, C.,** Oral retinoid treatment of human papillomavirus type 5-induced epidermodysplasia verruciformis, *N. Engl. J. Med.,* 302, 1091, 1980.
80. **Burge-Bottenbley, A. and Shklar, G.,** Retardation of experimental oral cancer development by retinyl acetate, *Nutr. Cancer,* 5, 121, 1983.
81. **Koch, H. F.,** Biochemical treatment of precancerous oral lesions: the effectiveness of various analogues of retinoic acid, *J. Maxillofac. Surg.,* 6, 59, 1978.
82. **Koch, H. F.,** Effect of retinoids on precancerous lesions of oral mucosa, in *Retinoids: Advances in Basic Research and Therapy,* Orfanos, C. E., Braun-Falco, O., and Farber, E. M., Eds., Springer-Verlag, Berlin, 1981, 307.
83. **Hong, W. K. and Doos, W. G.,** Chemoprevention of head and neck cancer, *Otolaryngol. Clin. North Am.,* 18, 543, 1985.
84. **Mathé, G., Guoveia, J., Hercend, T., Gros, F., Hazon, J., Misset, J., Ribaud, P., and Gaget, H.,** Correlation between precancerous bronchial metaplasia and cigarette consumption, the preliminary results of retinoid treatment, *Cancer Detect. Prev.,* 5, 461, 1982.
85. **Band, P. R., Feldstein, M., and Saccomanno, G.,** Reversibility of bronchial marked atypia: implication for chemoprevention, *Cancer Detect. Prev.,* 9, 157, 1986.
86. **Bichler, E.,** The role of aromatic retinoid in treatment of laryngeal keratinizing disorders and dysplasias, in *Proc. 13th Int. Congr. Chemother.,* Spitzy, K. H. and Karrer, K., Eds., V. H. Egermann, Vienna, 1983, 201.
87. **Wylie-Rosett, J. A., Romney, S. L., Slagle, N. S.,Miller, G., Palan, P., and Duttagupta, C.,** Influence of Vitamin A on cervical dysplasia and carcinoma *in situ, Nutr. Cancer,* 6, 49, 1984.
88. **Weiner, S. A., Surwit, E. A., Graham, V., and Meyskens, F. L.,** A Phase I trial of topically applied trans-retinoic acid in cervical dysplasia, *Invest. New Drugs,* 4, 241, 1986.
89. **Romney, S. L., Dwyer, A., and Slagle, N. S.,** Chemoprevention of cervix cancer: Phase I-II; a feasibility study involving the topical vaginal administration of retinyl acetate gel, *Gynecol. Oncol.,* 20, 109, 1985.

90. **Koeffler, H. P.**, Preleukemia, *Clin. Haematol.*, 15, 829, 1986.

91. **Bagby, G. C. Jr.**, *The Preleukemic Syndrome* (hematopoietic dysplasia), CRC Press, Boca Raton, FL, 1985, 219.

92. **Picozzi, V. J., Swanson, G. F., Morgan, R., Hecht, F., and Greenberg, P. L.**, 13-*cis*-retinoic acid treatment for myelodysplastic syndromes, *J. Clin. Oncol.*, 4, 589, 1986.

93. **Clark, R. E., Lush, C. J., Jacobs, A., and Smith, S. A.**, Effect of 13-*cis*-retinoic acid on survival of patients with myelodysplastic syndrome, *Lancet*, 1, 763, 1987.

94. **Sporn, M. B., Squire, R. A., and Brown, C. C.**, 13-*cis*-retinoic acid: inhibition of bladder carcinogenesis in the rat, *Science*, 195, 487, 1977.

95. **Tyler, H. A., Notley, R. G., Schweizer, F. A., and Dickerson, J.**, Vitamin A status and bladder cancer, *Eur. J. Surg. Oncol.*, 12, 35, 1986.

96. **Fagg, S. L., Hughes, A., Fielding, J. W., Hughs, M., and Howie, A.**, Retinoic acid receptor in human bladder tumors, *Clin. Oncol.*, 8, 329, 1982.

97. **Studer, U. E., Biedermann, C., Chollett, D., Karrer, P., Kraft, R., and Vonbank, F.**, Prevention of recurrent superficial bladder tumors by oral etretinate: preliminary results of a randomized, double-blind multicenter trial in Switzerland, *J. Urol.*, 131, 47, 1984.

98. **Soloway, M. S.**, Rationale for intensive intravesical chemotherapy for superficial bladder cancer, *J. Urol.*, 123, 461, 1980.

99. **Flamm, J. and Grof, F.**, Adjuvante lokale instillations Therapie mit vitamin A in der Nachbehandlung transurethral resezierter Harnblasen tumoren, *Urologe (A)*, 21, 229, 1982.

100. **Pichler, E. and Fritsch, P.**, Xeroderma pigmentosum: tumorprophylaxe mit etretinate *Hautarzt*, 35, 159, 1984.

101. **Kummet, T. and Meyskens, F. L.**, Vitamin A: a potential inhibitor of human cancer, *Semin. Oncol.*, 10, 281, 1983.

102. **Lippman, S. M., Kessler, J. F., and Meyskens, F. L., Jr.**, Retinoids as preventive and therapeutic anticancer agents (Part II), *Cancer Treat. Rep.*, 71, 493, 1987.

103. **Giguere, V., Ong, E. S., Segui, P., and Evans, R. M.**, Identification of a receptor for the morphogen retinoic acid, *Nature (London)*, 330, 624, 1987.

104. **Lippman, S. M., Shimm, D. S., and Meyskens, F. L., Jr.**, Nonsurgical treatments for skin cancer: retinoids and α-interferon, *J. Dermatol. Surg. Oncol.*, 14, 862, 1988.

105. **Sankowski, A., Janik, P., and Bogacka-Zatorska, E.**, Treatment of basal cell carcinoma with 13-*cis*-retinoic acid, *Neoplasma*, 31, 615, 1984.

106. **Grupper, C. H. and Berretti, B.**, Cutaneous neoplasia and etretinate, in *Proc. 13th Int. Congr. Chemother.*, Spitzy, K. H. and Karrer, K., Eds., V. H. Egermann, Vienna, 1983, 201.

107. **Braun-Falco, O., Galosi, A., Dorn, M., and Plewig, G.**, Tumor prophylaxe bei xeroderma Pigmentosum mit aromatischem Retinoid (Ro10-9359), *Hautarzt*, 33, 445, 1982.

108. **Kim, J. S., Lee, J. S., and Blick, M.**, Effects of retinoic acid (RA) on the gene expression, autophosphorylation, and EGF binding properties of the EGF-receptor in human head and neck squamous cells (HHNSCC), *Proc. Am. Cancer Res. Assoc.*, 29, 42, 1988.

109. **Lippman, S. M. and Meyskens, F. L.**, Treatment of advanced squamous cell carcinoma of the skin with isotretinoin, *Ann. Intern. Med.*, 107, 499, 1987.

110. **Roach, M.**, A malignant eccrine poroma responds to isotretinoin (13-*cis* retinoic acid), *Ann. Intern. Med.*, 99, 486, 1983.

111. **Lotan R., Neumann, G., and Lotan, D.**, Characterization of retinoic acid-induced alterations in the proliferation and differentiation of a murine and a human melanoma cell line in culture, *Ann. N.Y. Acad. Sci.*, 359, 150, 1981.

112. **Felix, E. L., Cohen, M. H., and Loyd, B. C.**, Immune and toxic and antitumor effects of systemic and intralesional Vitamin A, *J. Surg. Res.*, 21, 307, 1976.

113. **Meyskens, F. L., Edwards, L., and Levine, N.**, Role of topical tretinoin in melanoma and dysplastic nevi, *J. Am. Acad. Dermatol.*, 15, 822, 1986.

114. **Kessler, J. F., Jones, S. E., Levine, N., Lynch, P. J., Booth, A. R., and Meyskens, F. L. Jr.**, Isotretinoin and cutaneous helper T-cell lymphoma (mycosis fungoides), *Arch. Dermatol.*, 123, 201, 1987.

115. **Mahrle, G., Thiele, B., and Ippen, H.**, Chemotherapie Kutaner T-zell lymphome mit arotinoid, *Dtsch. Med. Wochenschr.*, 108, 1753, 1983.

116. **Tousignant, J., Raymond, G. P., and Light, M. J.**, Treatment of cutaneous T-cell lymphoma with the arotinoid Ro13-6298, *J. Am. Acad. Dermatol.*, 16, 167, 1987.

117. **Flynn, P. J., Miller, W. J., Weisdorf, D. J., Arthur, D. C., Brunning, R., and Branda, R. F.**, Retinoic acid treatment of acute promyelocytic leukemia: *in vitro* and *in vivo* observations, *Blood*, 62, 1211, 1983.

118. **Fontana, J. A., Rogers, J. S., and Durham, J. P.**, The role of 13-*cis*-retinoic acid in the remission induction of a patient with acute promyelocytic leukemia, *Cancer*, 57, 209, 1986.

119. **Arlin, A. Z., Mertelsmann, R., Berman, E., Gee, T., Kurland, E., Chaganti, R. S., Jhanwar, S. C., Moore, M. A., and Clarkson, B. D.,** 13-*cis*-retinoic acid does not increase the true remission rate and the duration of true remission (induced by cytotoxic chemotherapy) in patients with chronic phase chronic myelogenous leukemia, *J. Clin. Oncol.,* 3, 473, 1985.

120. **Meyskens, F. L., Gilmartin, E., Alberts, D. S., Levine N., Brooks, R., and Surwit, E.,** Activity of isotretinoin against squamous cell cancers and preneoplastic lesions, *Cancer Treat. Rep.,* 66, 1315, 1982.

121. **Komiyama, S., Hiroto, I., Ryu, S., Kuwano, M., and Endo, H.,** Synergistic combination therapy of 5-fluorouracil, Vitamin A and cobalt-60 radiation upon head and neck tumors, *Oncology,* 25, 253, 1978.

122. **Micksche, M., Cerni, C., Kokron, O., Titscher, R., and Wrba, H.,** Stimulation of immune response in lung cancer patients by Vitamin A therapy, *Oncology,* 34, 234, 1977.

123. **Millan, S. B., Flowers, F. P., and Sherertz, E. F.,** Isotretinoin, *South. Med. J.,* 80, 494, 1987.

124. **Windhorst, D. B. and Nigra, T.,** General clinical toxicity of oral retinoids, *J. Am. Acad. Dermatol.,* 6, 675, 1982.

125. **Edwards, L., Alberts, D. S., and Levine, N.,** Clinical toxicity of low-dose isotretinoin, *Cancer Treat. Rep.,* 70, 663, 1986.

126. **Ellis, C. N. and Voorhees, J. J.,** Etretinate therapy, *J. Am. Acad. Dermatol.,* 16, 267, 1987.

127. **Brazzell, R. K. and Colburn, W. A.,** Pharmacokinetics of the retinoids, isotretinoin and etretinate, *J. Am. Acad. Dermatol.,* 6, 643, 1982.

128. **Meyskens, F. L., Goodman, G. E., and Alberts, D. S.,** 13-*cis*-retinoic acid: pharmacology, toxicology, and clinical application for the prevention and treatment of human cancer, *Crit. Rev. Oncol. Hematol.,* 3, 75, 1985.

129. **Stern, R. S.,** The case of isotretinoin, *N. Engl. J. Med.,* 320, 1007, 1989.

130. **Shroot, B.,** Pharmacology of topical retinoids, *J. Am. Acad. Dermatol.,* 15, 748, 1986.

131. **Tannenbaum, A. and Silverstone, H.,** The genesis and growth of tumors. Effects of varying the level of B vitamins in the diet, *Cancer Res.,* 12, 744, 1952.

132. **Boutwell, R. K., Brush, M., and Rusch, H. P.,** The influence of vitamins of the B complex on the induction of epithelial tumors in mice, *Cancer Res.,* 9, 747, 1949.

133. **Rivlin, R. S.,** Riboflavin, in *Essential Nutrients in Carcinogenesis,* Poirier, L., Newberne, P. M., and Pariza, M. W., Eds., Plenum Press, New York, 1986, 349.

134. **Kensler, C. J., Sugiura, K., Young, N. F., Halter, C. R., and Rhoads, C. P.,** Partial protection of rats by riboflavin with casein against liver cancer caused by dimethylaminoazobenzene, *Science,* 93, 308, 1941.

135. **Morris, H. P. and Robertson, W. B.,** Growth rate and number of spontaneous mammary carcinomas and riboflavin concentration of liver, muscle, and tumor of C3H mice as influenced by dietary riboflavin, *J. Natl. Cancer Inst.,* 3, 479, 1943.

136. **Stoerck, H. C. and Emerson, G. A.,** Complete regression of lymphosarcoma implants following temporary induction of riboflavin deficiency in mice, *Proc. Soc. Exp. Biol. Med.,* 70, 703, 1949.

137. **Aposhian, H. V. and Lambooy, J. P.,** Retardation of growth of Walker rat carcinoma 256 by administration of diethyl riboflavin, *Proc. Soc. Exp. Biol. Med.,* 78, 197, 1951.

138. **Nizami, H. M. and Nizami, F.,** On the protective role of Vitamin B_2 in mice administered dimethylnitrosamine, *J. Prev. Med. Assoc.,* 29, 141, 1979.

139. **Ohkoshi, M., Ohta, H., and Ito, M.,** Effect of Vitamin B_2 on tumorigenesis of 3-methylcholanthrene in the mouse skin, *Gann,* 73, 105, 1982.

140. **Lane, M., Smith, F. E., and Alfrey, C. P.,** Experimental dietary and antagonist-induced human riboflavin deficiency, in *Riboflavin,* Rivlin, R. S., Ed., Plenum Press, New York, 1975, 325.

141. **Lu, S. H. and Lin, P.,** Recent research on the etiology of esophageal cancer in China, *Z. Gastroenterol.,* 20, 361, 1982.

142. **Rensburg, S. J., Benade, A. S., and Rose, E. F.,** Nutritional status of African populations predisposed to esophageal cancer, *Nutr. Cancer,* 4, 206, 1983.

143. **Metz, S. A., McRae, J. R., and Robertson, R. P.,** Prostaglandins as mediators of paraneoplastic syndromes: review and update, *Metabolism,* 30, 299, 1981.

144. **Carruthers, C. and Baumler, A.,** Distribution of ligandin in normal and azocarcinogen-treated rat liver and azocarcinogen-induced liver tumors, *Oncology,* 36, 265, 1979.

145. **Reynolds, R. D.,** Vitamin B_6 deficiency and carcinogenesis, in *Essential Nutrients in Carcinogenesis,* Poirier, L. A., Newberne, P. M., and Pariza, M. W., Eds., Plenum Press, New York, 1986, 339.

146. **Panush, R. S. and Delafuente, J. C.,** Vitamins and immunocompetence, *World Rev. Nutr. Diet.,* 45, 97, 1985.

147. **Mihich, E. and Nichol, C. A.,** The effect of pyridoxine deficiency on mouse sarcoma 180, *Cancer Res.,* 19, 279, 1959.

148. **DiSorbo, D. M. and Nathanson, L.,** High-dose pyridoxal supplemented culture medium inhibits the growth of a human malignant melanoma cell line, *Nutr. Cancer,* 5, 10, 1983.

149. **Gridley, D. S., Stickney, D. R., Nutter, R. L., Slater, J. M., and Shultz, T. D.,** Suppression of tumor growth and enhancement of immune status with high levels of dietary Vitamin B_6 in BALB/c mice, *J. Natl. Cancer Inst.*, 78, 951, 1987

150. **Ha, C., Kerkvliet, N. I., and Miller, L. T.,** The effect of Vitamin B_6 deficiency on host-susceptibility to Moloney sarcoma virus-induced tumor growth in mice, *J. Nutr.*, 114, 938, 1984.

151. **Potera, C., Rose, D. P., and Brown, R. R.,** Vitamin B_6-deficiency in cancer patients, *Am. J. Clin. Nutr.*, 30, 1677, 1977.

152. **Chabner, B. A., DeVita, V. T., and Livingston, D. M.,** Abnormalities of tryptophan metabolism and plasma pyridoxal phosphate in Hodgkin's disease, *N. Engl. J. Med.*, 282, 838, 1970.

153. **Yoshida, O., Brown, R., and Bryan, G. T.,** Relationship between tryptophan metabolism and heterotopic recurrences of human urinary bladder tumors, *Cancer*, 25, 773, 1970.

154. **Wagner, R. F., Di Sorbo, D. M., and Nathanson, L.,** Topical application of Vitamin B_6 significantly retards the growth of locally recurrent malignant melanoma, *Am. Soc. Clin. Oncol.*, 2, 232, 1983.

155. **Herbert, V.,** The role of Vitamin B^{12} and folate in carcinogenesis, in *Essential Nutrients in Carcinogenesis*, Poirier, L. A., Newberne, P. M., and Pariza, M. W., Eds., Plenum Press, New York, 1986, 293.

156. **Day, P. L., Payne, L. D., and Dinning, J. S.,** Procarcinogenic effect of Vitamin B_{12} on *p*-dimethylaminoazobenzene-fed rats, *Proc. Soc. Exp. Biol. Med.*, 74, 854, 1950.

157. **Poirier, L. A., Wenk, M. L., Madison, R. M., Thompson, D., and McKay, W.,** Vitamin B_{12} acceleration of hepatocarcinogenesis, *Proc. Am. Assoc. Cancer Res.*, 15, 51, 1974.

158. **Yamamoto, R. S.,** Effect of Vitamin B_{12}-deficiency in colon carcinogenesis, *Proc. Soc. Exp. Biol. Med.*, 163, 350, 1980.

159. **Ostryanina, A. D.,** Effect of Vitamin B_{12} on the induction of skin tumors in mice, *Patol. Fiziol. Eksp. Ter.*, 15, 48, 1971.

160. **Blackburn, E. K., Callender, S. T., Dacie, J. V., Doll, R., Mollin, D., and Wetherley-Mein, G.,** Possible association between pernicious anaemia and leukaemia: a prospective study of 1,625 patients with a note of a very high incidence of stomach cancer, *Int. J. Cancer*, 3, 163, 1968.

161. **Bodian, M.,** Neuroblastoma: an evaluation of its natural history and the effects of therapy, with particular reference to treatment by massive doses of Vitamin B_{12}, *Arch. Dis. Child.*, 38, 606, 1963.

162. **Koop, C. E. and Hernandez, J. R.,** Neuroblastoma: experience with 100 cases in children, *Surgery*, 56, 726, 1964.

163. **Eto, I. and Krumdieck, C. L.,** Role of Vitamin B_{12} and folate deficiencies in carcinogenesis, in *Essential Nutrients in Carcinogenesis*, Poirier, L. A., Newberne, P.M., and Pariza, M. W., Eds., Plenum Press, New York, 1986, 313.

164. **Heimburger, D. C., Alexander, C. B., Birch, R., Butterworth, C. E., Bailey, W. C., and Krumdieck, C. L.,** Improvement in bronchial squamous metaplasia in smokers treated with folate and Vitamin B_{12}, *JAMA*, 259, 1525, 1988.

165. **Rosenberg, M. R., Novicki, R. L., Jirtle, R. L., Novotny, A., and Michalopoulos, G.,** Promoting effect of nicotinamide on the development of renal tubular cell tumors in rats initiated with diethylnitrosamine, *Cancer Res.*, 45, 809, 1985.

166. **Pamucku, A. M., Milli, U., and Bryan, G. T.,** Protective effect of nicotinamide on bracken-fern induced carcinogenicity in rats, *Nutr. Cancer*, 3, 86, 1981.

167. **French, F. A.,** The influence of nutritional factors on pulmonary adenomas in mice, in *Inorganic and Nutritional Aspects of Cancer*, Schrauzer, G. N., Ed., Plenum Press, New York, 1978, 281.

168. **Bryan, G. T.,** The influence of niacin and nicotinamide on *in vivo* carcinogenesis, in *Essential Nutrients in Carcinogenesis*, Poirier, L. A., Newberne, P. M., and Pariza, M. W., Eds., Plenum Press, New York, 1986, 331.

169. **Van Rensburg, S. J.,** Epidemiologic and dietary evidence for a specific nutritional predisposition to esophageal cancer, *J. Natl. Cancer Inst.*, 67, 243, 1981.

170. **Glatthaar, B. E., Hornig, D. H., and Moser, U.,** The role of ascorbic acid in carcinogenesis, in *Essential Nutrients in Carcinogenesis*, Poirier, L. A., Newberne, P. M., and Pariza, M. W., Eds., Plenum Press, New York, 1986, 357.

171. **Chen, L. H., Boissonneault, G. A., and Glauert, H. P.,** Vitamin C, Vitamin E and cancer, *Anticancer Res.*, 8, 739, 1988.

172. **Mirvish, S. S., Cardesa, A., Wallcave, L., and Shubik, P.,** Induction of mouse lung adenoma by amines or urea plus nitrite and by *N*-nitroso compounds: effect of ascorbate, gallic acid, thiocyanate, and caffeine, *J. Natl. Cancer Inst.*, 55, 633, 1975.

173. **Llehr, J. G., Wheeler, W. J., and Ballatore, A. M.,** Influence of Vitamin C on estrogen-induced renal carcinogenesis in Syrian hamsters, in *Modulation and Mediation of Cancer by Vitamins*, Prasad, K.N. and Meyskens, F. L., Eds., S. Karger, Basel, 1983, 132.

174. **Gruber, H. E., Tewfik, H. H., and Tewfik, F. A.,** Cytoarchitecture of Ehrlich ascites carcinoma implanted in the hind limb of ascorbic acid-supplemented mice, *Eur. J. Cancer*, 16, 441, 1980.

175. **Banič, S.,** Vitamin C acts as a cocarcinogen to methylcholanthrene in guinea pigs, *Cancer Lett.,* 11, 239, 1981.

176. **Abul-Hajj, Y. J., and Kelliher, M.,** Failure of ascorbic acid to inhibit growth of transplantable and dimethylbenzanthracene induced rat mammary tumors, *Cancer Lett.,* 17, 67, 1982.

177. **Soloway, M. S., Cohen, S. M., and Dekernion, J. B.,** Failure of ascorbic acid to inhibit FANFT-induced bladder cancer, *J. Urol.,* 113, 483, 1975.

178. **Benedict, W. F., Wheatley, W. L., and Jones, P. A.,** Inhibition of chemically-induced morphological transformation and reversion of the transformed phenotype by ascorbic acid in C3H/10T$^{1}/_{2}$ cells, *Cancer Res.,* 40, 2796, 1980.

179. **Park, C. H., Amare, M., Savin, M. A., and Hoogstraten, B.,** Growth suppression of human leukemic cells *in vitro* by L-ascorbic acid, *Cancer Res.,* 40, 1062, 1980.

180. **Stich, H. F., Wei, L., Whiting, R. F.,** Enhancement of the chromosome-damaging action of ascorbate by transition metals, *Cancer Res.,* 39, 4145, 1979.

181. **Prasad, K. N. and Rama, B. N.,** Modification of the effect of pharmacological agents on tumor cells in culture by Vitamin C and Vitamin E, in *Modulation and Mediation of Cancer by Vitamins,* Prasad, K. N. and Meyskens, F. L., Eds., S. Karger, Basel, 1983, 244.

182. **Zannoni, V. G., Sato, P. H., and Rikans, L. E.,** Ascorbic acid and drug metabolism, in *Nutrition and Drug Interrelations,* Hathcock, J. N. and Coon, J., Eds., Academic Press, New York, 1978, 245.

183. **Reddy, B. S., Hanson, D., Mathews, L., and Sharma, C.,** Effect of micronutrients, antioxidants and related compounds on the mutagenicity of 3,2′-dimethyl-4-aminobiphenyl, a colon and breast carcinogen, *Food Chem. Toxicol.,* 21, 129, 1983.

184. **Kensler, T. W. and Taffe, B. G.,** Free radicals in tumor promotion, *Adv. Free Radical Biol. Med.,* 2, 347, 1986.

185. **Peterkofsky, B. and Prather, W.,** Cytotoxicity of ascorbate and other reducing agents towards cultured fibroblasts as a result of hydrogen peroxide formation, *J. Cell Physiol.,* 90, 61, 1977.

186. **Anthony, H. M. and Schorah, C. J.,** Severe hypovitaminosis C in lung cancer patients: the utilization of Vitamin C in surgical repair and lymphocyte-related host resistance, *Br. J. Cancer,* 46, 354, 1982.

187. **Kallistratos, G., Donos, A., and Fasske, E.,** The paradoxical effect of Vitamin C on benzo(a)pyrene-induced tumors and malignancy, *Naturwissenschaflen,* 71, 160, 1984.

188. **Mettlin, C., Graham, S., Priore, R., Marshall, J., and Swanson, M.,** Diet and cancer of the esophagus, *Nutr. Cancer,* 2, 143, 1981.

189. **Cook-Mozaffari, P. J., Azordegan, F., Day, N. E., Ressicaud, A., Sabai, C., and Aramesh, B.,** Oesophageal cancer studies in the Caspian litoral of Iran: results of a case control study, *Br. J. Cancer,* 39, 293, 1979.

190. **Higginson, J.,** Etiological factors in gastrointestinal cancer in man, *J. Natl. Cancer Inst.,* 37, 527, 1966.

191. **Bjelke, E.,** Dietary factors and the epidemiology of cancer of the stomach and large bowel, *Aktuel. Ernährungsmed. Klin. Prax.,* Suppl. 2, 10, 1978.

192. **Kolonel, L. N., Nomura, A. M., Hirohata, T., Hankin, J. H., and Hinds, M. W.,** Association of diet and place of birth with stomach cancer incidence in Hawaii Japanese and Caucasians, *Am. J. Clin. Nutr.,* 34, 2478, 1981.

193. **Fontham, E., Zavala, D., Correa, P., Hunter, F., Haenszel, W., and Tannenbaum, S.,** Diet and chronic atrophic gastritis: a case control study, *J. Natl. Cancer Inst.,* 76, 621, 1986.

194. **Ghosh, J. and Das, S.,** Evaluaiton of Vitamin A and C status in normal and malignant conditions and their possible role in cancer prevention, *Jpn. J. Cancer Res.,* 76, 1174, 1985.

195. **Hank, A. B.,** Vitamin C and cancer, *Prog. Clin. Biol. Res.,* 259, 307, 1988.

196. **Graham, S., Mettlin, C., Marshall, J., Priore, R., Rzepka, T., and Shedd, D.,** Dietary factors in the epidemiology of cancer of the larynx, *Am. J. Epidemiol.,* 113, 675, 1981.

197. **Wassertheil-Smoller, S., Romney, S. L., Wylie-Rosett, Slagle, S., Miller, G., Lucido, D., Duttagupta, C., and Palan, P. R.,** Dietary Vitamin C and uterine cervical dysplasia, *Am. J. Epidemiol.,* 114, 714, 1981.

198. **Jain, M. G., Cook, G. M., Davis, F. G., Grace, M. G., Howe, G. R., and Miller, A. B.,** A case-control study of diet and colorectal cancer, *Int. J. Cancer,* 26, 757, 1980.

199. **Cameron, E. and Pauling L.,** The orthomolecular treatment of cancer. I. The role of ascorbic acid in host resistance, *Chem. Biol. Interact.,* 9, 273, 1974.

200. **Murata, A., Morishige, F., and Yamaguchi, H.,** Prolongation of survival times of terminal cancer patients by administration of large doses of ascorbate, *Int. J. Vitam. Nutr. Res.,* 23 (Suppl.), 103, 1982.

201. **Cameron, E., Pauling, L., and Leibowitz, B.,** Ascorbic acid and cancer; a review, *Cancer Res.,* 39, 663, 1979.

202. **Cameron, E. and Pauling, L.,** Supplemental ascorbate in the supportive treatment of cancer: prolongation of survival times in terminal human cancer, *Proc. Natl. Acad. Sci. U.S.A.,* 73, 3685, 1976.

203. **Cameron, E., Campbell, A., and Jack, T.,** The orthomolecular treatment of cancer. III. Reticulum cell sarcoma: double complete regression induced by high-dose ascorbic acid therapy, *Chem. Biol. Interact.,* 11, 387, 1975.

204. **Creagan, E. T., Moertel, C. G., O'Fallon, J. R., Schutt, J., O'Connell, M. J., Rubin, J., and Frytak, S.,** Failure of high-dose Vitamin C (ascorbic acid) therapy to benefit patients with advanced cancer, *N. Engl. J. Med.,* 301, 687, 1979.

205. **Moertel, C. G., Fleming, T. R., Creagan, E. T., Rubin, J., O'Connell, M. J., and Ames, M. M.,** High-dose Vitamin C versus placebo in the treatment of patients with advanced cancer who have had no prior chemotherapy: a randomized double-blind comparison, *N. Engl. J. Med.,* 312, 137, 1985.

206. **Bussey, H. J., DeCosse, J. J., Deschner, E. E., Eyers, A. A., Lesser, M. L., Morson, B. C., Ritchie, S. M., Thomson, J. P., and Wadsworth, J.,** A randomized trial of ascorbic acid in polyposis coli, *Cancer,* 50, 1434, 1982.

207. **Reichel, H., Koeffler, H. P., and Norman, A. W.,** The role of Vitamin D endocrine system in health and disease, *N. Engl. J. Med.,* 320, 980, 1989.

208. **DeLuca, H. F. and Ostrem, V.,** The relationship between the Vitamin D system and cancer, in *Essential Nutrients in Carcinogenesis,* Poirier, L. A., Newberne, P. M., and Pariza, M. W., Eds., Plenum Press, New York, 1986, 413.

209. **Bell, N. H.,** Vitamin D-endocrine system, *J. Clin. Invest.,* 76, 1, 1985.

210. **Manolagas, S. C.,** Vitamin D and its relevance to cancer, *Anticancer Res.,* 7, 625, 1987.

211. **Norman, A. W., Roth, J., and Orci, L.,** The Vitamin D endocrine system: steroid metabolism, hormone receptors, and biological response (calcium binding protein), *Endocrinol. Rev.,* 3, 331, 1982.

212. **Gibbs, P. E. and Dugaiczyk, A.,** Origin of structural domains of the serum albumin gene family and a predicted structure of the gene for Vitamin D-binding protein, *Mol. Biol. Evol.,* 4, 364, 1987.

213. **Haddad, J. G.,** Nature and function of the plasma binding protein for Vitamin D and its metabolites, in *Vitamin D: Basic and Clinical Aspects,* Kumar, R., Ed., Martinius Nijhoff, The Hague, 1984, 383.

214. **McDonnell, D. P., Mangelsdorf, D. J., Pike, J. W., Haussler, M. R., and O'Malley, B. W.,** Molecular cloning of complementary DNA encoding the avian receptor for Vitamin D, *Science,* 235, 1214, 1987.

215. **Barsony, J. and Marx, S. J.,** A very rapid receptor mediated action of 1.25-dihydroxycholecalciferol: increase of intracellular cyclic GMP in human skin fibroblasts, in *Vitamin D: Molecular, Cellular and Clinical Endocrinology,* Norman, A. W., Ed., Walter de Gruyter, Berlin 1988, 767.

216. **Garland, C., Barrett,-Conor, E., Rossoff, A. H., Shekelle, R. B., Criqui, M. H., and Paul, O.,** Dietary Vitamin D and calcium and risk of colorectal cancer: a 19-year prospective study in men, *Lancet,* 1, 307, 1985.

217. **Eisman, J. A., Koga, M., Sutherland, R. L., Barkla, D. H., and Tutton, P. J.,** 1,25-Dihydroxy Vitamin D_3 and the regulation of human cancer cell replication, *Proc. Soc. Exp. Biol. Med.,* 191, 221, 1989.

218. **Frampton, R. J., Omond, S. A., and Eisman, J. A.,** Inhibition of human cancer cell growth by $1\alpha,25$-dihyroxy Vitamin D_3 metabolites, *Cancer Res.,* 43, 4443, 1983.

219. **Lointiér, P., Wargovich, M. J., Saez, S., Levin B., Wildrick, D. M., and Boman, B. M.,** The role of Vitamin D_3 in the proliferation of a human colon cancer line *in vitro, Anticancer Res.,* 7, 817, 1987.

220. **Cunningham, D., Gilchrist, N. L., Cowan, R. A., Forrest, G. J., McArdle, C. S., and Soukop, M.,** Alfacalcidiol as a modulator of growth of low grade non-Hodgkin's lymphomas, *Br. Med. J.,* 291, 1153, 1985.

221. **Noguchi, S., Tahara, H., Miyauchi, K., and Koyama, H.,** Influence of $1\alpha,25$-dihydroxy Vitamin D_3 on the development and steroid hormone receptor contents of DMBA-induced rat mammary tumors, *Oncology,* 46, 273, 1989.

222. **Colston, K., Colston, M. J., and Feldman, D.,** $1\alpha,25$-dihydroxy Vitamin D_3 and malignant melanoma: the presence of receptors and inhibition of cell growth in culture, *Endocrinology,* 108, 1083, 1981.

223. **Smith, E. L., Walworth, N. C., and Holick, M. F.,** Effect of $1\alpha,25$-dihydroxy Vitamin D_3 on the morphologic and biochemical differentiation of cultured human epidermal keratinocytes grown in serum-free conditions, *J. Invest. Dermatol.,* 86, 709, 1986.

224. **Morimoto, S. and Yoshikawa, K.,** Psoriasis and Vitamin D_3, *Arch. Dermatol.,* 125, 231, 1989.

225. **Abe, E., Miyaura, C., Sakagami, H., Takeda, M., Yoshika, S., and Suda, T.,** Differentiation of mouse myeloid leukemia cells induced by $1\alpha,25$-dihyhydroxy Vitamin D_3, *Proc. Natl. Acad. Sci. U.S.A.,* 78, 4990, 1981.

226. **Suda, T.,** The role of $1\alpha,25$-dihydroxy Vitamin D_3 in the myeloid cell differentiation, *Proc. Soc. Exp. Biol. Med.,* 191, 214, 1989.

227. **Weinberg, J. B., Misukonis, M. A., Hobbs, M. M., and Borowitz, M. J.,** Cooperative effects of gamma interferon and $1\alpha,25$-dihydroxy Vitamin D_3 in inducing differentiation of human promyelocytic leukemia (HL-60) cells, *Exp. Hematol.,* 14, 138, 1986.

228. **Colston, K. W., Berger, U., Coombes, R. C.,** Possible role for Vitamin D in controlling breast cancer cell proliferation, *Lancet,* 1, 188, 1989.

229. **Reichel, H., Koeffler, H. P., Tobler, A., and Norman, A. W.,** $1\alpha,25$-dihydroxy Vitamin D_3 inhibits γ-interferon synthesis by normal human peripheral blood lymphocytes, *Proc. Natl. Acad. Sci. U.S.A.,* 84, 3385, 1987.

230. **Manolagas, S. C., Hustmyer, F. G., and Yu, X. P.,** 1α,25-dihydroxy VitaminD₃ and the immune system, *Proc. Soc. Exp. Biol. Med.,* 191, 238, 1989.

231. **Mudde, A. H., Van Den Berg, H., Boshuis, P. G., Breedveld, F. C., Markusse, H. M., Kluin, P. M., Bijovet, O. L., and Papapoulos, S. E.,** Ectopic production of 1α,25-dihydroxy Vitamin D by B-cell lymphoma as a cause of hypercalcemia, *Cancer,* 59, 1543, 1987.

232. **Walters, M. R.,** 1α,25-dihydroxy Vitamin D₃ receptors in the seminiferous tubules of the rat testis increase at puberty, *Endocrinology,* 114, 2167, 1984.

233. **Haussler, M. R., Mangelsdorf, D. J., Komm, B. S., Terpening, C. M., Yamaoka, K., Allegretto, E. A., Baker, A. R., Shine, J., McDonnell, D. P., Hughes, M., Weigel, N. L., O'Malley, B. W., and Pike, J. W.,** Molecular biology of the Vitamin D hormone, *Rec. Progr. Horm. Res.,* 44, 263, 1988.

234. **Simpson, R. U. and Arnold, A. J.,** Calcium antagonizes 1α,25-dihydroxy Vitamin D₃ inhibition of breast cancer cell proliferation, *Endocrinology,* 119, 2284, 1986.

235. **Munker, R., Norman, A., and Koeffler, H. P.,** Vitamin D compounds: effect on clonal proliferation and differentiation of human myeloid cells, *J. Clin. Invest.,* 78, 424, 1986.

236. **Koeffler, H. P., Hirji, K., Itri, L., and the Southern California leukemia group,** 1α,25-dihydroxy Vitamin D₃: *in vivo* and *in vitro* effects on human preleukemic and leukemic cells, *Cancer Treat. Rep.,* 69, 1399, 1985.

237. **Robert, K. H., Hellström, E., Einhorn, S., and Gahrton, G.,** Acute myelogenous leukemia of unfavorable prognosis treated with retinoic acid, Vitamin D₃, D₃, alpha interferon and low doses of cytosine arabinoside, *Scand. J. Haematol.,* 34(Suppl. 44), 61, 1986.

238. **Prasad, K. N.,** Mechanism of action of Vitamin E on mammalian tumor cells in culture, in *Nutrition, Growth, and Cancer,* Tryfiates, G. P. and Prasad, K. N., Eds., Alan R. Liss, New York, 1988, 363.

239. **Bright-See, E.,** Role of Vitamins C and E in the etiology of human cancer, in *Vitamins, Nutrition, and Cancer,* Prasad, K. N., Ed., S. Karger, Basel, 1984, 68.

240. **Knekt, P., Aromaa, A., Maatela, J., Aaran, R.K., Nikkari, T., Hakulinen, M., Peto, R., Saxon, E., and Teppo, L.,** Serum Vitamin E and risk of cancer among Finnish men during a 10-year followup, *Am. J. Epidemiol.,* 127, 28, 1988.

241. **Rama, B. N. and Prasad, K. N.,** Alpha-tocopheryl acid succinate effects on melanoma, glioma, and neuroblastoma cells, in culture, *Proc. Soc. Exp. Biol. Med.,* 174, 302, 1983.

242. **Helson, L., Verma, M., and Helson, C.,** Vitamin E and human neuroblastoma, in *Modulation and Mediation of Cancer by Vitamins,* Prasad, K. N. and Meyskens, F. L., Eds., S. Karger, Basel, 1983, 258.

243. **Kagerud, A. and Paterson, H. I.,** Tocopherol in tumor irradiation, *Anticancer Res.,* 1, 35, 1981.

244. **Takenaga, K., Honma, Y., and Hozumi, M.,** Inhibition of differentiation of mouse myeloid leukemia cells by phenolic antioxidants and alpha-tocopherol, *Gann,* 72, 104, 1981.

245. **Smalls, E. and Patterson, R. M.,** Reduction of benzo(a)pyrene induced chromosomal aberrations by dl-alpha-tocopherol, *Eur. J. Cell. Biol.,* 28, 92, 1982.

246. **Chen, J., Goetchius, M. P., Combs, G. F., and Campbell, T. C.,** Effects of dietary selenium and Vitamin E on covalent binding of aflatoxin to chick liver cell macromolecules, *J. Nutr.,* 112, 350, 1982.

247. **Radner, B. S. and Kennedy, A. R.,** Suppression of x-ray induced transformation by Vitamin E in mouse C3H10T¹/₂ cells, *Cancer Lett.,* 32, 25, 1986.

248. **Borek, C., Ong, A., Mason, H., Donahue, L., and Biaglow, J. E.,** Selenium and Vitamin E inhibit radiogenic and chemically-induced transformation in vitro via different mechanisms, *Proc. Natl. Acad. Sci. U.S.A.,* 83, 1490, 1986.

249. **Pacht, E. R., Kaseki, H., Mohammed, J. R., Cornwell, D. G., and Davis, W. B.,** Deficiency of Vitamin E in the alveolar fluid of cigarette smokers, *J. Clin. Invest.,* 77, 789, 1986.

250. **Jandak, J., Steiner, M., and Richardson, P. D.,** α-tocopherol, an effective inhibitor of platelet adhesion, *Blood,* 73, 141, 1989.

251. **Jaffe, W. G.,** The influence of wheat germ oil on the production of tumors in rats by methylcholanthrene, *Exp. Med. Surg.,* 4, 278, 1946.

252. **Wattenberg, L. W.,** Inhibition of carcinogenic and toxic effects of polycyclic hydrocarbons by phenolic antioxidants and ethoxyquin, *J. Natl. Cancer Inst.,* 48, 1425, 1972.

253. **Sadek, I.,** Vitamin E and its effect on skin papilloma, in *Vitamins, Nutrition, and Cancer,* Prasad, K.N., Ed., S. Karger, Basel, 1984, 118.

254. **Cook, M. G. and McNamara, P.,** Effect of dietary Vitamin E on dimethylhydrazine-induced colonic tumors in mice, *Cancer Res.,* 40, 1329, 1980.

255. **Trickler, D. and Shklar, G.,** Prevention by Vitamin E of experimental oral carcinogenesis, *J. Natl. Cancer Inst.,* 78, 165, 1987.

256. **Nesbitt, J. A., Smith, J., McDowell, G., and Drago, J. R.,** Adriamycin-Vitamin E combination therapy for treatment of prostate adenocarcinoma in the Nb rat model, *J. Surg. Oncol.,* 38, 283, 1988.

257. **Lupulescu, A.,** Ultrastructural and cell surface studies of cancer epidermal cells following Vitamin E administration, in *Proc. Electr. Microsc. Soc. Am.,* Bailey, G. W., Ed., San Francisco Press, 1986, 120.

258. **Lupulescu, A.,** Hormonal regulation of epidermal tumor development, *J. Invest. Dermatol.,* 77, 186, 1981.

259. **Tengerdy, R. P., Mathias, M. M., and Nockels, C. F.,** Effect of Vitamin E on immunity and disease resistance, in *Vitamins, Nutrition and Cancer,* Prasad, K. N., Ed., S. Karger, Basel, 1984, 123.

260. **Prasad, K. N. and Rama, B. N.,** Modification of the effect of pharmacological agents, ionizing radiation and hyperthermia on tumor cells by Vitamin E, in *Vitamins, Nutrition and Cancer,* Prasad, K. N., Ed., S. Karger, Basel, 1984, 76.

261. **Helson, L.,** A Phase-I study of Vitamin E and neuroblastoma, in *Vitamins, Nutrition and Cancer,* Prasad, K. N., Ed., S. Karger, Basel, 1984, 274.

262. **Ernster, V. L., Goodson, W. H., Hunt, T. K., Petrakis, N. L., Sickless, E. A., and Miike, R.,** Vitamin E and benign breast "disease": a double-blind, randomized clinical trial, *Surgery,* 97, 490, 1985.

263. **Newberne, P. M. and Suphakarn, V.,** Nutrition and Cancer: a review with emphasis on the role of Vitamins C and E and selenium, *Nutr. Cancer,* 5, 107, 1983.

264. **Chlebowski, R. T., Dietrich, M., Akman, S., and Block, J. B.,** Vitamin K_3 inhibition of malignant murine cell growth and human tumor colony formation, *Cancer Treat. Rep.,* 69, 527, 1985.

265. **Taper, H. S., DeGerlache, J., Lans, M., and Roberfroid, M.,** Nontoxic potentiation of cancer chemotherapy by combined C and K_3 vitamin pretreatment, *Int. J. Cancer,* 40, 575, 1987.

266. **Krishanamurthi, S., Shanta, V., and Sastri, D.,** Combined therapy in buccal mucosa cancers, *Radiology,* 99, 409, 1971.

267. **Israels, L. G., Walls, G. A., Ollmann, D. J., Friesen, E., and Israels, E. D.,** Vitamin K as a regulator of benzo(a)pyrene metabolism, mutagenesis, and carcinogenesis, *J. Clin. Invest.,* 71, 1130, 1983.

268. **Zacharski, L., Henderson, W. G., Rickles, F. R., Forman, W., Cornell, C., Forcier, R., Edwards, R., Headley, E., Kim, S., O'Donnell, J., Tornyos, K., and Kwaan, H.,** Effect of warfarin anticoagulation on survival in carcinoma of the lung, colon, head and neck and prostate, *Cancer,* 53, 2046, 1984.

269. **Chlebowski, R. T., Akman, S. A., and Block, J. B.,** Vitamin K in the treatment of cancer, *Cancer Treat. Rev.,* 12, 49, 1985.

270. **Gallin, J. I., Seligmann, B. E., Cramer, E. B., Schiffmann, E., and Fletcher, M. P.,** Effects of Vitamin K on human neutrophil function, *J. Immunol.,* 128, 1399, 1982.

271. **Shoyab, M. and Todaro, G. J.,** Vitamin K_3 (menadione) and related quinones, like tumor promoting phorbol esters, alter the affinity of epidermal growth factor for its membrane receptors, *J. Biol. Chem.,* 255, 8735, 1980.

272. **Holm, L. E., Callmer, E., Hjalmar, M. L., Lidbrink, E., Nilsson, B., and Skoog, L.,** Dietary habits and prognostic factors in breast cancer, *J. Natl. Cancer Inst.,* 81, 1218, 1989.

273. **Dakshinamurti, K. and Chauhan, J.** Biotin, *Vitamins and Hormones,* 45, 337, 1989.

Chapter 6

ADVANTAGES AND DISADVANTAGES OF HORMONOTHERAPY AND VITAMIN THERAPY AS COMPARED TO OTHER CANCER THERAPIES

I. GENERAL CONSIDERATIONS

Even more than half a century ago when endocrine therapy was in its empirical stage, this method was judged to be superior to surgery and radiation therapy. During that time, cancer was assumed to be a systemic disease caused by glandular imbalance or dysfunction of endocrine glands, especially gonads, thyroid, thymus, and adrenal secretions. In 1925 Cummings stated that the importance of the endocrine glands in cancer is such that "no progressive physician or surgeon can afford to ignore their role either in etiology or therapeutics". To eliminate cancer it is not sufficient to extirpate the local growth; we must correct the constitutional and metabolic conditions.[1,2]

At present the biologic complexity of cancer has led us to conclude that there is no longer reason to believe that the primary therapy for cancer should be confined only to the operating room.[3] This conclusion is due to recent progress in cancer biology and endocrine pharmacology as well as other factors, such as: (1) development of new hormone antagonists and agonists (tamoxifen, aminoglutethimide, luteinizing hormone-releasing hormone [LHRH] agonists), which can provide similar or even identical therapeutic effects as endocrine ablative therapy; (2) cytotoxicity and occurrence of secondary cancers, which follow chemotherapy and radiation therapy; (3) multidrug resistance (MDR), a phenomenon which frequently occurs following cytotoxic or chemotherapeutic agents; (4) cytotoxic drugs, which kill indiscriminately the cancer cells as well as their normal counterparts; (5) decrease or depression of immune host defense system, which follows chemotherapy and radiation therapy; (6) toxic, disfiguring, and psychologic consequences, some of them life-threatening, which make it difficult for patients to accept; (7) dependence on endocrine replacement therapy for life; (8) development of new synthetic vitamin agonists, which are more active than natural vitamins, and improved knowledge regarding the action of vitamins at the cellular level; (9) chemotherapy and radiation therapy reached a plateau; and (10) surgery is also invasive, irreversible, and not always feasible.

All these new developments in endocrine and vitamin pharmacology make the conventional cancer surgery, radiation, and chemotherapy less acceptable and, in some cases, even obsolete. These recent events have led to a resurgence of hormonotherapy and vitamin therapy in cancer patients. Since these new therapeutic approaches are much less toxic and less carcinogenic and produce similar therapeutic effects, they are more often acceptable for cancer patients. Both hormones and vitamins produce a better palliation and improve the quality of life. These are important factors in cancer treatment. We must always be aware that we are treating not only the cancer, but also the patient. It is not desirable for the patient and his physician to use combined cytotoxic and radiation procedures in order to gain and keep the patient alive for a few months, but in deteriorating and miserable condition. Hence, hormonotherapy and vitamin therapy are important therapeutic approaches and will constitute the "fourth arm" of cancer therapy, often replacing the conventional therapeutic methods.[4] The discovery and isolation of several hormone receptors and certain vitamin receptors make patient selection more feasible and more specific. The pool of patients can be divided into many subsets based on suitability for each type of therapy. In addition, we will be able to predict more accurately the relapses, the outcome and, in general, the survival of cancer patients.

II. ADVANTAGES AND DISADVANTAGES OF HORMONOTHERAPY AND VITAMIN THERAPY

We will review in this chapter the advantages and disadvantages of hormonotherapy and vitamin therapy over the conventional cancer therapies, such as chemotherapy, radiation therapy, immunotherapy, and surgery.

A. HORMONOTHERAPY AS COMPARED TO CHEMOTHERAPY

There is no evidence that chemotherapy causes a meaningful prolongation of survival in cancer patients. Chemotherapy adds considerable toxicity, and reported trials have not adequately assessed its overall impact on quality of life. Most patients with metastatic carcinoma of the breast or of the prostate are at high risk for myelosuppression after cytotoxic chemotherapy, making it difficult to evaluate response to treatment. Because of these factors there is little evidence that chemotherapy provides palliation for patients with metastatic advanced carcinoma, and it should not always be regarded as part of standard management. Mainly patients who are no longer responding to hormones may be considered for trials of chemotherapy. Future trials should randomize patients to chemotherapy, with assessment of quality and quantity of survival for all patients made by an observer who is unaware of the treatment. Thus, the major challenge for future trials of palliation will be inclusion of quality of life assessment.

Most patients experience dramatic relief of symptoms when first treated by endocrine therapy, and the toxicity of this treatment is low compared with that of chemotherapy.[5] It seems inappropriate to introduce toxic chemotherapy in the management of a minimally symptomatic patient who is responding to hormonotherapy. A critical review of the literature shows that there is no convincing evidence to suggest that chemotherapy is of benefit to a meaningful proportion of cancer patients. Chemotherapy has a high potential for toxicity in the patients with extensive bone metastases or visceral metastases (brain, liver) and should not be regarded as part of standard management for prostate or breast cancer. Clinical trials of chemotherapy are appropriate for selected patients with hormone-resistant metastatic disease, and these trials should compare chemotherapy with best supportive care. Clinical trials of chemotherapy at the earlier stages of disease are unlikely to demonstrate benefit until drugs are identified that greatly prolong survival for patients with hormone-refractory metastatic cancer. Therefore, hormonotherapy always should be tried first; then combined chemohormonotherapy or chemotherapy alone should be used in patients who did not respond to previous therapies. Chemotherapy should never be tried first. There is no evidence to justify the use of more toxic and expensive cytotoxic drugs instead of standard treatment, and if the patient does not respond favorably to chemotherapy in 3 to 6 months, this should be discontinued. A true comparison between chemotherapy and hormonotherapy would state that chemotherapy is detrimental since it adds toxicity, but does not cause significant prolongation of survival.

Despite 30 years of research and development, the role of chemotherapy in the adjuvant treatment of primary and metastatic cancer remains controversial. Thus, at least 12 different drugs have been tested alone or in combination in at least 31 published randomized control trials. Although almost 10,000 patients have been enrolled in these trials, the degree to which chemotherapy improves the overall health of patients with primary breast cancer and increases life expectancy remains undecided. Thus, results from combining data for other types of trials are inconclusive.[6] The list of side effects is rather formidable and includes nausea, vomiting, alopecia, bone marrow depression, and organ damage. In addition, some chemotherapeutic agents are themselves carcinogenic. Renal, cardiac, hepatic, neurologic, and ototoxic side effects are associated more often with a specific commonly used drug than with a series of drugs. Recently it has been shown that some chemotherapeutic drugs may be carcinogenic by themselves. Patients with multiple myeloma or Hodgkin's disease have a greater chance of developing acute leukemia after being treated with chemotherapy, and in several other cancers, increased incidence of acute leukemia may result secondary to the use of drug therapy.[7] Hence, only 10% of all cancers can be cured with chemotherapy, and chemotherapy often is met with significant opposition by physicians and patients alike, who fear its well-publicized toxic effects.[8]

The incidence of most cancers increases with age; 50% of all cancers occur in people older than age 65, and the incidence of distant metastases at the time of diagnosis may also increase with age. These observations imply that elderly patients with cancer are more susceptible than younger patients to complications of chemotherapy; especially, myelotoxicity with increased severity and duration of myelodepression reported in patients over 65 who received adjuvant chemotherapy.[9] Age-related decrements in glomerular filtration rate and cardiac reserve suggest that doses of renally excreted drugs and cardiotoxic anthracyclines should be reduced in elderly patients. Another very important aspect of chemotherapy and radiation therapy is carcinogenicity of antineoplastic agents in man. Since chemotherapeutic drugs were first introduced there has been an increasing number of reports of second malignancies following their use.

Review of the literature shows several important facts. Anticancer drugs are in all probability mostly also carcinogenic. Alkylating agents, such as melphalan, chlorambucil, and cyclophosphamide, seem to lead to the highest rate of second malignancies, the most common being leukemias, lymphomas, and bladder carcinomas. Cytotoxic drugs given to cancer patients may cause secondary neoplasms either by a direct carcinogenic effect or, indirectly, through depression of immunity. Cancer chemotherapeutic agents seriously interfere with the genetic and metabolic machinery of cells; thus, the alkylating agents and those that bind tightly to DNA are most likely to be followed by new malignancies. Data obtained from animal studies incriminate cyclophosphamide, procarbazine, BCNU, CCNU, and decarbazine as carcinogens, and also cast suspicion on cisplatin, chlorambucil, and azathioprine. Also, an enormous amount of human data have revealed sufficient evidence that cyclophosphamide, treosulphan, and azathioprine are carcinogenic in humans; limited evidence implicates chlorambucil. In addition, a number of drug combinations are known to be carcinogenic, for example, mechlorethamine, vincristine, procarbazine, and prednisone. Increasing numbers of second tumors that develop after cancer chemotherapy are being reported; this is important, especially in children treated for various cancers. The overall risk of developing a new tumor is estimated to be 3 to 20% at 20 years.

After chemotherapy treatment, the most common second tumors are a variety of acute leukemias. Non-Hodgkin lymphomas (NHLs), carcinomas of the urinary bladder, and other malignancies are less common. Conditions which could influence the carcinogeneity of an antitumor drug are its carcinogenic potency, long-term administration, the total dose used, and long-term survival of the patient. Secondary leukemias now constitute approximately 10% of all leukemias; the most common type is acute myeloid leukemia (AML). A wide variety of other malignancies has developed after cancer chemotherapy. There is usually a longer latent period between the initial treatment and the appearance of second solid tumors (approximately 10 years) than between treatment and secondary leukemia (approximately 4 to 6 years). In many cases the secondary tumors occur following chemotherapy combined with radiotherapy; the cancers most frequently encountered are carcinomas of the lung, skin, breast, colon, pancreas, Kaposi's sarcoma, and soft tissue sarcomas. Immunity is severely impaired by the immunosuppressive agents. The major cancer chemotherapeutic drugs also suppress both humoral and cell-mediated immune functions. Depression of immunity is less profound with intermittent therapy than with continuous prolonged chemotherapy. Immunosuppressed patients are prone to infections, some of which may be caused by viruses with oncogenic potential. Epstein-Barr virus is strongly implicated in causing NHLs, as well as

AIDS. However, it is not certain if immunosuppression acts as a cocarcinogenic factor. Another possibility is that immunosuppressive or chemotherapeutic drugs may act synergistically with various carcinogens to cause neoplasms. In general, various cancers probably arise from a complex interplay of multiple factors, including a direct cellular effect (somatic mutation); synergistic effects of various treatments with other carcinogens, such as sunlight, smoking, food additives, and depression of host immunity; and liberation of oncogenic viruses and genetic susceptibility. Finally, certain cancer chemotherapeutic agents, particularly the alkylating agents, form electrophilic reactants and damage cells by binding to nucleophilic cellular macromolecules including DNA. Neoplastic change occurs if the cellular damage cannot be repaired. Therefore, the findings from recent studies emphasize the need for lifetime followup of cancer patients who have been treated with chemotherapy, radiotherapy, or both. Prolonged followup is particularly important in children who have a potentially long life expectancy.

In the future, fewer carcinogenic chemotherapeutic agents should be developed and methods should be studied for delivering lethal doses of chemotherapeutic agents to cancer cells with minimal damage to adjacent normal cells or to the immune system.[10,11] Compared to cytotoxic drugs, hormones and vitamins are much less toxic, are not carcinogenic, and are not immunosuppressors. In fact, certain vitamins (A, C, D, E) are immunoaugmentators; they increase cell-mediated and humoral immunity with an increase of antibody formation. Thus, they increase the host-immune defense of cancer patients and should always be preferred to chemotherapy and radiation therapy as adjuvant therapy for hormone-responsive cancers.

Hormones and vitamins also should be used in combination therapy with cytotoxic agents — chemohormonotherapy or palliation therapy. Why some cancers are curable by chemotherapy, while most are not, is an enigma and a major challenge for clinical oncologists. The ability of cancer cells to develop resistance to cytotoxic drugs poses a major obstacle to the ultimate success of chemotherapy, and drug resistance still remains the major unsolved problem in chemotherapy. Multidrug resistance (MDR), or pleiotropic drug resistance, is a phenomenon by which cells are resistant to several structurally unrelated agents, most of which are natural products; subsequently, cells protect themselves from the toxic effects of drugs.

MDR has been strongly linked to the overexpression of a membrane-associated glycoprotein, called P-glycoprotein, which appears to play a role in drug efflux. This 170,000-kDa protein, termed P170 or P-glycoprotein, is consistently seen in all highly multidrug-resistant rodent and human lines studied. P-glycoprotein is thought to function as an energy-dependent, drug efflux pump of broad specificity, mediating resistance to unrelated agents. Because P-glycoprotein is located in the plasma membrane, antibodies can be used to alter or kill cells containing the protein; these cells are extremely sensitive to killing by this agent.[12,13] The discovery that P-glycoprotein is present in several normal cells should not necessarily affect the utility of this treatment because in the gastrointestinal tract, liver, and kidney, the protein is present on the apical or lumenal surface of cells. The lumenal surface is not exposed to the blood. An atypical pattern of MDR has been characterized and related to altered topoisomerase activity. The situation is further complicated by the discovery that human cells contain two P-glycoprotein genes, mdr2 (also known as MDR1) and mdr3 (also known as MDR2); these are differently expressed in normal tissues.[14]

Cellular resistance to cytotoxic drugs is thought to occur in different ways. One assumes that a neoplastic cell is resistant to chemotherapy at the time of its malignant transformation, or is then said to be *de novo* resistant (Skipper model)[15]; or it is assumed to become resistant only after exposure to therapeutic cytotoxic agents, and is then considered to have acquired resistance (Goldie and Coldman model).[16] It is not certain if P-glycoprotein can predict response to chemotherapy. Tumor heterogeneity precludes a simple answer at this time.

Neoplasms that exhibit *de novo* or resistance at the beginning are refractory to chemotherapy and carry the worst prognosis. Hence, even using multidrug regimens it is difficult to overcome drug resistance and predict the outcome, due to the existence of various subclones with a broad distribution of drug sensitivities within the same tumor.

Reversal of MDR has been accomplished *in vitro* by a variety of agents, including verapamil, reserpine, quinidine, anthracycline and vincristine, vinblastine, and cyclosporine.[17] The mechanism of reversing MDR includes competition with cytotoxic drug binding sites on the energy-dependent efflux pump and on alterations in cell membrane lipid integrity. Most agents reversing MDR suffer from a common problem, e.g., concentrations of unbound drug necessary to reverse MDR *in vitro* cannot be maintained in humans without exceeding the maximum tolerated dose of the sensitizing agent. Recently, tamoxifen and other analogs have been shown to possess activity for reversing MDR. However, their mechanism of reversing MDR does not appear to be related to an antiestrogenic effect. Recent evidence has been presented that toremifene, a new triphenylethylene with a longer half-life (5 to 6 d), has activity as a chemosensitizing agent in MCF-7 doxorubicin-resistant cells at clinical concentrations. This effect is dose dependent. The *N*-desmethylmetabolite appears to be as equally active as toremifene in reversing drug resistance. Thus, toremifene may be uniquely suited for use as a clinical modulator of tumor drug resistance in combination with other cytotoxic agents in humans.[18]

Multiple attempts have been made in the past few years to increase the efficacy of chemotherapy. A considerable body of evidence has suggested that an apparent plateau of response rates (in the range of 55 to 65%) and of median duration of response (generally <1 year) has occurred in advanced breast cancer treatment. Most efforts to improve therapeutic effectiveness by increasing dose intensity, by using "noncross-resistant" drugs or by using more drugs have been unsuccessful. While a small minority of patients treated with cytotoxic chemotherapy may achieve a complete remission, the eventually relapse and death of virtually all of these patients suggest that drugs alone have not been able to eradicate sufficient numbers of tumor cells to result in cure of more than an occasional patient. Given the general safety and palliative potential of hormonotherapy, many investigators have attempted to combine hormonal and drug treatment for improving clinical outcome. Although no difference in some response parameters was seen between two chemotherapeutic schedules, one including Cytoxan, Adriamycin, and 5-fluorouracil (5-FU) and the second including methotrexate and tamoxifen, a limited number of patients with inflammatory breast cancer had a signficantly higher response rate (93 vs. 61%) than patients with recurrent metastatic disease. Time to progression (13 vs. 17 months) and survival (17 vs. 23 months) of responders significantly favored the treatment arm including tamoxifen and premarin. Hence, further efforts to increase the efficacy of chemotherapy by combining with endocrine therapy to temporarily perturb DNA synthesis in hormonally responsive cancer cells is worthwhile.[19]

Thus, the benefit of combined chemo- and hormonal therapy, as opposed to their sequential use for cancer patients, continues to be disputed. Hormones mediate many cellular events, including cell growth and differentiation, which mainly concern the oncologist. Most growth inhibitory hormones and antihormones decrease tumor growth fraction by retaining and diverting cells in the G_0-phase, while growth stimulatory hormones, e.g., mitogenic hormones, increase tumor growth fraction by recruiting G_0-cells into cell cycle. Hence, by modulating tumor growth fraction hormones can further enhance the tumor-cytotoxic potential of highly effective chemotherapeutic regimens. It is also possible, but not certain, that for patients with growing ER-negative tumors, the effects of chemotherapy can only be inproved minimally by hormonal therapies. Interestingly, some effects of corticosteroid and peptide hormones (prolactin) may be elicited independently from ER at the plasma cell membrane. Some advantages of chemotherapy, hormone therapy, and vitamin therapy are listed in Table 1.

TABLE 1

Comparison between Chemotherapy, Hormonotherapy, and Vitamin Therapy

	Chemotherapy	Hormonotherapy	Vitamin therapy
Toxicity (side effects)	+ + +	+	±
Carcinogenicity and mutagenicity	+ + +	±	−
Tumor steroid receptors	±	+ + +	+
Immunosuppression	+ + +	±	±
Immunoaugmentation	±	+ +	+ +
Multidrug resistance (MDR)	+ + +	+	+
Combination better than sequential	+ +	±	±
General safety and quality of life	±	+ +	+ +

Certain cell membrane effects may, in turn, modulate cell responsiveness to peptide hormones. Most cytotoxic drugs act primarily on rapidly growing, poorly differentiated cell subpopulations, while hormones act primarily on slow-growing, well-differentiated cell subpopulations. However, hormones and cytotoxic drugs do not combine their effects in cell clones of intermediate differentiation, which are the majority of clones in most tumors. Thus, some oncologists conclude that there is no theoretical advantage to the combined use of growth-inhibitory hormones and cytotoxic drugs over their sequential use.[20] However, chemohormonotherapy in combination drugs, such as prednimustine (ester of chlorambucil and prednisolone) or estramustine (ester phosphate of nitrogen mustard and estradiol), is more efficient than treatment with chlorambucil and prednisolone, nitrogen mustard or estradiol or even with each drug alone.

B. HORMONOTHERAPY AS COMPARED TO RADIATION THERAPY

The use of radiation therapy either preoperatively or postoperatively in the treatment of operable cancer remains a controversial issue despite decades of experience with its use. Some investigators remain firmly convinced as to its value, even though prospective randomized clinical trials have failed to demonstrate a survival benefit resulting from adjuvant radiation therapy. A gradual decline in the routine use of postoperative radiation has been seen over the past decade.[21] To understand normal tissue radiation biology, an estimation of the kinetics of cell renewal tissues is vital.[22] The radiation effects on organ function depend on the reproductive requirements of the irradiated cells. For instance, tissues (muscle and neurologic tisue) whose functional activity does not require cell renewal are "resistant" to radiation, whereas many tissues of the body require continued cellular proliferation for their function. These renewal tissues, including the skin and its adnexa, the gastrointestinal mucosa, bone marrow, reproductive organs, and many exocrine glands are "sensitive" to radiation. Tissues, such as the liver and bone, require little or no proliferation during the steady state, and normal function can be maintained despite large doses of radiation.

Following large doses of radiation, the prodromal syndrome of nausea, vomiting, diarrhea, cramps, fatigue, sweating, fever, and headache occurs. Three distinct modes of death may occur. The first, with very high doses of radiation (>10,000 rad), is seen within hours and appears to result from neurologic and cardiovascular damage. Being so quick, it probably is caused by extranuclear events within these organs. At intermediate doses of radiation (500 to 1000 rad), death occurs within days, and it is associated with extensive gastrointestinal mucosal damage, resulting in prolonged, severe, bloody diarrhea, dehydration, and secondary infection. At lower doses of radiation (around the LD_{50}), death is caused by hematopoietic failure. This has a latency period.

The most important adverse effects of radiation are on the immune response. In general, the following conclusions concerning the effect of radiation on the immune response can be made: (1) B-lymphocytes are radiosensitive and undergo both interphase and mitotic death following radiation; (2) all functional T-cell subpopulations have sensitive precursor cells, and suppressor T-cell precursors may undergo interphase death; (3) the homing potential of cells is affected by radiation; (4) resting cells are more sensitive to interphase death than are the same cells when stimulated to divide before irradiation; and (5) the effects of whole-body irradiation are qualitatively and quantitatively different from those caused by localized or regional irradiation.

Clearly, regional irradiation of the lymph nodes adjacent to tumors has been associated with increased curability in head and neck tumors in adults without adverse effects. Examples of such radiocurable tumors are carcinomas of the cervix, larynx, breast, and prostate, in addition to Hodgkin's disease and seminomas. Radiation can be combined with surgery and chemotherapy. Combination of radiation with surgery and chemotherapy may improve the therapeutic effects and survival, such as adjuvant chemotherapy with irradiation for breast cancer or with surgery and radiation for colon cancer. Also, association with hormones, vitamins, and interleukins (IL-1, IL-3) reduces the toxic effects and increases the effectiveness. One of the greatest disadvantages of radiation is the occurrence of malignancies following cancer radiotherapy. Experiments in animals have shown that carcinogenesis is a long-term effect of radiation exposure. When given in sufficiently high doses, radiation acts as a complete carcinogen in that it acts as both an initiator and promoter.[11] Ionizing radiation causes cancer, either by a direct carcinogenic effect on cells in the radiation field, or indirectly by depressing immunity. The most common malignancies are leukemias and bone sarcomas followed by thyroid cancer, skin cancers, breast cancer, and central nervous system and other cancers.

Thus, an almost unending variety of other neoplasms has followed radiotherapy of various primary tumors. For instance, of 226 patients who underwent postoperative radiotherapy for breast cancer, 4 developed sarcomas of the chest wall, 3 SCC's (2 of the esophagus), 2 angiosarcomas of the arm, and 1 patient, multiple BCC's. In a control group of 503 patients treated without radiation, only 1 patient developed a myxosarcoma of the arm.[23] Radiotherapy of carcinomas of the uterine cervix has been followed by the development of endometrial adenocarcinomas, carcinomas of the colon, rectum, anus, bladder, peritoneal mesotheliomas, and osteosarcomas of the pelvic bones.[24] The risk of radiation carcinogenesis is affected by the type of exposure (X-rays, gamma rays, neutron irradiation), total dosage, dose rate, and dose fractionation. Tissue sensitivity and other host factors (age and endocrine function) also play a role in determining whether cancer occurs following exposure.

Possible causes of neoplasms following radiation therapy are that radiation may damage one or both strands of DNA, purine or pyrimidine bases, or other possible targets in the cell. Defective DNA repair may progress to malignant change. While direct cellular damage is the most likely cause of second cancers following radiotherapy, some neoplasms occur well outside the radiation field. Other possible factors, such as immunosuppression, may play a role. Genetic factors may affect susceptibility or resistance to cancer by affecting carcinogen metabolism, regulation of the immune response, level of interferon secretion, or response to virus infection. Radiation therapy may also act as a sensitizer or may induce dormant malignant change that is subsequently activated, e.g., as in patients with psoriasis treated with radiotherapy initially, in whom squamous cell carcinoma develops after treatment with psoralen and ultraviolet radiation years later. The initial point of action of ionizing radiation in the induction of cancer is not known. Specific locus mutation seems improbable, but chromosomal damage and healing could be involved, at least in some cases. Other cellular organelles may be the target.

Lifetime followup of the exposed cohort appears essential to estimate the complete differential distribution of radiogenic neoplasia over time. The following variables are important factors that affect the outcome: genetic constitution, nongenetic constitutional factors, age at exposure, interaction with other carcinogens, and reactions during the latency period.

Thus, in the mouse, irradiated breast or ovarian cells may remain dormant until stimulated by a change in hormonal balance that leads to neoplasia. In avoiding the induction of secondary cancer, radiation therapy has the advantage over chemotherapy in that it involves partial rather than whole-body exposure. However, the carcinogenicity of radiation relative to chemotherapeutic agents is not known. Certainly, a combination of radiation therapy with chemotherapy increases the incidence of malignancies (leukemia) as compared to each therapy alone.[25] Hence the long-term carcinogenic risks of radiotherapy should be kept in mind when it is used as adjuvant therapy to surgical resection of tumors. When using such treatments, the physician must carefully weigh the risks of inducing new cancers or of increasing the incidence of recurrences of the original cancer, against the possible benefits of completely eradicating any residual neoplastic cells.

C. HORMONOTHERAPY AS COMPARED TO IMMUNOTHERAPY

Approaches to immunotherapy of cancer are rapidly changing. However, in spite of many clinical studies in the past decades, virtually no immunotherapeutical approach has emerged as an obligatory treatment of any type or stage of malignancy. To date, the results of immunotherapy of tumors have been disappointing. When surgery, radiotherapy, and chemotherapy were hardly expected to add more to what had already been accomplished in cancer treatment, it is no surprise that immunotherapy became the new hope in the fight against cancer. Without much fundamental background many clinical trials were started in which all kinds of nonspecific immunostimulants were tested, but the results of the randomized trials were so disappointing that today many clinicians no longer believe in any role of the immune response of the host to his tumor. The only exceptions seem to be hairy cell leukemia (HCL), for which there is no better drug than α-interferon, and three other human tumors, melanoma, renal cancer, and superficial bladder cancer (intravesical instillation of BCG vaccine), which occasionally have been treated by some form of active immunization; however, it has not yet been proven that this is the best available choice.[26]

The main objectives of immunotherapy are (1) to restore immunocompetence of immunodeficient patients; (2) to prevent or reverse immunosuppression induced by chemotherapy, radiotherapy, and surgery; (3) to induce specific tumor immunity; (4) to increase specific tumor immunity if weak; and (5) to modulate immune response for selected objectives (increase cytotoxic antibody, activate macrophages, and augment cell-mediated immunity). Despite several clinical trials, immunotherapy is still in its developmental stage, and its role as compared to hormonotherapy, chemotherapy, or radiotherapy cannot be determined at this time. However, clinical research using interferons (INFs), interleukins (ILs), and monoclonal antibodies (MoAbs) is starting. It is hoped that these antibodies may mediate nonspecific immune responses, particularly if "cocktails" of antibodies become available to cover all possible antigens that a tumor may carry, or if used to bring appropriate toxic drugs to the tumor cell thus improving the specificity of cytotoxic drugs.

Nevertheless, interleukins and interferons are highly toxic compounds; at best, the patients develop an influenza-like disease, or, at worst, a comatose state can be induced. Interleukin-2 causes circulatory disturbances, and some patients require admission to intensive care units for support (see Chapter 4). Intravenous infusion of unlabeled antibodies is the most widely used method, and transient responses have been demonstrated. However, monoclonal antibodies conjugated to radionuclides (^{131}I) have been quite successful in localizing tumors (carcinoma of the bronchus, colorectal, and ovarian cancers) of <1 cm diameter (radioimmunoscintigraphy). Therapy trials with MoAbs conjugated to isotopes, toxins, and drugs have shown some promise. Purging of autologous bone marrow with monoclonal antibodies and complement *in vitro* has been used in ALL and non-Hodgkin's lymphoma, and preliminary data suggest that this approach may be an effective therapy. Reviewing the literature, it seems that monoclonal antibodies have potential uses in clinical medicine (see Table 2). Thus, the most successful area for exploitation has been in diagnosis.

TABLE 2
Clinical Uses of Monoclonal Antibodies

Diagnosis

Tumor markers
Cytology
Histology
Immunopathology
Radioimmunoscintigraphy (for detection of primary or metastatic lesions)

Therapy

Systemic therapy
Direct cytotoxicity of MoAb
Bone marrow clearance
Antibody conjugated to
  Drugs
  Radionuclides
  Toxins

Prognosis

Subclassification of tumors
Differentiation antigens: antigens associated with low or high metastatic potential
Predicted response (or lack thereof) to specific therapeutic regimens

Although the greatest excitement with monoclonal antibodies is their potential for therapy (delivering high doses of drug, toxin, or radioactivity to the site of the tumor), there are several problems limiting their use at present. The first problem is their specificity or lack of specificity; they cannot discriminate completely between tumor and normal cells. The second problem is their affinity; although they bind to tumors, they do not stick tightly enough. The third problem is that most antibodies are of mouse origin and when injected into a patient induce a secondary antibody anti-mouse response. Innovations in monoclonal antibody tumor targeting may offer novel clinical opportunities in the treatment of human carcinoma.[27,28]

There are some critical factors for successful monoclonal antibody therapy, such as: (1) cross reactivity with normal tissues; (2) affinity of antibody; (3) distribution of surface membrane antigens; (4) tumor vascularization; (5) tumor size; (6) circulating antigens, and (7) degree of tumor necrosis. Some hormones (corticosteroids, diethylstilbestrol (DES), tamoxifen, toremifene, and thymosin fractions), vitamins (A, E, D), and growth factors (CSF, EGF) are immunomodulators. During the past decade, renewed interest in immunotherapy has been stimulated by genetic engineering and mass cell culture, which have made available highly purified molecules of interferons, interleukins, tumor necrosis factors, and hematopoietic growth factors (HGFs), but the great hopes have remained largely unfulfilled, and much remains to be learned.[29,30] All these new factors (interferons, interleukins, and growth factors) are generically termed "biologic response modifiers" (BRM); they are newer approaches to immunotherapy, and may be considered the "fourth modality or fourth arm of cancer treatment".

Three major species of human interferon are identified: α, β, and γ. α-Interferon is produced by leukocytes (B-cells, T-cells, null cells, and macrophages) following exposure to B-cell mitogens, foreign cells, viruses, and tumor cells. β-Interferon is produced by fibroblasts following exposure to viruses or foreign nucleic acids. γ-Interferon is produced by T-lymphocytes following stimulation of T-cell mitogens, specific antigens, or IL-2. Their therapeutic applications are thoroughly described in Chapter 4 of this book. Interleukin-2

(IL-2) is active during the early stages of tumor growth (day 3) in both immunogenic and nonimmunogenic murine tumors; IL-2 is active in the advanced stages of tumor growth (day 10), but only in animals with weakly immunogenic tumors. The antitumor effect in nonimmunogenic tumors is primarily mediated by LAK cells and in weakly immunogenic tumors by T-cells as well as LAK cells or TIL cells (adoptive immunotherapy).

Early trials with growth factors have demonstrated their potentially important clinical role. Cell-surface receptors for hormones and growth factors are attractive alternatives to tumor-specific antigens as targets for monoclonal antibodies. Clinical trials with these reagents will be essential to study toxicity and side-effects, and to optimize the method and schedule of delivery, as well as to determine whether combinations of growth factors are more effective than single growth factors.[29] Recent studies revealed that the neuroendocrine and immune systems are now recognized to be intimately linked in bidirectional communication. A common molecular basis for neuroendocrine and immune systems has been recently provided. Thus, the immune system and its products can modulate neuroendocrine functions and neuroendocrine peptide hormones, and their receptors are now included as endogenous components of the immune system.

Evidence for this bidirectional link includes (1) cells of the immune system can synthesize biologically active neuroendocrine peptide hormones (ACTH, endorphins, and GH), and it is possible that these immunocytes may also influence their own function in an autocrine-like fashion; (2) immune cells also possess receptors for many of these peptides; (3) the same neuroendocrine hormones can influence immune function; and (4) lymphokines can influence neuroendocrine tissues. The findings that both the hormones and the hormone receptors on leukocytes and pituitary cells are common, provide evidence that the immune system has the capacity to react at the molecular level similarly to a neuroendocrine organ, and may provide new clues to define better the pathologic states of tumor pathophysiology.[31] Although immunotherapy is very effetive in certain animal models and has been used to treat human cancers for several decades, unfortunately none of these approaches has been shown to be effective in controlled trials. Newer approaches using biologic response modifiers, such as interferons, interleukins, and monoclonal antibodies, will be more promising in the future for cancer treatment. This will be an exciting new area of cancer research which will generate important clinical data over the next few years.

D. HORMONOTHERAPY AS COMPARED TO SURGERY

Recent advances in cancer biology have led to the practical conclusion that there is no longer reason to believe that surgery should be the only primary treatment for cancer. This conclusion is a major departure from standard practice. Surgery in the premodern era was based on empiric observation and natural history rather than scientific concepts. Generally, surgery alone cannot be considered curative except in cases with very small tumors and no lymph node involvement. Radiation therapy, chemotherapy, and especially hormonal and vitamin therapy are used to prevent, delay, or lessen the recurrence and spread of disease. Due to recent advances in endocrine pharmacology and cancer biology, surgical ablation of endocrine glands or endocrine ablative therapy (adrenalectomy, hypophysectomy, oophorectomy, and orchiectomy), which formerly were used as the initial therapy in many patients with metastatic cancer (breast, prostate), are much less commonly employed today. This is due primarily to the introduction into clinical practice of new pharmacologic agents (antiestrogens — tamoxifen, aminoglutethimide, LHRH antagonists), which induce remissions as often as do the surgical procedures. Thus, "medical or chemical" oophorectomy, adrenalectomy, and hypophysectomy induce similar or almost identical therapeutic results, but with a lower morbidity and virtually no mortality, and make the previous surgical ablative procedures less used or even obsolete. Hence, at present either of these therapies seems preferable to surgical adrenalectomy, oophorectomy, or hypophysectomy.[32]

TABLE 3
Comparison between Surgery, Hormonotherapy, and Vitamin Therapy

	Surgery	Hormonotherapy	Vitamin therapy
Invasive, disfigurement	+ +	−	−
Feasible difficult	+ +	−	−
Replacement therapy	+ +	±	−
Spread of disease (metastasis) following treatment	+	−	−
Psychologic consequences	+ +	−	−
Response rate	+	+	±
Tumor receptors	+	+	+
Host-immune defense	−	+	+
Health status and quality of life	−	+	+
Morbidity and mortality	+ +	−	−
More costly	+	±	±
Local disease	+	±	±
Systemic disease	±	+ +	+

Endocrine ablation therapy for advanced cancer is usually irreversible. Oophorectomy, adrenalectomy, and hypophysectomy not only involve problems associated with the intra-operative and postoperative periods, but also result in endocrine hypofunction and its sequelae. This is particularly true with adrenalectomy and hypophysectomy procedures in which life-long hormone replacement therapy is required. Medical or chemical oophorectomy, adrenalectomy, and hypophysectomy are more safe, reversible, and more acceptable for patients with metastatic hormone-sensitive cancer. Surgery, an invasive procedure, by squeezing the tumor accelerates the spread of cancer cells in the circulation, and subsequently increases the changes of the metastatic process. Surgery can weaken the host immune defenses and deteriorate the health status. Surgery is also invasive, irreversible, sometimes disfiguring and not always feasible. Thus, ideally, medical or chemical ablative surgery is effective, convenient, and not associated with significant side effects. In reviewing the literature, it appears that there are significant advantages of hormonotherapy and vitamin therapy over surgery (see Table 3).

Since in most cancer patients presenting at diagnosis the disease has already spread (systemic disease), at present cancer is more a medical than a surgical disease. Hence, treatment should be mainly an adjuvant systemic therapy (hormone, vitamins, growth factors) rather than surgical. Surgery in the treatment of cancer patients should be reserved for: (1) definitive treatment for primary cancer, appropriate local therapy, and integration of surgery with other modalities (chemotherapy, radiation, or hormone therapy); (2) resection of metastatic disease with curative intent (e.g., pulmonary metastases in sarcoma patients, metastases from colorectal cancer); (3) treatment of oncologic emergencies; (4) the reduction of the residual disease (e.g., Burkitt's lymphoma, ovarian cancer); (5) palliation; (6) solid tumors, and (7) reconstruction and rehabilitation.

Surgery also should be done in preneoplastic or precancer conditions for preventing cancer, such as cryptorchidism, polyposis coli, ulcerative colitis, multiple endocrine neoplasia (Types II and III), familial colon cancer, familial breast cancer, and familial ovarian cancer.[33] Surgery also has a role in diagnostic pathologic states in cancer patients by using excision biopsy or needle biopsy for cytologic analysis of the removed material and thus can provide a tentative diagnosis of the presence of malignant cells. It is important for precise staging of patients when planning treatment. Despite improvements and significant progress in screening and early diagnosis of cancer, unfortunately, when patients with solid tumors present to the physician for the first time, approximately 70% already have micrometastases beyond the primary site. Hence, surgery should be combined with radiotherapy or adjuvant chemotherapy or hormonotherapy. The survival rate at 5 years will significantly increase to 70 to 80% as compared to surgery alone (10%) in certain solid tumors, such as child rhabdomyosarcoma. Some surgical procedures, such as transurethral resection of prostate (TURP) increase long-term mortality by occurrence of myocardial infarction. This is a greater risk factor, possibly related to absorption of irrigation fluid.[34] With regard to costs and benefits measured by Q-TWIST (time without symptoms and toxicity) between different adjuvant therapies, it was found in a recent study that following mastectomy, in postmenopausal women with node-positive breast cancer and treated with endocrine therapy alone, chemoendocrine therapy, or no treatment, chemoendocrine therapy provides better results.[35]

III. COMMENTS AND CONCLUSIONS

In the past decade, important advances in endocrine pharmacology and tumor biology have been made, and hormones and vitamins have proven to exert significant therapeutic effects over conventional therapies, such as chemotherapy, radiation therapy, and surgery. Due to the fact that both hormones and vitamins are less toxic, have fewer side effects, and can provide the same beneficial therapeutic effects, they are replacing, in many cases, surgical procedures, cytotoxic agents, and radiation therapy. They are noninvasive, reversible, and nondisfiguring and have fewer psychologic consequences; also they are more acceptable to patients, providing the same therapeutic and palliative effects as other therapy and improving the quality of life. They are used more often as a systemic adjuvant therapy in patients with advanced metastatic cancer alone or in combination with chemotherapy (chemohormonotherapy) and with radiation as well as with immunotherapy. They are significant biologic response modifiers (BRM). They can significantly enhance the therapeutic effects of chemotherapeutic drugs and radiation and decrease their toxic side effects. Since hormones and vitamins exert their therapeutic effects mainly by changing hormone receptor status, they act more specifically on cancer cells by inducing damage on cell membranes, and nuclear chromatin, leaving the normal replicating cells sometimes undamaged. Thus, they are primarily cytostatic or tumoristatic as compared to cytotoxic drugs or radiation, which are mainly cytotoxic for both neoplastic and normal cells. Cytotoxic drugs and radiation indiscriminately kill both cancer cells and normal cells. Hormones and vitamins act on specific cell cycle phases, particularly the G_0/G_1-phase; they are cell cycle specific (CCS) agents and can shift cancer cells into a dormant stage (G_0) where they can stop for months or years, reducing the pool of dividing cells and subsequently the "growth fraction" or rapidly dividing cells. Also, they can make the dormant cells from G_0 re-enter the cell cycle thus exposing them to chemotherapeutic, radiation, or hormone therapy. Hence, both hormones and vitamins play an important role in "cellular therapy" of cancer.

By estimation of hormone receptor and tumor markers, the oncologist can better select the patients and divide them in various subgroups suitable for each therapy. Thus, he can better "tailor" hormonotherapy and vitamin therapy and predict more accurately the outcome of cancer treatment as compared to chemotherapy or radiation therapy. Furthermore, new hormone agonists and antagonists, which are more active (10 to 300 times) as compared to natural hormones, increase the effectiveness of hormonotherapy dramatically over the use of natural or synthetic hormones. By blocking the binding of hormones to their cellular receptor, they antagonize their biologic response and thus decrease the steroid hormone levels close to "castrate" levels including a "medical" castration, which is reversible and nondisfiguring and has fewer psychologic consequences. Hence, new antiestrogens (tamoxifen and its derivatives) and LHRH antagonists are replacing the conventional surgical castration (oophorectomy, orchiectomy).

Also, the use of steroid synthesis inhibitors, such as aminoglutethimide (AG) or 4-OHA, can produce a "chemical adrenalectomy" or "chemical hypophysectomy", which is more acceptable and less life-threatening to cancer patients. Hormones and vitamins are chemo-suppressor and chemopreventive and can halt the evolution of micrometastases, which is undetectable to surgeons. Since hormones and vitamins are used in large or pharmacologic doses in order to elicit their antitumor effects, they can disrupt the hypothalamus-pituitary gonadal or hypothalamopituitary adrenal axis, the feedback mechanism, and induce some toxic or side effects; however, their toxic effects are fewer compared to those of cytotoxic drugs or radiation therapy. Due to the presence of steroid hormone receptors, most hormone-dependent cancers (breast, prostate cancer, lymphoproliferative disease) respond dramatically to hormones; other cancers (endometrial, ovarian, exocrine, pancreas, colorectal), also quite often improve following hormone or vitamin therapy. Therefore, in hormone responsive neoplasms, hormonotherapy should always be tried first, and then chemohormonotherapy or chemotherapy alone.

Carcinogenicity and occurrence of secondary cancers, which can be seen following chemotherapy and radiation therapy, are virtually nonexistent after hormonotherapy and vitamin therapy. Also, the occurrence of multiple drug resistance (MDR), which quite frequently follows cytotoxic agents, is seen less often in patients treated with hormones and vitamins. The effectiveness of hormonotherapy and vitamin therapy is potentiated by a concomitant administration of hormonotherapy, immunotherapy, and vitamin therapy. Some interleukins (IL-1, IL-3) have radioprotective effects, mainly in laboratory animals following wholebody irradiation. Certain hormones, especially antiestrogens (tamoxifen and toremi-fene), can reverse the phenomenon of MDR (multidrug resistance), which is the main obstacle or the main reason for chemotherapy failure. Hormonotherapy and vitamin therapy are the first choice as palliative therapy in terminally ill patients, in whom palliation and improving quality of life are more important than using aggressive therapy in order to gain a few months, at best, in a patient with deteriorating life. Physicians should always keep in mind when making therapeutic decisions that they are treating not only the cancer, but also the patient; the hippocratic advice "primum non nocere" (first do not harm) should be remem-bered. Despite recent advances in cancer chemotherapy regarding reduction of toxicity and improving quality of life by new drugs, such as carboplatin, etoposide, and ifosfamide, still it is hoped that better drugs less toxic and carcinogenic will be developed.[36] Also, the use of chemotherapeutic drugs in the treatment of node negative breast cancer patients has become a very controversial matter. Currently, it is a trend that adjuvant chemotherapy should be reserved only for patients at high risk of relapse, and tamoxifen which has minimal toxocity, should be the treatment of choice for patients at low risk.[37] Always, the physician should weigh the potential benefits of chemotherapy and its toxicity. Generally, hormonotherapy and vitamin therapy offer new approaches and provide many advantages over the conventional therapies; they are less toxic and more acceptable to the patients and will become the ideal therapeutic methods in cancer management.

REFERENCES

1. **Cummings, C.**, The endocrine evolution and therapy of cancer, *Am. J. Cancer*, 2, 143, 1925.
2. **Cummings, C.**, The endocrine vs. surgery in the treatment of cancer, *Clin. Med.*, (Chicago), 31, 693, 1924.
3. **Bonadonna, G.**, Conceptual and practical advances in the management of breast cancer, *J. Clin. Oncol.*, 7, 1380, 1989.
4. **Goldie, J. H.**, Scientific basis for adjuvant and primary (neoadjuvant) chemotherapy, *Semin. Oncol.*, 14, 1, 1987.
5. **Tannock, I. F.**, Is there evidence that chemotherapy is of benefit to patients with carcinoma of the prostate?, *J. Clin. Oncol.*, 3, 1013, 1985.

6. **Himel, H. N., Liberati, A., Gelber, R. D., and Chalmers, T. C.,** Adjuvant chemotherapy for breast cancer: a pooled estimate based on published randomized control trials, *JAMA,* 256, 1148, 1986.
7. **Kyle, R. A.,** Second malignancies associated with chemotherapeutic agents, *Semin. Oncol.,* 9, 131, 1982.
8. **Pauli, J. W., Coombs, P. A., and Allegra, J. C.,** Cancer chemotherapy: a current perspective, *Med. Times,* 114, 29, 1986.
9. **Balducci, L., Phillips, D. M., Wallace, C., and Hardy, C.,** Cancer chemotherapy in the elderly, *Am. Fam. Physician,* 35, 133, 1987.
10. **Rieche, K.,** Carcinogenicity of antineoplastic agents in man, *Cancer Treat. Rev.,* 11, 39, 1984.
11. **Penn, I.,** Secondary neoplasms as a consequence of transplantation and cancer therapy, *Cancer Detect. Prev.,* 12, 39, 1988.
12. **Moscow, J. A. and Cowan, K. H.,** Multidrug resistance, *J. Natl. Cancer Inst.,* 80, 14, 1988.
13. **Pastan, I. H. and Gottesman, M. M.,** Molecular biology of multidrug resistance in human cells, in *Important Advances in Oncology, 1988,* DeVita, V. T., Hellman, S., and Rosenberg, S. A., Eds., Lippincott, Philadelphia, 1988, 3.
14. **Ling, V.,** Does P-glycoprotein predict response to chemotherapy?, *J. Natl. Cancer Inst.,* 81, 84, 1989.
15. **Skipper, H. E., Schabel, F. M., and Lloyd, H. H.,** Experimental therapeutics and kinetic: selection and overgrowth of specifically and permanently drug-resistant tumor cells, *Semin. Hematol.,* 15, 207, 1978.
16. **Goldie, J. and Coldman, A.,** Quantitative model for multiple levels of drug resistance in clinical tumors, *Cancer Treat. Rep.,* 67, 923, 1983.
17. **Zamora, J. M., Pearce, H. L., and Beck, W. T.,** Physical-chemical properties shared by compounds that modulate multiple drug resistance in human leukemic cells, *Mol. Pharmacol.,* 33, 454, 1988.
18. **DeGregorio, M. W., Ford, J. M., Benz, C. C., and Wiebe, V.,** Toremifene: pharmacologic and pharmacokinetic basis of reversing multidrug resistance, *J. Clin. Oncol.,* 7, 1359, 1989.
19. **Lippman, M. E., Cassidy, J., Wesley, M., and Young, R. C.,** A randomized attempt to increase the efficacy of cytotoxic chemotherapy in metastatic breast cancer by hormonal synchronization, *J. Clin. Oncol.,* 2, 28, 1984.
20. **Hug, V., Thames, H., and Clark, J.,** Chemotherapy and hormonal therapy in combination, *J. Clin. Oncol.,* 6, 173, 1988.
21. **Lichter, A. S.,** Is radiation therapy in conjunction with mastectomy indicated for the treatment of operable breast cancer?, *Cancer Invest.,* 5, 243, 1987.
22. **Hellman, S.,** Cell kinetics, models, and cancer treatment: some principles for the radiation oncologist, *Radiology,* 114, 219, 1975.
23. **Ferguson, D. J., Sutton, H. G., and Dawson, P. J.,** Delayed hazards of adjuvant therapy for breast cancer, *Breast,* 11, 2, 1985.
24. **Penn, I.,** Second malignancies following radiotherapy or chemotherapy for cancer, in *Immunopharmacologic Effects of Radiation Therapy,* Dubois, J. B., Serrou, B., and Rosenfeld, C., Eds., Monograph Series Eur. Org. Res. Treat. Cancer, 8, 1981, 415.
25. **Kohn, H. I. and Fry, R. M.,** Radiation carcinogenesis, *N. Engl. J. Med.,* 310, 504, 1984.
26. **Rümke, P.,** Possibilities and limitations of immunotherapy, in *Tumor Immunology: Mechanisms, Diagnosis, Therapy,* W. den Otter and Ruitenberg, E. J., Eds., Elsevier, Amsterdam, 1987, 337.
27. **Schlom, J.,** Innovations in monoclonal antibody tumor targeting, *JAMA,* 261, 744, 1989.
28. **Foon, K. A.,** Laboratory and clinical applications of monoclonal antibodies for leukemias and non-Hodgkin's lymphomas, *Curr. Probl. Cancer,* 13, 57, 1989.
29. **Sato, G. H. and Sato, J. D.,** Growth factor receptor, monoclonal antibodies and cancer immunotherapy, *J. Natl. Cancer Inst.,* 81, 1600, 1989.
30. **Foon, K. A.,** Biological response modifiers: the new immunotherapy, *Cancer Res.,* 49, 1621, 1989.
31. **Weigent, D. and Blalock, J. E.,** Interactions between the neuroendocrine and immune systems: common hormones and receptors, *Immunol. Rev.,* 100, 79, 1987.
32. **Wells, S. A. and Santen, R. J.,** Ablative procedures in patients with metastatic breast carcinoma, *Cancer,* 53 (Supp. 3), 762, 1984.
33. **Rosenberg, S. A.,** Principles of surgical oncology, in *Cancer, Principles and Practice of Oncology,* DeVita, V. T., Hellman, S., and Rosenberg, S. A., Eds., Lippincott, Philadelphia, 1989, 236.
34. **Coppinger, S. W. and Hudd, C.,** Risk factor for myocardial infarction in transurethral resection of prostate?, *Lancet,* 2, 859, 1989.
35. **Goldhirsch, A., Gelber, R. D., Simes, R. J., Glasziou, P., and Coates, A. S.,** Costs and benefits of adjuvant therapy in breast cancer: a quality adjusted survival analysis, *J. Clin. Oncol.,* 7, 36, 1989.
36. **Yarbro, J. W., Bornstein, R. S., and Mastrangelo, M. J.,** Recent advances in cancer chemotherapy, *Semin. Oncol.,* 17 (Supp. 2), 1, 1990.
37. **O'Reilly, S. M. and Richards, M. A.,** Node negative breast cancer, *Br. Med. J.,* 300, 346, 1990.

Chapter 7

CHEMOPREVENTION OF CANCER BY HORMONES AND VITAMINS

I. PROSPECTS AND STRATEGIES FOR THE USE OF HORMONES AND VITAMINS AS PROPHYLACTIC AGENTS

Chemoprevention of cancer is a means of cancer control in which the occurrence of this disease is prevented by administration of one or several chemical compounds. The most desirable way of eliminating the impact of cancer in humans is by prevention. The first set of strategies for achieving this objective is to remove the causative agents. However, the causes in most human cancers are not known. Under some circumstances, the causative factors are known; neoplasia has already been initiated, and prevention then consists of suppressing the evolution of the neoplastic process. Individuals already exposed to carcinogens as well as individuals at high risk to cancer due to genetic factors fall into this category. While the removal of causative agents remains the primary objective of cancer prevention, this would be difficult to achieve in the foreseeable future, and is likely to be imcomplete. Thus, the development of a second line of prevention based on chemoprevention will be of considerable importance in the future.

To date, there are many compounds that have been demonstrated to prevent the occurrence of cancer, and over 20 different classes of chemicals have been shown to have chemopreventive properties; thus, the options for selecting optimal compounds will be many. Since experimental investigations demonstrate that chemoprevention can readily protect experimental animals against the occurrence of cancer, we now must learn to use this protection effectively for human cancers.[1] Studies in the U.S., as in other western countries, indicate that improvements in cancer treatment are unlikely to have a dramatic impact on overall cancer mortality, and consequently, a shift in research emphasis from research on treatment to research on prevention should be made in order to gain substantial progress against cancer.[2,3]

Although hormones and vitamins play a crucial role in the occurrence and development of several types of neoplasms in laboratory animals, which are histologically identical to that of humans, there is no direct evidence that hormones or vitamins, per se, are causative or etiologic factors of human cancers. However, there is ample evidence and literature mentioned in this book (see chapters 2 and 5) which strongly suggest that hormones and vitamins are factors which dramatically affect the incidence and development as well as propagation of several types of human cancers (breast, prostate, endometrial, ovarian, leukemia and lymphomas, esophageal, skin, lung, papillomas, endocrine, etc.). A rational basis for chemoprevention of human cancers will be to use chempreventive agents which are less toxic, such as hormones (endocrine prevention) and vitamins and their synthetic analogs (vitamin prevention).

A. ENDOCRINE PREVENTION OF CANCER

Endocrine prevention is based mainly on the use of hormones or hormone agonists or antagonists as prophylactic agents against cancer. Only progress in the understanding of the mechanisms by which hormones and their synthetic analogs act on cancer cells can lead to specific means of cancer prevention. The applicability of new laboratory methods for early detection to epidemiologic surveys will be very helpful, and a new epidemiology based on laboratory data will emerge. The success of endocrine prevention will depend principally on early detection of hormonally sensitive cancers called hormone-dependent cancers, which

TABLE 1
Most Frequent Cancer-Causing Factors

Factors	Type of Cancer
Chemicals	Stomach, kidney, bladder skin, lung
Viruses	Burkitt's lymphoma
Ionizing radiation (X-ray); γ-radiation (atomic blast, disaster, etc.)	Leukemia, thyroid cancer
	Leukemia, thyroid cancer
Genetic predisposition	Xeroderma pigmentosum
Hormones	Hormone-dependent cancers
Immunosuppression	Organ transplantation
Different treatments (cytostatics)	Leukemia; other secondary neoplasms
Ultraviolet radiation	Skin cancer
Diet	Colon cancer, breast cancer
Socioeconomic conditions (smoking)	Lung cancer
Oral contraceptives	Endometrial cancer, breast cancer, hepatocellular cancer

cannot develop or propagate in the absence of hormones. These neoplasms will soon shrink and finally die after the hormone source is removed. On the contrary, in the presence of hormones, they will continue to grow and metastasize and finally kill the host.

For early detection, the use of sensitive procedures, such as tumor markers (oncofetal, ectopic hormones, enzymes) and screening procedures (Pap smears, mammography, ultrasonography), are needed. They should be used in conjunction with one another; the determination of a single marker is not accurate enough to diagnose or rule out the presence of a tumor. Their accuracy will be significantly increased when they are used in combination (tumor markers, oncogenes, DNA content, and screening procedures). The idea of hormones as chemopreventative or prophylactic agents against cancer started in 1916, when Lathrop and Loeb[4] found that the hormonal milieu of multiple pregnancies predisposed to carcinoma formation and that an early ovariectomy prevented the occurrence of mammary carcinomas in large numbers of mice. Although this was important experimental evidence suggesting that estrogens can act as carcinogens, while their removal or using estrogen-antagonists can act as prophylactic agents, it was overlooked for many years.

At present, there is a general belief that most cancers, almost 90%, originate from environmental factors; thus, they have an environmental origin.[5] Hence, hormones, both exogenous (taken as drugs or coming from dietary sources) and endogenous (abnormally produced by endocrine glands), are significant factors in cancer prevention. The most frequent cancer-causing factors at present are listed in Table 1.

Recent data regarding international epidemiology of hormone-dependent cancers (HDC) suggest that the distribution of the endocrine-dependent cancers (breast, prostate, colon, and thyroid) is related to dietary factors and micronutrients, including vitamins and some minerals (selenium, cadmium, and iodine). For example, a predominantly high-protein, high-fat diet imposed in early life can make individuals susceptible to the development of these cancers.[6] Clinical evidence shows associations among breast cancer, colon cancer, and endemic goiter. Caloric restriction has a generally inhibitory effect on carcinogenesis, while dietary fat tends to promote tumor growth, but only of mammary tumors. On the contrary, a high-fiber, low-fat, and vitamin-rich diet decreases the occurrence of cancers. Diet can also influence the synthesis of some hormones (growth hormone (GH), steroid hormones, and thyroid hormones). Thus there is a correlation between hormones, vitamins, nutrition, and carcinogenesis (See Table 2). However, there are difficulties in classifying certain hormones and vitamins as chemopreventive and prophylactic agents for different types of cancers since most epidemiologic studies use different doses, biologic parameters, and socioeconomic factors. The epidemiologic evidence and the role of chemopreventive agents will differ if hormones intervene in the early stages of cancer development, when they are more effective or if they intervene in the later stages, when they exert an adjuvant or secondary role.[7]

TABLE 2
Chemopreventive Hormones and Vitamins for
Cancer

Compound	Findings		
	Epidemiologic	Experimental	Clinical
Hormones			
Tamoxifen	+	+ +	+ + +
Progesterone	±	+ +	+
Danazol	±	±	+
LHRH	±	±	+
DHEA	+	+ +	ND
OC and HRT	±	±	±
Vitamins			
β-carotene	+	±	+
Vitamin A	+	+	+
4-HPR	−	+ + +	−
Vitamin E	+	+	±
Vitamin D	−	+	ND

Note: HRT (hormone-replacement therapy); DHEA (dehydroepiandrosterone); OC (oral contraceptives); 4-HPR (retinamide; synthetic retinoid); ± (weak) evidence; ND = not determined.

1. Tamoxifen

Tamoxifen is an antiestrogen which exerts important chemosuppressive and chemopreventive effects on neoplasms. Its chemosuppressor, or cancerostatic activites, are thoroughly described in chapters 2 and 3. Chemopreventive effects of tamoxifen are of great significance, in addition to breast cancer, to the management and prevention of other potentially hormone-dependent tumors. It has been demonstrated that tamoxifen can prevent the induction of rat mammary carcinomas by carcinogens. Therefore, there are experimental data to support its application in patients at high risk for breast cancer. Some investigators believe that tamoxifen prevents the occurrence of cancer by chemosuppression of an occult disease rather than true chemoprevention.[8] Mice with a high incidence of mammary cancer can be protected from developing tumors by ovariectomy in early life, and both animal and human evidence suggests that early oophorectomy can inhibit phenotypic expression of malignancy.[4,9] It has long been postulated that an antagonistic hormone should be developed to prevent breast cancer. The discovery and development of antiestrogens for clinical use apparently could make chemoprevention a reality, and thus in 1986, tamoxifen was used for the first time as a chemopreventive agent.[10] A large body of evidence in women and in rodents has shown consistently that tamoxifen is a partial estrogen agonist, inducing elevation of sex hormone-binding globulin and cortisol-binding globulin, reduction of low-density lipoprotein (LDL), and elevation of high-density lipoprotein (HDL).[11]

Tamoxifen appears to exert its chemopreventive and suppressive activities by causing a G_1 block in cell culture. Its ability to prevent disease recurrence in postoperative patients could also be interpreted as a G_1 block of existing malignant cells.[12] Based on its physiologic and pharamacologic properties tamoxifen is proposed as a preventive chemosuppressive agent of subclinical breast cancer. Its primary action in producing a G_1 progression block suggests that prolonged treatment duration would be necessary.[12] The use of an antiestrogen for preventive chemosuppression in premenopausal patients raises concern about the effects of the drug upon the pituitary-ovarian axis. Tamoxifen also inhibits the neoplastic cell replication. It can bind to nuclear estrogen receptors (ER) to block estrogen action. It causes an increase in TGF-β and decreases other autocrine growth factors. Tamoxifen can increase sex hormone-binding globulin (SHBG) and may interact with other cellular components of cancer cells (calmodulin, protein kinase-C (PKC), and antiestrogen-binding sites (AEBS).

Experimental investigations have been carried out in DMBA-induced mammary carcinomas in rats at different periods or with different doses of tamoxifen to eradicate the microfoci and transform cells into mammary tissue. After 30 d a dose-related delay in the appearance of palpable mammary tumors was observed compared to nontreated animals. However, the continuous administration of tamoxifen resulted in more than 90% tumor-free animals. The problem is that the timing of the carcinogen damage must be known in order to prevent it from occurring. In the carcinogen-induced mammary cancers, prevention by tamoxifen is effective only in the early life of animals (up to 100 d of age), and only in that time will the concomitant administration prevent the occurrence of mammary tumors.[8] Similarly, only the ovariectomy of young animals will prevent the development of mouse mammary tumors.[4]

In human breast cancer, unfortunately we are ignorant about when the carcinogenic insult started and the nature of carcinogenic insult. Thus, prospective chemopreventive trials should be conducted only in a small number of women, those who are at high risk of developing breast cancer (about 1 in 12 women). This small group should be carefully identified (women with relatives in their family having diagnosed breast cancer). Also the drug used for chemoprevention should be simple and nontoxic as well as affordable for countries with limited health resources. The greatest challenge is the identification of this group of women at high risk for breast cancer, and the family history is one of the few reliable risk indicators. Thus, if 40% of high-risk women will take tamoxifen and assuming a 50% reduction in incidence, then 1 in 5 of the high-risk group might be prevented from developing breast cancer. Therefore, a 1% reduction in breast cancer incidence might be effected by this approach, using family history as a risk indicator.[13] Tamoxifen is a less toxic, almost nontoxic, drug. Chemoprevention trials should be conducted mainly in premenopausal women at high risk of developing breast cancer. They should use 20 mg/d of tamoxifen with placebo, to be given for probably a minimum of 10 years. These trials will be expensive, but they are worthwhile. It would be more costly not to prevent these high-risk patients than to allow them to develop breast cancer. Thus, tamoxifen may prevent recurrence of hormone-dependent disease and potentially retard the drift toward hormone-independent clones by preventing cell division.

Tamoxifen may exert its chemopreventive effects by several different mechanisms; it (1) prevents the induction of rat mammary carcinoma by carcinogens, (2) blocks (reversibly) the cancer cells in the G_1-phase, (3) prevents the cell division of independent clones, (4) inhibits ER and breast cancer cell line (MCF-7) growth after transplant in athymic mice, (5) has been successful as adjuvant therapy during clinical trials. The pilot trial does provide supportive evidence for the value of tamoxifen as a preventive agent. There was a significant reduction in new primary breast cancers in the treated group compared to nontreated (18 vs. 30). The lack of toxicity of tamoxifen has been a consistent feature of adjuvant trials in both postmenopausal and premenopausal women.[13] In premenopausal women with mastalgia, tamoxifen was well tolerated, and the incidence of minor side-effects, particularly hot flushes and menstrual irregularities, can be easily controlled by dose reduction; this can also be true for cancer prevention. In addition to breast cancer, other tumors (endometrial, ovarian, renal, and colorectal cancer, and malignant melanoma) had responded to tamoxifen. However, with the exception of endometrial carcinoma, objective responses to tamoxifen treatment are low.

Thus, all of the laboratory and clinical evidence suggest that tamoxifen may be prescribed indefinitely and make a significant impact upon the survival of castrate premenopausal and postmenopausal patients. The constant presence of tamoxifen within the cancer cells will be necessary to prevent the synthesis of estrogen-stimulated autocrine growth factors, and also may stimulate the synthesis of an inhibitory factor (TGF-β). Tamoxifen may act both as an autocrine and a paracrine growth regulator and thus prevent the development of suboccult tumors or the transformation of premalignant into malignant cells. Others propose a more complex approach to prevention. They suggest a total ablation of ovarian function with LHRH-agonist followed by the replacement of estrogen, possibly with additional intermittent progestin, to protect the uterus. The advantage of LHRH is its reversibility, but this kind of trial will be very costly (at least tenfold more than tamoxifen alone).[14] Although tamoxifen is the current drug of choice, other agents may be developed in the future with even fewer side effects or toxicological implications, and thus make significant improvements in cancer prevention by the end of this century.

2. Progesterone

Progesterone exerts protective effects on breast and endometrial carcinoma formation. It was previously reported that progesterone administration can reverse endometrial hyperplasia and can protect against the development of endometrial cancer in postmenopausal woman. The mechanism of this antiestrogenic effect can be explained by the changes induced by progesterone in steroid receptor metabolism and enzyme activity. Thus, in a 10-year, prospective double-blind study of 84 postmenopausal women who received cyclically estrogen-progesterone therapy, no endometrial cancer was observed.[15] More recent studies revealed that the "unopposed estrogen hypothesis" explains the epidemiology of uterine endometrial cancer as the effects of estrogens "unopposed" by progesterone on endometrial cell proliferation. The other hypothesis, "estrogen plus progesterone hypothesis" for breast cancer, also indicates the role of estrogens and progesterone in the epidemiology and prevention of breast cancer. Both hypotheses suggest that the risk of breast cancer could be reduced and, thus, occurrence of breast cancer prevented by delaying the onset of regular ovulatory menstrual cycles and by minimizing the therapeutic use of estrogens in postmenopausal women.[15]

Another prospective study was designed to evaluate the risk of endometrial cancer after treatment with estrogens alone or in conjunction with progesterones. In a large cohort study of 23,244 patients observed for 5 to 7 years, some treated with estrogens alone, others with combination of estrogens and progestogens, it was found that the use of estrogens without progestogens is associated with a two- to threefold increase in risk of endometrial neoplasia.[16] Use of progestogens either removes this increased risk, or delays its onset. In a case-control study including 41 women with breast cancer and 119 controls, all premenopausal women revealed that breast cancer was associated with high plasma estradiol and prolactin and with low progesterone. Similar but weaker associations were observed for urinary estrogens and pregnandiol in the luteal phase. Thus, the high risk of breast cancer is associated with changes in endogenous hormones, such as high levels of estradiol and prolactin and low levels of progesterone.

However, most epidemiologic and clinical studies regarding the use of exogenous hormones as either oral contraceptives (OC) or hormone replacement therapy (HRT) and breast cancer risk are conflicting. Some of them showed an increased two- to fourfold risk of breast cancer; others showed little effect or no effect. A large prospective study of exogenous hormone use and breast cancer in Seventh-Day Adventists in California revealed no substantial increase in breast cancer risk associated with the use of oral contraceptives in this population; although among women with exposure to both oral contraceptives and hormone replacement treatment, there was a suggested increase in risk.[17] Also, previous studies of exogenous hormone use, either as OC or as HRT, after the menopause generally have not shown great increases in breast cancer risk associated with exposure to these agents. Other studies of OC use, however, indicate that certain subgroups of women may be at increased risk of breast cancer (those with history of benign breast disease or of maternal breast cancer). Risk of breast cancer is also reduced in women who have had their ovaries removed before menopause, and oophorectomy at an earlier age is associated with lower breast cancer risk.

Experimental investigations showed that a concomitant administration of progesterone and estradiol-17β extinguishes cancer in almost 52% of DMBA-treated rats.[18] The same combination has produced long-lasting beneficial effects in human cancers. Although the antitumorigenic effect of progesterone is known in estrogen-dependent tumors, little is known regarding the role of progesterone in cancer development in non-estrogen-dependent tissues. We studied the chemopreventive effect of progesterone on the development of chemically induced carcinomas (squamous cell carcinomas in mice and basal cell carcinomas in rats) by 3-methylcholanthrene (3-MCA). Progesterone administration decreased the average number, size, and weight of tumors by 45 to 50% compared to those tumors treated with MCA alone, at any time interval. DNA synthesis studied by autoradiography with the use of [³H]-thymidine showed a decrease of DNA synthesis in the cancer cell nuclei following a combined administration of progesterone and MCA (18.4%) compared to the DNA synthesis following administration of MCA alone (35.0%).

Electron microscopic observations revealed salient ultrastructural findings following progesterone administration, with advanced cytolysis, tumefied mitochondria, large populations of secondary lysosomes, and autophagic formations. Cell differentiation tended to be of a glandular-adenomatoid type following progesterone and MCA administration as compared to the characteristic squamous cell and basal cell carcinomas after treatment with MCA alone. Scanning electron microscopic observations revealed advanced cytolytic areas with several disintegrated neoplastic cells and cell debris intermingled with red blood cells, following progesterone and MCA administration. Hence, these experimental observations demonstrate that progesterone in pharmacologic doses exerts significant chemopreventive effects on carcinoma formation, possibly by interfering with MCA metabolism and inhibiting DNA synthesis in the epithelial cancer cells. This is an interesting fact since almost 90% of cancers are of epithelial origin.[19]

3. Danazol

Danazol, an isoxazole derivative of the synthetic steroid, ethisterone, has a complex endocrine pharmacology. Recent studies demonstrate that danazol: (1) prevents the midcycle surge of luteinizing hormone (LH) and follicle-stimulating hormone (FSH); (2) does not significantly suppress basal LH and FSH in gonadally intact human beings; (3) can prevent the compensatory increase in LH and FSH in castrated animals; and (4) does not bind to the estrogen receptor. Hence, danazol is a steroid which has direct effects on hypothalamic function, mulitple classes of steroid receptors, gonadal steroidogenesis, and endogenous steriod metabolism. Oral administration of danazol to hemicastrated female rats prevented the compensatory ovarian hypertrophy that would normally have occurred. Danazol exerts an antitumorigenic activity. Thus, a 66% objective response rate to danazol in the treatment of DMBA-induced mammary carcinomas in rats has been reported.

The results of LHRH stimulation tests in subjects receiving danazol remain controversial. Some authors claim that LHRH administration to subjects receiving danazol results in normal LH and FSH responses; it has been concluded that danazol has important biologic actions at the hypothalamic level, while others have reported that danazol blunts the LH and FSH responses to LHRH.[20] Danazol appears to have little or no effect on the nongonadotropic anterior pituitary hormones and does not change basal levels of thyroid-stimulating hormone (TSH), or prolactin.[20]

Studies regarding the effects of estrogens, progesterone, or no hormone replacement on the growth of peritoneal endometriotic implants in castrated monkeys showed that in a hypoestrogenic, hypoprogestational environment, the endometrial tissue is atrophied. Danazol produces a hypoestrogenic-hypoprogestational state, and thus prevents "reseeding" of the endometrial tissue, and ultimately prevents the evolution of endometriosis. In four large studies, danazol at a dose of 800 mg/d for almost 6 months produced a significant symptomatic improvement (72 to 100%), and also a laparoscopic improvement (85 to 94%).[21] The recurrences were uncommon after completion of treatment and the rates are very low (between 5 and 15% of treated patients per year). These studies suggest that danazol is an effective drug in the treatment and prevention of endometriosis. The recurrence of endometriosis should be ruled out only by laparoscopic examination. Danazol therapy should always be started only during menstruation, at doses of 400 mg and then increase to 800 mg, to be sure that the patient is not pregnant.[21]

4. Luteinizing Hormone-Releasing Hormone (LHRH)

These are a new class of synthetic agonists and antagonists which recently have proven to be an effective means in the treatment and prophylaxis of breast cancer and prostate cancer, and less effective in endometrial and ovarian neoplasms. Since it is well demonstrated that breast cancer is an estrogen-dependent cancer and prostate cancer is an androgen-dependent tumor, it is a good rationale to use these new drugs in human cancer treatment and prevention. Almost one third of patients with breast cancer have a hormone-dependent cancer. Hormone-dependent cancer, when compared to its hormone-independent counterpart, is characterized by its more indolent clinical evolution, better histologic differentiation, less mitotic activity, and a tendency to spread to bone and soft tissues rather than to visceral sites.

From several humoral factors that regulate the growth of human breast cancer, estrogens appear to be the most important. Estrogen acts at the cellular level through its specific receptor. Hormone-receptor interaction subsequently induces the formation of other proteins, including progesterone receptor (PR), and growth factors which act by an autocrine and paracrine mechanism and can influence the growth of the tumor. Thus, the management and prophylaxis of breast cancer is more complex.[22] All endocrine therapies of breast cancer have the main goal of decreasing the estrogen levels, and this can be achieved by different methods, including ablative surgery (oophorectomy), use of antiestrogens (tamoxifen), inhibition of estrogen biosynthesis (aminoglutethimide), or inhibition of LH and FSH (LHRH agonists and antagonists).

From all these strategies, aminoglutethimide is ineffective in premenopausal women. On the other hand, tamoxifen therapy of breast cancer in premenopausal women does lead to tumor regression, but in several instances does not produce a complete "medical castration" since some of premenopausal women still continue to menstruate. Furthermore, tamoxifen can stimulate the pituitary-ovarian axis in young women, and this leads to an increase in the levels of circulating estrogens. Surgery is also invasive, irreversible, and not always feasible. Ideally, the treatment and prevention should be effective, convenient, and not associated with significant side effects. These criteria might be fulfilled by this new class of compounds, namely, the LHRH analogs.[22] The discovery that LHRH analogs could inhibit LH and FSH and so cause suppression of ovarian and testicular function led investigators to study their potential application in the treatment and prevention of hormone-dependent tumors in animals and humans.

Animal studies have revealed that LHRH analogs, e.g., leuprolide, cause a tumor regression rate by 50% in 7,12-dimethylbenz(a)anthracene (DMBA)-induced mammary carcinoma in rats. Similarly, twice daily i.m. injection of Zoladex in rats with the DMBA-induced breast carcinoma produced a high tumor reduction rate comparable to that seen with surgical castration in this model system. Nitrosomethylurea (NMU)-induced breast cancer in rats has also responded to long-term LHRH agonist treatment. Hormonal measurements in these animal studies showed that long-term treatment with LHRH analogs produced an effective "chemical castration" which is the rational basis for tumor regression and prevention. Also, administration of adequate doses to premenopausal women with breast cancer does indeed induce a complete "medical castration". Similar results were achieved in the management and prevention of prostate cancer, and the findings are thoroughly described in Chapter 3.

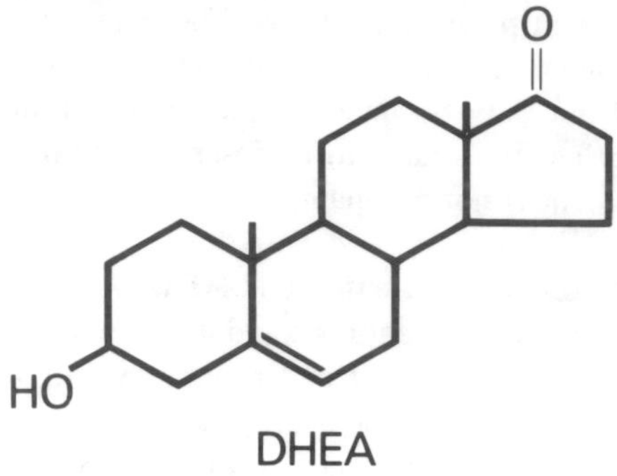

FIGURE 1.   Chemical structure of dehydroepiandrosterone (DHEA).

These exciting early results suggest that we may now have indeed a modality of breast cancer therapy capable of producing a specific, physiologic inhibition of ovarian function, and probably a cancer prophylaxis. Interestingly, carcinoma of the male breast, a rare tumor with an incidence only 1% of that in females, is more responsive to LHRH analogs than to traditional orchiectomy, which is considered an effective palliative measure in 60 to 70% of males with breast cancer. Complete remission of pulmonary metastases have been reported after daily injections of leuprolide or nasal inhalation of buserelin. The effectiveness of LHRH agonists is due to their inhibition of testicular androgens, thereby decreasing their conversion to estrogens. This treatment should be considered as a more acceptable way to induce a medical castration (orchiectomy) and to manage this rare cancer.[22]

5. Dehydroepiandrosterone (DHEA) and Structural Analogs

This is a new class of cancer chemopreventive agents. DHEA was first isolated in 1934 by Butenandt and Tscherning,[23] from human urine, and later it was suggested that DHEA is secreted by the adrenal gland (see Figure 1) since its synthesis increased after adrenocorticotropic hormone (ACTH) administration and decreased after ACTH suppression. DHEA is secreted by the human adrenal gland primarily as the sulfate ester; over 99% of the circulating DHEA in humans is sulfated, with less than 1% representing the free steroid.[24] Recently, it has been demonstrated in laboratory animals (mice and rats) that DHEA exerts cancer preventive effects, and it is possible that DHEA exerts these preventive effects by inhibiting the enzyme, glucose-6-phosphate dehydrogenase (G_6PDH), a major rate-limiting enzyme in the pentose phosphate pathway, and a major source of cytosolic NADPH; this appears to be the central mechanism of the cancer preventive action of DHEA.[25]

Treatment with the steroid also inhibits the rate of metabolism of [³H]-DMBA to water-soluble products by the cultured fibroblasts. Epiandrosterone, a more effective inhibitor of G_6PDH than DHEA, is also more active in inhibiting the rate of metabolism of [³H]-DMBA to water-soluble products. DHEA produces two biologic effects that suggest it might demonstrate cancer preventive activity *in vivo*. The steroid protected cultured cells against chemical carcinogen-induced cytotoxicity and transformation, and DHEA treatment of mice induced a striking antiweight effect, primarily through a reduction in caloric deficiency. Spontaneous, chemically induced, and radiation-induced tumors in many different organs are all reduced in frequency in food-restricted rodents.

The data from several human epidemiologic studies also suggest a positive correlation of high relative body weight and incidence of cancer of the breast, colon, rectum, prostate, endometrium, kidney, cervix, ovary, thyroid, and gallbladder.[26] In contrast, lung, bladder, and stomach cancer appear to be inversely associated with body weight. It was also found that long-term DHEA treatment inhibited the development of spontaneous breast cancer in mice, of DMBA- and urethane-induced lung adenomas in mice, and of 1,2,dimethyl hydrazine (DMH)-incuded colon tumors in BALB/c mice. Also, DHEA administration to F344 rats previously treated with dihydroxy-di-*n*-propyl nitrosamine inhibited the development of thyroid tumors and preneoplastic lung foci.[27] In the two-stage procedure for induction of skin tumors (DMBA initiation and TPA promotion) in mice, it was found that DHEA exerts a direct anticarcinogenic action. In the mouse, either topical application of DHEA to the skin at 100 or 400 μg, or oral administration in the diet at 0.6% for 2 weeks, inhibits the rate of binding of [³H]-DMBA to skin DNA.[25]

DHEA inhibits also DNA synthesis in epidermal cancer cells and abolishes the [³H]-thymidine incorporation following TPA stimulation in epidermal cells. The inhibition of DNA synthesis is likely to be induced by G_6PDH inhibition. Hence, DHEA and related steroids repress DNA synthesis in neoplastic cells by reducing ribonucleotide and deoxy-ribonucleotide synthesis as a result of G_6PDH inhibition; and the administration of these nucleosides will reverse the DHEA-induced inhibition. Therefore, if DHEA exerts its cancer preventive action by decreasing G_6PDH activity, it is anticipated that individuals who are carriers of hereditary G_6PDH deficiency will have a lowered cancer incidence. Studies on cell lines showed that G_6PDH deficiency is a sex-linked hereditary defect occurring with a high frequency in certain populations (Sephardic Jews and Sardinians) and is also common in black populations. It was first proposed that the lowered cancer rates in Israelis of North African or Asian origin, relative to the higher rates in those of Western European or American origin, might be due to the higher frequency of G_6PDH deficiency in the former population. A lower frequency of G_6PDH deficiency was observed in both male (4.5%) and female (0.57%) cancer patients, relative to that in male (9.4%) and female (3.8%) controls. Thus, these studies suggest that G_6PDH deficiency may protect against cancer. However, additional work is needed to establish a causal relationship between the incidence of G_6PDH (glucose-6-phosphate dehydrogenase) and cancer development.

Some investigations showed that the oral treatment of mice and rats with DHEA protects against the development of a broad spectrum of tumors. Although long-term DHEA treatment of mice and rats is without apparent side effects, its conversion into estrone and testosterone and its uterotropic effect can limit the usefulness of DHEA as a cancer chemopreventive agent. Recently, two new synthetic steroids, 16α-fluoro-5-androstan-17-one(8354) and 16α-fluoro-5α-androstan-17-one(8356), which lack the uterotropic and seminal vesicle enlarging effects of DHEA, have shown 15 times greater efficacy than DHEA when given orally in blocking both [³H]-DMBA binding to skin DNA and TPA stimulation in epidermal [³H]-thymidine incorporation. The lack of estrogenic and androgenic activity of these steroids 8354 and 8356, along with their greater potency, suggest that such compounds may find application in chemoprevention of human cancer.[25]

6. Oral Contraceptives (OC) and Hormone Replacement Therapy (HRT): Their Risk for Human Cancer

In recent years, there has been a great controversy over the long-term risks and benefits regarding the use of oral contraceptives (OC) and hormone replacement therapy (HRT), and the incidence of breast cancer, cervical cancer, and liver cancer. The possible relationship of oral contraceptives (OC) and development of cancer is an issue which has profound public health significance. Oral contraceptives are potent drugs which are being taken electively by a large and healthy young population. This has recently stirred a great concern and controversy in the medical journals as well as in the media, regarding the long-term risk of oral contraceptive use, hormonal replacement therapy, and cancer development. However, epidemiologic studies regarding the use of oral contraceptives or hormone replacement therapy for the symptoms of menopause have given conflicting results.[28-35] Some studies showed an overall excess risk,[28-31] whereas others recently have failed to show an increased risk of breast cancer after long-term use.[32-35] Thus, there is still no general consensus among clinicians and researchers concerning their safety or health hazards, mainly neoplasia in the long-term.

Some studies conducted in Great Britain and Sweden showed a great risk, with a significant increase in risk of breast cancer between 2.2 and 17.1 among those ever exposed in parity I compared to controls from the same parity. A strong dose-response effect (duration of use) among users of parity I greatly increases the likelihood that the observation is associated with pill usage.[28,29] Two recent studies in Sweden revealed that early users of OC have larger primary breast tumors than later users and never users, and more often axillary metastases.[29,30] The finding in the Royal College of General Practitioners (RCGP) study of a higher percentage with tumors of greater invasiveness among women aged 35 and younger at diagnosis supports this opinion. Estrogen (ER) and progesterone receptor (PR) content are lower among early users vs. later users, who themselves show lower levels than never users, after adjusting for age and diagnosis. The survival of early OC users is significantly poorer than later users, and survival of never users is in agreement with findings of the RCGP study in women younger than 35 years old.[28]

Other studies also show that all women taking OC before age 36 had a highly significant relative risk of breast cancer with total duration of OC use and relative risks of 1.43 for 49 to 96 months use, and 1.74 for 97 or more months use. The relative risks were similar for use before and after first full-term pregnancy. There is evidence that oral contraceptive pills containing less than 50 µg estrogen have a lower risk associated with their use than higher estrogen dose of OC and that there may be some protective effect of use of progestogen-only pills. Thus, the exposure-response relationship between duration of OC use and risk of breast cancer is dependent on the age at first use of OC. The risk of breast cancer increased with a younger starting age of OC use. Both the duration of OC use before 25 years of age and commencement of OC use before the first full-term pregnancy were associated with an increased risk of breast cancer.[30] The use of OC by young women with a family history of breast cancer increased the breast cancer risk.

Studies in a large cohort group regarding the risk of breast cancer after estrogen and estrogen-progestin replacement, showed that long-term perimenopausal treatment with estrogens (or at least estradiol compounds) seems to be associated with a slightly increased risk of breast cancer, which is not prevented and may even be increased by the addition of progestins.[31] In contrast, other studies conducted on a large group of women aged 25 to 39 years, more than half of whom were using oral contraceptives, found no evidence of any adverse effect of oral contraceptive use on the risk of breast cancer.[32] Thus, the oral contraceptive use by mature women does not increase breast cancer risk. A recent study in Australia, one of the first countries in which oral contraceptive agents became available for use, showed that women aged 20 years to 69 years, who used oral contraceptives, showed no overall relationship between the use of OC and the risk of breast cancer.[33]

Also, studies conducted in women aged 20 to 54 years who used oral contraceptives and had a family history of breast cancer, there was no evidence that use of oral contraceptives, even long-term, contributed to their risk of the disease. Analyses designed to reveal a potential latent effect also showed no evidence of an adverse effect. Hence, detailed analyses of oral contraceptives formulation, the characteristic of the women involved, and the pattern of the risk involved and duration of use suggest that there is no direct evidence between the use of oral contraceptives and the risk of breast cancer, even in women with a family history of breast cancer.[34] A recent study in a cohort of 3303 women, who had benign breast proliferative disease confirmed by biopsy and who took exogenous estrogens as a replacement hormone therapy for menopause, showed that exogenous estrogens are not associated with increased breast cancer risk in women with benign breast disease. There was no significant association between breast cancer risk and birth control pills, cigarette smoking, or alcohol consumption. Thus, a previous history of benign breast disease does not contraindicate replacement estrogen therapy.[35]

Since postmenopausal women and women who have undergone oophorectomy have a higher risk for developing osteoporosis and cardiovascular diseases than premenopausal women of similar ages, hormone replacement therapy is conventionally recommended for preventing these risks. Thus, prolonged hormone replacement therapy (HRT) is being used to prevent, not treat, disease. The beneficial effects of HRT are justified and should be offered to many more women for relief of adverse effects of menopause. Recent studies showed that women who had a natural menopause and did not receive hormone replacement therapy had an abnormal lipid metabolism, with a decline in their serum levels of high-density lipoprotein (HDL) cholesterol and an increase of low-density lipoprotein (LDL) cholesterol, which may contribute to an increase in the risk of coronary disease.[36]

Hormone replacement therapy may prevent some of these changes. HRT is conventionally given as natural estrogens. The addition of a progestin to estrogen is widely recommended for long-term use on the grounds that this combination is necessary to prevent endometrial hyperplasia and uterine cancer. However, the real concern of hormone replacement treatment is the risk of cancer, and data are conflicting on the effects of HRT on breast cancer. Some show that the risk is reduced, whereas other data suggest a slight increase. The concern is real because it may be a long time before the effect is seen clinically. Estrogens are no longer given alone in women with an intact uterus because of the link with endometrial carcinoma. Fortunately this risk is virtually abolished by giving sufficient progestogen cyclically for 10 to 12 d each month.

Studies regarding the risk of breast cancer in postmenopausal women who have used estrogen replacement therapy (ERT) revealed that the risk of breast cancer did not appear to increase appreciably with increasing ERT duration or latency, even for durations and latencies of 20 years or longer. Data are still conflicting. Some studies support the hypothesis that estrogens plus progestin would be more carcinogenic than estrogen alone. They are also compatible with a large population-based case-control study from Denmark, which found sequential therapy with estrogen and progestin to be possibly associated with an increased risk of breast cancer, but no increased risk with estrogen use overall.[37]

In contrast, other studies suggest that an estrogen-progestin regimen reduces the risk of breast cancer. Women who received both estrogen and progestin had a significantly reduced risk of breast cancer as compared with women not receiving hormone treatment. In the only randomized placebo-controlled trial of extended hormone replacement and breast cancer risk, 168 women received a daily placebo or a conjugated estrogen (2.5 mg) and a cyclic medroxyprogesterone (10 mg); after 10 years there was no breast cancer in the women treated with the hormone as compared with a 5% incidence in the women given the placebo.

A recent study analyzed the association between survival in breast cancer and menopausal hormone treatment prior to diagnosis; out of 6,617 estrogen-treated women, 261 developed the disease compared with a control group without estrogen treatment. Both groups were observed for a period of 0 to 9 years. The relative survival rate was significantly higher (by about 10% at 8 years) in patients who had received estrogen treatment corresponding to an approximately 40% reduction in excess mortality. The more favorable course could be confirmed only in patients aged 50 years or more at diagnosis and was most pronounced in recent users. Thus, exogenous female sex hormones affect survival in women with breast cancer. It is possible that several mechanisms might have contributed to the higher survival rate in breast cancer patients with recent exposure to menopausal hormone treatment. It is assumed that female sex hormones interact favorably with the complex process of tumor cell dissemination and establishment of distant metastases even late during the preclinical phase.[38]

A case-control study of male breast cancer in patients aged 20 to 74 years at diagnosis investigated the role of a number of suspected risk factors and showed that the only statistically significant risk factor identified was greater weight of the cases at age 30; a man who weighed 80 or more kg at age 30 had twice the risk of breast cancer of a man weighing less than 60 kg at that age. Serum estrone levels were positively, and sex-hormone-binding globulin levels were negatively, related to body weight, and this suggests that the underlying risk factor is an increased exposure to bioavailable estrogens.[39] Risk of breast cancer is approximately 100 times greater in women than in men. In women, breast cancer does not occur before puberty. Excess endogenous or exogenous estrogens can enhance risk by stimulation proliferation of epithelial cells that have undergone partial malignant transformation. The breast, however, is much less responsive to the tumor-promoting effects of estrogens than the endometrium, and estrogens probably play a less important role in the later stages of mammary than endometrial carcinogenesis. Generally, hormones are not mutagenic and are likely to exert their carcinogenic effect not by causing DNA damage, but by increasing or decreasing the rate of cell proliferation, atrophy, or differentiation of stem or intermediate cells.

Furthermore, premenopausal oophorectomy, without exogenous estrogen replacement therapy, reduces risk; and the degree of prevention is inversely related to the age at which the ovaries are removed. Child-bearing also alters risk: parous women are at lower risk than multiparous women, and the risk in women who had children increases with the age at which their first child was born. Having additional children may also be weakly protective. Hence, probably the risk of breast cancer is mediated through hormonal alterations in mammary cell kinetics.

The possible association between endometrial cancer risk and oral contraceptive (OC) use has been the subject of many investigations, but the results from retrospective as well as prospective studies that have already been published are not consistent. Thus, several case-control and prospective cohort studies have shown an increased risk of noninvasive cervical intraepithelial neoplasia (dysplasia and carcinoma *in situ*) or invasive cervical cancer for long-term pill users.[40,41] However, other studies have noted a decreased risk of endometrial cancer among women who used combination OC.[42-44] Thus, pill associations prevailed for both adenocarcinomas and squamous cell tumors, and risks were highest for those using pills containing high estrogen potencies.

In addition, there was some evidence that pill associations were most pronounced among women who had never used barrier methods of contraception or who had genital infections, suggesting that oral contraceptives may act a cocarcinogens with transmissible agents. Thus, long-term use of OC may have a carcinogenic effect on cervical epithelium. Another study also showed a statistically significant, or borderline significance of invasive cervical cancer, in particular, for long-term use (≥ 7 years) and early onset of use (≤ 24 years) with relative risks of 1.8 and 3.0, respectively.[40] A large cohort study of women aged 44 to 100 years showed that women who had used estrogen replacement therapy had a relative risk of endometrial cancer of 10 compared to women who had never used estrogens. Risk increased with increasing duration of use; thus, women who had used estrogens for 15 or more years had a relative risk of 20 compared to nonusers, while current and recent users (i.e., those who had used estrogens within 1 year) had the greatest risk of 25; women who had last used estrogens 15 or more years ago still had a significantly increased risk of 5.8.

Interestingly, women who smoked at the time of menopause had a significantly reduced risk of endometrial cancer.[41] This study used almost exclusively oral estrogens as conjugated equine preparations. Combination hormone replacement therapy (estrogen plus progestin) was used only in 1% of women. Cigarette smoking is protective against the development of endometrial cancer, and this may be due to an antiestrogenic effect of smoking. Women who smoke have lower urinary excretion rates of endogenous estrogens, and lower serum concentrations of estrogens during estrogen therapy.[42]

In contrast, other studies showed that women who had used a combination of oral contraceptives for at least 12 months had a protective effect which persisted for at least 15 years after the cessation of OC use. Examination of the eight most frequently used OC formulations revealed little difference in the age-adjusted risks, which ranged from 0.2 to 0.7 for women who had ever used a formulation compared with women who had never used OC. Use of OC for 12 months or longer conferred protection against all three major histologic subtypes (adenocarcinoma, adenocanthoma, and adenosquamous cancer) of endometrial cancer. An international epidemiologic study regarding the relationship of combined oral contraceptives to risk of endometrial cancer from a multinational hospital-based case-control of various steroid contraceptives and five different cancers in seven developing countries and two participating centers in two developed countries, showed a protective effect at least as great in the developing countries with low incidence rates as in the developed countries with higher rates. The reduction in risk was observed for adenocarcinomas with and without squamous elements.[43] Also, an international, hospital-based, case-control study regarding the relative risk of liver cancer in women who had ever used combined oral contraceptives and liver cancer showed no evidence that short-term use of oral contraceptives enhances risk of liver cancer in countries where the determinant of this disease are similar to those observed in the countries where this study was conducted (Chile, China, Colombia, Israel, Kenya, Nigeria, Philippines, Thailand, United Kingdom).[44]

A possible relationship between hormone factors (exogenous hormones, such as DES, oral contraceptives) and risk of ovarian germ cell cancer showed an increased risk for ovarian cancer in young women, and a hormonal etiology for germ cell tumors is suspected. Recent evidence also shows that estrogen therapy or endogenous estrogen stimulation may increase the risk of endometrial sarcomas, granulosa cell tumors and thecomas of the ovary, polycystic ovarian disease (Stein-Leventhal syndrome), and stromal hyperthecosis, all of which may be accompanied by continuous exposure of the endometrium to estrogens in the absence of progesteron stimulation, and are associated with a high risk of endometrial carcinomas and endometrial sarcomas.[45]

B. VITAMIN CHEMOPREVENTION OF CANCER

Cancer is the second most common cause of death in the U.S. and appears unlikely to diminish in importance as a cause of morbidity and mortality. Despite a dramatic improvement in treatment of hematologic cancers, there is a great lack of progress among neoplasms of epithelial origin, such as lung, prostate, breast and bladder, cervical, colon, and head and neck cancers, which account for more than 90% of cancer mortality.[46] One promising area of current research in nutrition and cancer relates to the possibility that vitamins and micronutrients may decrease the incidence of epithelial cancers, and thus reduce the cancer risk and ultimately the number of cancer deaths by an order of 10 to 30%, which will be a large number of prevented cancers each year.

Vitamins are essential components of an adequate diet and exert important cellular functions, such as coenzymes, cellular antioxidants, and/or regulators of gene expressions; thus, the integrity of physiologic systems, including cellular repair, detoxification, immune processes, and neural and endocrine function, depends upon the vitamin status of the host. For these reasons, it is anticipated that the vitamin supply to cells and tissues would affect the development and evolution of cancer. Various naturally occurring and synthetic agents cause regression of premalignant or malignant changes *in vivo* or *in vitro*, both in animals and in humans, by inhibiting or preventing the development or progression of cancer.[47] Among promising chemopreventive agents are certain vitamins, including Vitamin A and β-carotenoids, Vitamin E, C, and possible B$_2$ (riboflavin), selenium salts, prostaglandin synthesis inhibitors, and antiproteases. These various agents cause regression of premalignant changes and therefore may prevent the subsequent development of cancer.[48] From 14 vitamins recognized in human nutrition, only Vitamin A, retinoids and β-carotene, Vitamin E, C, and possible B$_2$ play an important role in cancer chemoprevention and prophylaxis. Evidence from laboratory animals as well as from human populations suggest that vitamins can modulate the development and outcome of animal tumors as well as human neoplasms, and thus influence human carcinogenesis.[49-51]

Although the ideal chemoprevention has to start in the premalignant stage for occult malignancy, which may require the reversal of the premalignant state, and has to provide an absolute prevention of malignancy, this is very difficult, if not practically impossible at present. Hence, most chemoprevention clinical trials are started in the late stage of human cancer and mainly suppress or regress the tumor development (chemosuppression), instead of preventing or delaying their initial development and progress, which is the main reason for chemoprevention. A number of specific micronutrients have been suggested as possible late-stage inhibitors of human cancer, including Vitamin A and its synthetic derivatives (retinoids), β-carotenes, Vitamins C and E, and possibly B_2 and selenium.

The role of vitamins in cancer development and therapy are summarized in chapters 1 and 5. Their mechanism(s) at the cellular or molecular level, namely, in cancer cell physiology, are complex and not yet clearly defined. Further investigations are required in order to better understand their role in controlling the premalignant cell populations, their transformation into malignant cells, their pharmacokinetics and toxicity, and in general, their role in cancer cell biology and pharmacology, which are crucial factors for chemoprevention. In human cancer prevention, vitamins have been most effective for cutaneous malignancies, including actinic keratosis, keratoacanthoma, dysplastic nevus syndrome, epidermodysplasia verruciformis, basal cell carcinoma, and possibly squamous cell carcinoma. Also, vitamins have been effective in several noncutaneous precancers and cancers, such as oral leukoplakia, cervical dysplasia, bronchial metaplasia, laryngeal papillomatosis, superficial bladder carcinoma, preleukemia, breast cancer, prostate cancer, colon cancer, lung cancer, esophageal cancer, atrophic gastritis, and endometrial and ovarian cancers as well as head and neck squamous cell carcinoma.[51,52]

1. Vitamin A (Retinol), Retinoids, and β-Carotene

The largest body of evidence regarding retinoids as chemopreventive agents has accumulated for cutaneous lesions. Skin cancers and premalignant dermatologic conditions lend themselves to the study of chemoprevention because it is easy to diagnose them in the early stages (precancer lesions), and these lesions are most likely to respond to therapeutic interventions. Also, retinoids are concentrated in the skin, and thus, systemic administration and topical applications have proven effective.[51] With respect to Vitamin A and retinoids, it has been shown in experimental animals that Vitamin A deficiency leads to an increased susceptibility to cancer formation, due to the occurrence of atypical squamous metaplasia, that may be prevented by normal or moderately increased dietary Vitamin A levels, but without adding high doses of Vitamin A.

Similarly, epidemiologic studies have shown an inverse relation between the frequent consumption of food rich in Vitamin A and/or β-carotene and cancer risk. Thus, maintenance dietary levels of Vitamin A and retinoids protect against early tumor development, and this protective effect is decreased whenever premalignant changes occur. Hence, in the early stages, long-term administration of physiologic levels of Vitamin A or β-carotene against cancer formation is justified, but in the more advanced stages of tumor devleopment, especially in the presence of premalignant lesions, only the pharmacologic doses will be effective.[53]

The most effective chemopreventive action of Vitamin A and retinoids are in dermatologic malignancies (actinic keratosis, keratoacanthoma, basal cell carcinoma, and dysplastic nevi) and nondermatologic malignancies (oral leukoplakia, bronchial metaplasia, cervical dysplasia, preleukemia, and myelodysplastic syndroms [MDS], as well as colon, lung, breast, prostate, endometrial, and ovarian cancers). Some of these preventive effects are described in chapter 5. Since it has recently been shown that many effects of Vitamin A are due to its precursors, carotenoids, β-carotenes, or provitamin A, which are also less toxic than synthetic retinoids, the focus of this chapter will be on the chemopreventive effects of carotenoids and β-carotene.

In contrast to retinoids, about which much is known, the function and the mechanism of action of carotenoids are less clearly understood. The carotenoids, chiefly β-carotene, are found in yellow and green vegetables and fruits. A proportion is converted to retinol in the body (mainly liver) so that ingestion of large amounts of β-carotene could reduce cancer risk in an indirect way by preventing retinoid deficiency. However, some dietary carotenoids are absorbed directly from the intestine without undergoing transformation to retinol; they circulate in the blood and are stored in the adipose tissue, whereas retinoids are under a homeostatic control being regulated by feedback mechanism. Carotenoids exert important antioxidant activities. They have the ability to trap certain organic free radicals and to deactivate excited molecules, particularly excited or singlet oxygen; these molecules are generated as by-products of some normal metabolic processes. Thus, carotenoids may also exert a direct protective effect against carcinogenesis by deactivating these types of molecules, or by preventing damage caused by oxidation.[54]

It is assumed that free radicals may play a role in the etiology of cancer, and carotenoids prevent cancer by the antioxidant mechanism. About 70% of the absorbed carotenoids are converted into retinol and the rest is transported in the lipoprotein fraction of plasma, low-density lipids (LDL), and is taken up by adipose tissue and liver. The plasma level of carotenoids changes in direct relation to diet and is diet dependent; in contrast, the plasma level of retinol is largely diet-independent except in the deficient state. By comparison, retinol is present exclusively in animal products, such as liver, meat, eggs, and milk products, but not in plant-derived foods. After absorption in the small intestine, retinol is transported as retinyl ester in chylomicrons to the liver, where it is stored. From the liver, it is transported to the tissues through the blood, bound to a specific retinol-binding protein (RBP). RBP is a single polypeptide chain with a molecular weight of about 21,000 and has one binding site for one molecule of all-trans retinol. In the blood, RBP circulates as a complex and another serum protein, transthyretin (formerly called prealbumin). Normal levels of RBP in human serum range between 40 and 60 μg/ml. Retinol is released from the liver at essentially constant rates and is hardly influenced by the intake of Vitamin A.[55]

Epidemiologic studies including large number of individuals showed no relationship between RBP levels and cancer incidence.[56] Retinol and the other retinoids have potent, hormone-like effects on cell growth and differentiation of epithelial tissues. The types of epithelial tissues that depend on retinoids to control normal cell growth and differentiation include most of the primary cancer sites, such as the lung, breast, colon, rectum, esophagus, and stomach. Because the development of cancer may be due to disruption of normal cell differentiation, the possibility of using retinoids to prevent cancer was explored shortly after the discovery of Vitamin A.[57] The major drawback to retinoids as possible prophylactic agents against cancer relates to their transport and storage in the body. The human body maintains strict homeostatic control over the amount of retinol that is bound to RBP and passed into circulation, so that blood levels of retinol are unrelated to intake of Vtiamin A. Long-term high intake of retinol, since it is stored in the liver, can lead to hepatotoxicity or other symptoms of hypervitaminosis A. In fact, in the average American diet, more than half of the Vitamin A is derived from β-carotene, the chief form of provitamin A.

Since retinoids and carotenoids behave very differently in the body, they exert their anticancer effects via different mechanisms. These kinetic facts make it difficult to see a role for retinol in dietary influences on carcinogenesis. Hence, retinoids and carotenoids act differently in cancer chemoprevention. Studies regarding the presumed mechanisms as preventive cancer agents show that retinol and the retinoids exert their action on the cell nucleus, involving the expression of genetic information in controlling cell differentiation.[58] Specific binding proteins for retinol and retinoic acid are responsible for the transport of retinol and retinoic acid into the cell, suggesting a hormone-like control of cell proliferation and/or differentiation. In addition, retinol has a variety of effects on the cell membrane, including membrane receptors for various hormones; it antagonizes some known tumor promoters, which suggests a protective role of retinoids in the promotion stage of carcinogenesis. Furthermore, retinol increases both the humoral and the cell-mediated immune responses, which are based on the induction of cytotoxic T-cells by retinol.[58] In contrast, carotenoids exert their chemopreventive effect as antioxidants. β-carotene is a very efficient single-oxygen scavenger and also inhibits the lipid peroxidation induced by free radicals.[54]

a. Experimental Studies in Cultured Cell Lines and Laboratory Animals

These studies have revealed that retinoids have the ability to inhibit the process of malignant transformation induced in cultured cells by different means, including radiation, testosterone, phorbolesters, and other chemical carcinogens.[59] In experimental animals, Vitamin A and retinoid deficiency enhances susceptibility to induce cancers of the oral cavity, lung, bladder, and colon.[49] With repsect to the effect of retinoids on pre-existing malignancies, their administration has been shown to cause regression of tumors induced by either chemical or viruses and to delay the appearance of transplanted tumors. In animal tumor models, both carotenoids and retinoids show cancer preventive effects. Comparative studies on skin tumors in mice induced by UV-B irradiation, by DMBA and croton oil application, or by DMBA and UV-B irradiation, show that carotenoids without Vitamin A activity are most effective in inhibiting UV-B induced tumors while Vitamin A is more active in inhibiting the tumors induced by DMBA and croton oil application.[60] Studies using retinol, β-carotene, and canthaxantin, a carotenoid which cannot be converted into retinol, to prevent genotoxic damage in exfoliated human oral mucosa cells show that retinol and β-carotene strongly reduces the genotoxicity, while canthaxantin has no effect.[61] These studies show that β-carotene exerts its anticancer effects by two different mechanisms: the first, in which conversion into retinol is required, and the second, in which carotenoids without Vitamin A activity exert a protective effect.

b. Epidemiologic Studies

These case-control studies and a few cohort studies, examining the effect of dietary Vitamin A, retinol and/or carotene on several types of cancer (lung, prostate, other sites) show in almost all cases an inverse relation between the intake of carotene and cancer; almost none of the studies shows a relationship with the retinol intake.[62] These studies clearly indicate that β-carotene is much more consistent in exerting the cancer prevention effect, and retinol intake is not associated with cancer prevention. This can be explained by the fact that carotene reaches the peripheral tissues while retinol is largely stored in the liver. Epidemiologic studies also have revealed that the protective effects of Vitamin A or β-carotene have been found most consistently and most strongly in cancers in which squamous cell histologic types predominate, such as oral, esophageal, laryngeal, lung, and cervical cancer.[63] In contrast, the effects of Vitamin A or carotene have been inconsistent for cancer of the stomach, colon, rectum, breast, ovary, or prostate, where adenocarcinoma is the predominant type. Although associations have been observed for breast cancer and cancer of the ovary, they are generally weak and seen only in certain age groups.

Thus, epidemiologic studies show a protective effect of a high intake of β-carotene on cancer, and no effect of retinol. This is due to the fact that a high intake of retinol does not result in a high plasma level since retinol is stored in the liver. In contrast, the intake of carotenoids is reflected in the plasma level of carotenoids and is therefore more likely to exert a cancer preventive effect in peripheral tissues. Hence, knowledge regarding the metabolism of retinol and carotene and results from epidemiologic studies strongly suggest the effect of carotene being most likely responsible for cancer prevention. This leads to the conclusion that a high intake of carotene most likely influences cancer incidence in humans, either via an effect exerted by carotene itself, or after conversion into retinol.[64] The main advantages of β-carotene as a potential cancer chemopreventive agent are related to its metabolism in the body. In contrast to retinol, dietary intake of β-carotene appears to be directly related to blood levels. Furthermore, excess carotene is stored in adipose tissues rather than in the liver so that consumption of even high doses of β-carotene for long periods does not seem to cause toxic symptoms. The major problem in assessing the role that β-carotene may play in cancer chemoprevention relates to the fact that some other component of vegetables, such as dietary fiber, or even lower intake of fat, could be responsible for part of the decreases in cancer risk. Nonetheless, the overall consistency of the findings for all cancer sites of epithelial cell origin show that carotenoids are important agents in cancer chemoprevention. They are also less toxic than retinoids. Since most preventive effects of Vitamin A (retinol) and synthetic retinoids on various premalignant conditions are described in chapter 5, in this chapter we will focus mainly on the protective action of carotenoids and/or some new retinoids on different cancer types, such as cutaneous premalignant and malignant conditions, lung cancer and bronchial metaplasia, head and neck squamous cells carcinoma, cervical dysplasia, and oral carcinoma as well as prostate, bladder, and esophageal cancer.

c. Cutaneous Premalignant and Malignant Diseases

These are the most used diseases in the study of chemoprevention because of their early diagnosis, and they are most likely to respond to therapeutic interventions, such as topical application or systemic administration. Retinoids possess antineoplastic activity in premalignant conditions (actinic keratosis) and cutaneous neoplasms (basal cell and squamous cell carcinomas, keratoacanthoma, mycosis fungoides, and malignant melanoma). In actinic keratosis, due to excessive exposure to ultraviolet light, a complete regression has been documented in about half of the patients treated with topical retinoic acid cream and partial regression has occurred in the remainder. The number of patients having complete regression is increased by oral retinoid therapy, but also the side effects increase. Keratoacanthomas are morphologically similar to squamous cell carcinoma and are capable of progressing to malignancy; these skin tumors completely regress following oral retinoid therapy without the need for maintenance treatment.[51]

Clinical trials using carotene for prevention of basal cell carcinoma of the skin among albino Africans, who are a high risk of dying from skin cancer before the age of 30, are now underway. Thus, Vitamin A (retinol), retinoids, and β-carotene cause regression of premalignant changes, may prevent the subsequent development of cancer, and reduce the risk of skin cancer in certain high-risk patients. Retinoid and carotenoid therapy appear promising for premalignant changes occurring in the skin as well as in other epithelial tissues.

d. Lung Cancer

Lung cancer has been the common cause of cancer deaths among men and is clearly associated with cigarette smoking. It is now recognized that smoking causes bronchial metaplasia, or dysplasia, premalignant conditions that can progress over time to invasive carcinomas. Epidemiologic studies found an inverse association of Vitamin A intake with lung cancer. Subjects having a higher intake of Vitamin A had a lower incidence of lung cancer, regardless of the number of cigarettes smoked. Recently, it has been found that etretinate, an oral retinoid, induces a highly significant decrease with degree of bronchial metaplasia, despite continued cigarette smoking. These findings were confirmed by bronchoscopy and endobronchial biopsy.[65] Also, retinol palmitate was used as preventive treatment in a randomized clinical trial activated in the Milan Cancer Institute in non-small-cell lung cancer, stage Ia. It was found that administration (p.o. 300,000 IU daily) after complete resection could reduce the occurrence of cancer relapses (within 3 years). At the time of the analysis, a total of 42 (23%) from 181 patients had relapsed; 16 (18%) in the treated patients, and 26 (28%) in the nontreated patients (controls). The largest difference between treated patients and controls was observed for bone metastases and brain metastases, and for squamous histology. Only two cases of new primary cancer were detected, both in controls.

Clinical application of retinol palmitate was more effective in lung carcinomas of the squamous type, compared to nonsquamous cell lung cancer. After a median followup of 14 months, only minor side effects were observed, such as skin and mucous membrane desquamation and dryness, headache, hair loss, itching, or dyspepsia, but at much lower frequency. Thus, high doses of oral retinol palmitate in emulsion was well tolerated with limited subjective and objective toxicity. The results, although preliminary, are promising for both tolerance and efficacy of treatment.[66]

Previous studies showed that increased consumption of green and yellow vegetables reduces the risk of cancer, especially lung cancer among cigarette smokers. The reduction in risk has generally been attributed to a greater intake of total carotenoids or β-carotene.[62,63,65,66] Also, a number of studies have reported that blood levels of β-carotene or total carotenoids are lower in cancer cases, again especially lung cancer, than in controls.[50,67] Retinol, retinol-binding protein (RBP), and Vitamin E are less consistently related to cancer risk. The possible protective effect of high dietary intake of retinoids and β-carotene for cancer also has been described in animal experimental and tissue culture studies.[51,68] In a recent multiple risk factor intervention trial (MRFIT) the relationship was evaluated between carotenoids and cancer in 156 initially healthy men, who subsequently died of cancer, and 311 controls individually matched for age, smoking status, randomization group, and clinical center. Both total carotenoids and β-carotene levels were lower in the 66 lung cancer cases than in their matched controls.

For all cancer deaths combined, there were no significant differences in total carotenoids or β-carotene between cases and controls. The relationship between lower serum carotenoid levels and lung cancer persisted after adjusting for the number of cigarettes, alcohol intake, and serum thiocyanate levels and cholesterol levels in the blood. Serum levels of retinol, α-tocopherol, and retinol-binding protein (RBP) were not related to any cancer site. These results provide further evidence for a possible protective effect of β-carotene against lung cancer among cigarette smokers.[63]

Other studies also reported an inverse relationship between serum β-carotene and subsequent lung cancer, such as in the prospective Basel study.[50] However, they did not report the relationship between the level of β-carotene and the time to development of lung cancer in the followup. In the BUPA study, significantly lower mean levels of β-carotene in serum specimens of men diagnosed with lung cancer (15.8 μg/dl for cancer cases vs. 20.3 μg/dl for controls) have been reported.[67] A significantly lower β-carotene level among 74 lung cancers in men of Japanese ancestry in Hawaii than in the controls (20 μg/dl in the cases as compared with 29 μg/dl for controls) has also been reported.[69] In conclusion, all these case-control studies based on stored serum specimens have indicated an inverse relationship between serum carotenoid levels and subsequent lung cancer. Thus, from these similar recent studies it has been concluded that there is a possible link between lung cancer and β-carotene, other carotenoids, and other nutrients found in green or yellow vegetables, and these are highly recommended in the diet by the National Cancer Institute.[70] It is possible that β-carotene dietary supplements are effective only in individuals at high risk for lung cancer who have low blood levels or low intake of carotenoids. It is also possible that the putative lung cancer protective effects of β-carotene are due to other micronutrients in green or yellow vegetables that are highly correlated with β-carotene.

e. Head and Neck Squamous Cell Carcinoma (HNSCC)

HNSCC includes cancers of the skin, salivary, and thyroid glands, as well as cancers of mucous membranes of the upper air and food passages, and accounts for 5% of all tumors, affecting approximately 42,000 persons in this country. Leukoplakia and erythroplasia of the oral mucous membranes are the premalignant lesions. Risk of malignant transformation is greatest in erythroplasia, intermediate in erythroleukoplakia, and lowest in leukoplakia. Thus, premalignant head and neck lesions present a unique opportunity for an investigation of the role of chemoprevention and the use of retinoids. Furthermore, patients with squamous cell carcinoma of the head and neck region are at increased risk for developing a second primary cancer, due to the existence of multiple premalignant lesions, a phenomenon called field cancerization.[71] Many patients, varying from 10% of patients with laryngeal cancer to 40% of patients with oropharyngeal cancer, will develop a secondary primary tumor.

Thus, patients with an early-stage cancer of the head and neck are another group likely to benefit from chemoprevention. The effective treatment of HNSCC patients should include not only the therapy of the first detected tumor, but also the prevention of the development of additional tumors from premalignant lesions. Vitamin A analogs (retinoids) might be useful for therapy and prevention of HNSCC. Retinoids have been found to inhibit the development of oral cancer in experimental animals and to suppress premalignant lesions (e.g., leukoplakia) in humans. They have also been found to exhibit a number of unique effects on the development, differentiation, and growth of normal and malignant epithelial cells as well as to augment host antitumor immune responses.[72]

There are several clinical studies in premalignant lesions of the head and neck, all reporting good response with retinoids in oral leukoplakia.[51,53] Treatment consisted of 6-month trial of a placebo, β-carotene, β-carotene plus Vitamin A, and Vitamin A alone for chemoprevention in Indian betel quid chewers having oral leukoplakia. A complete response was observed in 59% of patients with oral leukoplakia and treated with Vitamin A (200,000 IU/week), followed by patients treated with β-carotene (180 mg/week) and Vitamin A (100,000 IU/week) with complete response in 27%, then β-carotene alone (180 mg/week) having 14.8% complete response, and placebo only with 3%.[53] These promising results were recently confirmed in a randomized clinical trial, in which patients with oral leukoplakia were randomly selected to receive oral 13-cis-retinoic acid (CRA), brand name Accutane, at a daily dose of 1 to 2 mg/kg or placebo for 3 months. Complete or partial response occurred in 67% of patients receiving CRA compared with only 10% of patients receiving placebo.[73]

Although these results are highly significant, lesions relapsed and progressed once retinoid therapy was halted. It is possible that combined trials with CRA and β-carotene (provitamin A that has less toxicity than CRA) should be initiated in order to maintain these improvements. Reversal of dysplasia was also observed in 61% of the 13-cis-retinoic acid group vs. 16% in the placebo group. Metaplastic lesions in the lungs of heavy smokers were also reversed by retinoids. Aggressive laryngeal papillomatosis also showed response to 13-cis-retinoic acid with some complete response, and disappearance of papillomas were reported.[74] When used as a single agent 13-cis-retinoic acid caused partial response (50 to 70% decrease in tumor mass) in several patients with advanced squamous cell carcinoma of the nasopharynx or the epiglottis. The mechanism of retinoid action is probably mediated via modulation of the proliferation and differentiation of premalignant and malignant cells. Indeed, cytokinetic and ultrastructual changes that accompany this reversal indicated that retinoids, such as β-all-trans retinoic acid, inhibit basal cell proliferation, stimulate mucous cell proliferation, and redirect differentiation into mucous and ciliated cells, instead of into squamous cells, thereby restoring normal epithelial morphology.

f. Prostate Cancer

A positive relationship between prostatic cancer risk and the intake of Vitamin A and carotenoids was found in some case-control studies. An increased risk for prostatic cancer is somewhat associated with increasing intake of Vitamin A and is consistent with most of studies, which were all based on Vitamin A intake estimated from food consumption data.[75] One study suggests that particularly carotene intake is positively related with risk. Thus, Vitamin A and total carotenes were assessed in a large number of cases with prostate cancer in Hawaii, and it was found that in men <70 years of age, there were no significant associations with risk for prostate cancer. In the elderly men, over 70 years, however, risk increased directly with the amount of Vitamin A consumed. The findings were similar for the various components of Vitamin A, but were somewhat stronger for total carotenes than for total retinol. These results were generally consistent across the five ethnic groups and were not affected by statistical adjustment for dietary fat.[76] A protective effect of β-carotene in men consuming little fat was also found. More conclusive results were found *in vitro* studies regarding the effects of Vitamin A on carcinogen-induced effects in rodent prostate.[75] Treatment of mouse ventral prostate explant cultures with chemical carcinogens, such as benzo(a)pyrene, 3-methylcholanthrene, and the direct-acting agent N-methyl-N^1-nitro-N-nitrosoguanidine produced hyperplastic, squamous metaplastic and dysplastic changes in the prostatic epithelium. Vitamin A counteracts these effects when it is added to the medium with carcinogens, and it reverses these effects when it is administered to the explants after carcinogen exposure.

Both all-*trans*-retinol and β-retinoic acid, which are naturally occurring retinoids, have this protective effect, retinoic acid being more potent. Thus, in mouse ventral prostatic explants, Vitamin A inhibits the induction of morphological changes by chemical carcinogens, and it reverses these changes once they are induced. Most of the data from case-control studies discussed earlier suggest a positive relation between Vitamin A/β-carotene intake and human prostatic cancer risk, but there are conflicting data from some case-control studies. Furthermore, data from *in vitro* studies would support a protective role of Vitamin A. Therefore, a definitive conclusion as to whether Vitamin A and/or β-carotene intake is positively related with prostatic cancer risk is not yet possible. There seems, however, to be a certain pattern to the results of specific group studies. Thus, Vitamin A and/or carotenes may play a role in the genesis of prostatic cancer that develops at older age (70 years and over), but not when the disease develops earlier in life. A positive relationship between prostatic cancer risk was found in case-control studies only for older cases, and only when intake of Vitamin A and carotenes was estimated from food consumption data. Finally, if rather accurate measures of intake are used, Vitamin A and carotenes are positively associated with prostatic cancer risk, whereas if less reliable measures are used, there seems to be no association or a negative relation.

Vitamin A is generally suspected to be an anticarcinogen agent on the basis of both its activity in various cancer models and its cellular and biochemical actions, and carotenes are similarly regarded as anticarcinogens. Vitamin A is required for normal differentiation of prostatic glandular epithelium, as Vitamin A deficiency leads to prostatic squamous metaplasia. In addition, there are retinol and retinoic acid-binding proteins in the human prostate, and this suggests that Vitamin A can directly affect the prostate gland. The fact that there are great differences among young and old people with regard to the etiopathogenesis and risk of prostatic cancer, suggests there are two types of prostatic cancer which primarily differ in their etiology rather than in their clinical behavior or morphology. This "two-disease" hypothesis may explain why dietary association, i.e., Vitamin A and/or β-carotenes, is found only for the older patients (>70 years), and not for younger (<70 years). Also, endocrine changes are more frequent and different between younger and older patients, particularly plasma levels of testosterone and 5α-dihydro-testosterone are lower in older groups. Thus, environmental factors (hormones, vitamins) are related to prostatic cancer risk. They are likely to act as enhancers of progression of prostatic cancer, but they are not causative factors. Prevention may be particularly effective for prostatic cancer, and changes in diet, hormones, and vitamins may result in an absolute decrease in mortality and morbidity.[75]

g. Urinary Bladder Tumors

A dose-response decrease in risk with increases in the use of β-carotene was observed for male and female bladder cancer risk in 59 patients with bladder cancer. Retinoids have demonstrated varying degrees of antitumor and chemopreventive activity in superficial bladder tumors.[51]

Experimental studies showed a strong chemopreventive effect of retinoids in urinary bladder cancer induced in the rodents by the chemical carcinogen MNU and OH-BBN. Early work using the MNU and OH-BBN bladder cancer models focused on the inhibitory effects of 13-*cis*-retinoic acid. From a large number of retinoids, the synthetic *n*-alkyl amide derivatives of retinoic acid possess a greater acitivty to toxicity ratio than that seen with 13-*cis*-retinoic acid. Thus, changes of the basic retinoid structure can have a significant effect on anticancer activity. Addition of an ethylamide or a hydroxyethylamide group to all-*trans*-retinoic acid results in compounds which are highly effective chemopreventive agents for mammary carcinoma, while the onset of retinoid administration can be delayed after 1 week and retain its activity in inhibition of urinary bladder carcinogenesis. These studies demonstrate a retention of cancer inhibitory activity when retinoid administration is delayed and are particularly important for clinical use of retinoids in cancer prevention. Comparative studies showed a different target organ specificity for retinoids in cancer chemoprevention; thus, 13-*cis*-retinoic acid is most effective in urinary bladder cancer, whereas TMMP ethyl retinoate is more active in skin DMBA carcinogenesis, and retinyl acetate in NMU and DMBA mammary carcinogenesis.[77] It is apparent that a variety of retinoids possess anticancer activity in experimental models for urinary bladder cancer and breast cancer, and that minor modifications of the retinoid molecule can have striking effects in cancer chemoprevention.

h. Breast Cancer

Breast cancer is also sensitive to retinoids and hormone chemoprevention. Experimental studies show that retinyl acetate is extremely active in the NMU or DMBA mammary-induced carcinomas. Retinyl acetate and *N*-(4-hydroxypheryl) retinamide (4-HPR) are highly effective in reducing mammary cancer incidence and increasing the latency of induced mammary cancers. While retinyl acetate and 4-HPR are both effective inhibitors of chemical mammary rat carcinogenesis, their metabolism and organ distribution are quite different. Chronic dietary administration of high doses of retinyl acetate results in the accumulation of retinyl esters in the liver, a process frequently associated with significant hepatotoxicity, while administration of 4-HPR results in an accumulation in the mammary gland. Thus, it appears that 4-HPR is preferable to retinyl acetate for prevention of experimental breast cancer. Interestingly, the combination of hormones and retinoids enhances significantly cancer inhibition and prevention. Hence, the combination of ovariectomy plus 4-HPR is significantly more effective in cancer chemoprevention than is either treatment alone. Incidence of mammary tumors in the intact placebo group was 94%, as compared to 15% in the ovariectomized and retinyl acetate-treated group. Rates of tumor appearance in the single treated retinyl acetate or ovariectomy groups were intermediate between the intact placebo and ovariectomy-retinyl acetate group.[78] A similar synergistic inhibition was demonstrated in NMU-induced mammary carcinogenesis by concomitant administration of retinyl acetate and 2-bromo-α-ergocryptine (an inhibitory of pituitary prolactin secretion). Hence, "combination chemoprevention" between retinoids and hormones shows promise and practical implications for prevention of human cancer. Also, a combination between retinoids and cytostatics is possible.

Some toxic effects of retinoids may be prevented by inhibitors of prostaglandin synthesis such as aspirin; 4-hydroxyphenyl retinamide is also a potent inhibitor of prostaglandin synthesis. The mechanism(s) by which retinoids inhibit mammary carcinogenesis is presently unclear. It is likely that hormones are involved in the mediation of retinoid action at the molecular level. Some hormones influence the regulation of cytosolic retinoic acid-binding protein concentration in the mammary gland during differentiation. Both retinyl acetate and 4-HPR significantly inhibit terminal ductal hyperplasia, a precancerous lesion, and hyperplastic alveolar nodulogenesis by approximately 50%. They also inhibit DNA synthesis in mammary gland.[79] Fenretinide (4-HPR) may exert chemoprevention of contralateral human breast cancer.

Two recent prospective studies on human breast cancer showed that plasma Vitamin A (retinol) and its circulatory transport proteins, retinol-binding protein (RBP) and prealbumin, were measured in nine postoperative female breast cancer patients, and it was found that the values of Vitamin A, RBP, and prealbumin were all very low in patients who subsequently had cancer recurrence.[80] In an eight-year prospective study on breast cancer, serum samples were analyzed for Vitamins A and E and for retinol-binding protein (RBP); a significant correlation between increasing age and Vitamin A and RBP concentrations was observed. There was also a trend for increased blood concentrations of Vitamin E with age, but this was not significant. Only serum RBP and Vitamin A concentrations were highly correlated.[81]

i. Cervical Dysplasia and Cervical Cancer

It has been shown that cervical intraepithelial neoplasia progresses to microinvasive and invasive cervical cancer, in some cases, over several years. Women who are at risk of developing cervical dysplasia and cancer may be readily identified and monitored using cytology, colposcopy, and colposcopic biopsy; these premalignant cervical lesions provide an opportunity for chemoprevention in inhibiting or mitigating their evolution toward neoplasia. Previous studies have demonstrated that women with severe dysplasia or carcinoma *in situ* (CIS) of the cervix had significantly lower dietary intake of Vitamin A and β-carotene.

In a recent study the mean plasma β-carotene levels were significantly reduced in all women with cervical dysplasias, as well as in patients with cancer, compared to those in the control group. Statistical analyses of variances (ANOVA) demonstrated highly significant differences between the four study populations, and there was an inverse association between plasma levels of β-carotene and severity of dysplasia. The lowest mean plasma β-carotene value (7.4 μg/dl) was detected in patients with cancer. In contrast, all patients in different groups (controls, cervical dysplasia, CIS, and invasive cancer) had normal plasma retinol levels (63 μg/dl), with no difference between groups. Thus, β-carotene deficiency, independent of retinol, constitutes a risk factor for the development of cervix neoplasia.[82] Preliminary studies using tretinoin topical application by sponges and cervical caps with retinyl acetate have demonstrated good response rates with minimal systemic toxicity. Topical β-all-*trans* retinoic acid vs. placebo cream has also been used. Topical vaginal administration of retinyl acetate gel has also recently been used in chemoprevention of cervix cancer.[83]

j. Oral Carcinoma

Oral carcinoma experimentally induced in hamsters by dimethylbenzanthracene was successfully prevented by pretreatment with Vitamin A, or Vitamins A and E. It has previously been demonstrated in an oral carcinogenesis model that cotreatment with Vitamin A or E delayed tumor development. The mechanism of this prevention is early truncation of the ornithine decarboxylase response to dimethylbenzanthracene. Although Vitamins A and E alone stimulate ornithine decarboxylase, and this effect is additive with dimethylbenzanthracene, Vitamin A inhibits the late-phase ornithine decarboxylase response to dimethylbenzanthracene in all animals. It is well known that topical administration of dimethylbenzanthracene to the tongue or cheek pouch of the hamsters induced squamous cell carcinomas in 100% of the animals in 10 to 14 weeks. Coadministration of Vitamins A or E with DMBA significantly inhibits tumor development.

The most likely molecular mechanism of chemoprevention for Vitamin A is a direct inhibition of ornithine decarboxylase on mRNA formation and polyamine biosynthesis, although Vitamin A may also affect tumorigenesis by its effect on chromatin structure or on transglutaminase induction.[84] Oral administration of retinoids confers a beneficial effect on oral leukoplasia and a number of other precancerous conditions. In addition, a recent trial of supplements containing both retinol and β-carotene showed a threefold decrease in chromosome breakage in oral mucosal cells of Filipino betel nut and tobacco chewers. Testing separately retinol and carotene, the same reduction in chromosome breakage was found for each agent.[61] Hence, Vitamins A and E have a role in prevention, and it is possible that treatment of premalignant lesions may decrease the rate of malignant transformation.

k. Esophageal and Gastric Cancer

Esophageal and gastric cancer were found in a case-control study of black men in Washington, D.C. to have a higher risk among those with the lowest Vitamin A intake.[85] Also, patients who developed breast, gastrointestinal, lung, and skin cancer had lower plasma Vitamin A levels as compared to controls. In the prospective Basel study, β-carotene was significantly lower in lung cancer cases, followed by gastric cancer cases. Vitamin A was below average only in cases with gastric cancer, and the vitamin was consistently lower in cancer cases than in controls; the lowest value was found for cancer of the stomach, due to a below average consumption. Vitamin E was low in cancer of the colon. Plasma lipids were correlated strongly with Vitamin E and to a lesser extent with Vitamin A, whereas β-carotene is correlated poorly with β-lipoproteins, but significantly with total cholesterol. Thus, vitamins influence carcinogenesis in humans.[50]

2. Vitamin B₂ (Riboflavin)

A recent study regarding the role of Vitamin B_2 (riboflavin) in cancer prevention on a population in China with a high incidence of esophageal cancer, showed that a combined treatment with retinol, riboflavin, and zinc had no significant effect on prevalence of esophagitis, which is a precancerous lesion for esophageal cancer. It seems that riboflavin and retinol may not induce regression of the esophagitis due to the presence of other factors, but may prevent the induction of precancerous lesions (esophageal dysplasia, atrophic gastritis). This study, however, does not rule out the epidemiologic evidence for an involvement of vitamin deficiencies in the development of esophageal cancer.[52]

3. Vitamin C (Ascorbic Acid)

Some studies noticed a high incidence of stomach cancer when examining cancer reports in Colombia, South America resulting from harsh diets, which may have predisposed the stomach to nitrosamine-induced cancer. Atrophic gastritis and intestinal metaplasia were directly associated with corn ingestion and inversely with ingestion of lettuce which contains Vitamin C. A study regarding atrophic gastritis and Vitamin C status in two British towns with different stomach cancer death rates revealed that the prevalence of severe atrophic gastritis was significantly higher in the high-risk town than in the low-risk town. Plasma ascorbate concentration and fruit intake were lower in the high-risk area and lower social classes, suggesting a poorer Vitamin C status. However, no direct relationship between Vitamin C and severe atrophic gastritis was found.[86] This suggests that risk of stomach cancer is determined in two stages — a long-term effect, in which atrophic gastritis is produced, and a short-term effect, in which Vitamin C is protective. A significant negative association between Vitamin C intake and the risk of colon cancer was recently found. However, no significant association between intake levels of dietary fiber, vitamins, or food groups and rectal cancer risk was found.[87]

A randomized trial of Vitamin C and E in the prevention of recurrence of colorectal polyps, presumed precursors for colorectal cancer, showed only a small reduction in the rate of polyp recurrence associated with Vitamins C and E supplementation. Thus, consumption of fruits, natural sources of Vitamin C, might be associated with reduced cancer risk.[88] A recent hospital-based case-control study of lung cancer conducted in a high-risk region of Louisiana, regarding dietary intake of carotene, retinol, and Vitamin C, showed an inverse association between level of carotene intake and lung cancer risk, and this protective effect was specific for squamous and small cell carcinoma. A stronger protective effect for these tumors was associated with dietary Vitamin C intake. A significant inverse gradient in risk with retinol intake was limited to adenocarcinoma and more pronounced among blacks.[89] No conclusive evidence regarding the dietary intake of Vitamin C and prostate cancer risk has been found, although there are some conflicitng data.[75] In tissue culture, Vitamin C increases the survival of ovarian cell tumors that are exposed to radiation and reverses malignant changes in hamster lung cells that are induced by tobacco or marijuana smoke.

Many possible mechanisms for a preventive effect of Vitamin C in either human or animals have been proposed; these include maintenance of the integrity of the intercellular matrix, enhancement of immune mechanisms, promotion of tumor encapsulation, and formation of an antioxidative effect. Vitamin C blocks the conversion of nitrates to carcinogens, and this inhibition of carcinogen formation may be especially important with respect to gastric cancer.

4. Vitamin E (α-Tocopherol)

Vitamin E (α-tocopherol) and the risk of cancer has been the subject of many but conflicting experimental and epidemiologic studies. Like Vitamin C, Vitamin E received popular attention as a possible inhibitor of cancer. However, relevant epidemiologic data are limited. Although an inhibitory effect has been seen in a small number of experimental animals, such an effect has not been observed consistently. Since Vitamin E is an important intracellular antioxidant, is a free radical scavenger, and reduces mutations in some bacterial testing systems, it could be a potential inhibitor of carcinogenesis. The protective effect of Vitamin E might vary by type of cancer, which may account for the apparent contradictions. In a recent study regarding the serum Vitamin E level and risk of female cancers (cervix, uterus, breast, endometrium, and ovary), an inverse relation was observed between α-tocopherol level and risk of cancer. A low level of α-tocopherol, in general, strongly predicted epithelial cancers, but only slightly predicted elevated risk of cancers in reproductive organs exposed to estrogens. These results suggest that a low Vitamin E intake is a risk factor for cancer in many, but not all organs. The expression of Vitamin E protective effect may depend on the primary causes, which vary between different cancers.

The incidence of hormone related cancers is not associated with the serum α-tocopherol level.[90] Also previous findings show no association between α-tocopherol and prostate cancer, and suggest that hormonal exposure in some instances overrides the possible protective effect of Vitamin E. Dietary fat intake may influence the risk of breast cancer and possible of ovarian cancer. It has been suggested that obesity potentiates the conversion of plasma androstenedione to estrone, which then acts as a promoter for cancer.[91] Therefore, a low serum α-tocopherol level can predict the development of cancer in women. Its predictive capacity is rather strong for epithelial cancers, but weak or absent for hormone-related cancers. An association between serum Vitamin E and subsequent risk of cancer was found statistically significant for lung, colon and rectum, stomach, bladder, central nervous system, and skin, only in the first year from the date of blood collection; in these cases it was significantly lower than in matched controls. For subjects whose cancers were diagnosed one or more years after blood collection, the difference was not statistically significant. It is possible that the low Vitamin E levels were a metabolic consequence, rather than a precursor of cancer and subsequently can explain the overall inverse association between serum Vitamin E and risk of cancer observed in epidemiologic studies.[92]

A 10-year longitudinal epidemiologic study carried out in Finland established a strong inverse relationship between serum Vitamin E and risk of cancer. The strongest inverse association was observed for cancers of stomach, pancreas, and urinary tract organs, and for all cancers unrelated to smoking. Also, the strongest association between α-tocopherol and cancer risk was observed in the youngest groups, and to a lesser degree among people of age 70 or more. These findings support the hypothesis that high Vitamin E intake prevents cancer.[93] Interestingly, Vitamin B_{12} malabsorption was found to be a common finding in patients with AIDS and may be a very early manifestation of infection with human immunodeficiency virus Type I (HIV-I), and may be used for early detection of AIDS patients.[94]

II. COMMENTS AND CONCLUSIONS

There are several kinds of evidence supporting the belief that many, if not most, human cancers are avoidable or preventable, if their causes are detected and eliminated in the early stages of carcinogenesis, consequently altering the risk of developing the malignancy. Epidemiologists estimate that 75% of all cancer deaths in the U.S. potentially can be avoided by the elimination or minimization of cancer risk factors. Also, in the later stage, prevention can be achieved by inhibiting, retarding, or even reversing the premalignant or precancerous lesions and their transformation into malignant lesions or neoplasms. Chemoprevention of human cancers, which means prevention of cancer by the use of pharmacologic agents, such as hormones and vitamins, to inhibit, mitigate, or reverse the carcinogenic process, represents a promising new field for clinical oncology. Recent evidence regarding intrinsic mechanism(s) of human carcinogenesis suggests that there are several agents potentially able to interfere with the various steps of the carcinogenic process. Although there is no conclusive evidence that hormones and vitamins are etiologic or causative factors of cancer development, there is ample evidence that hormones and vitamins as well as their analogs, retinoids and carotenoids, are significant factors in promotion and modulation of several experimental and human cancers, and subsequently they exert important effects in cancer chemoprevention and prophylaxis. They can act alone, or in combination, having synergistic or additive effects, so-called combination prevention. Since hormones and vitamins are less toxic and have only minor side effects, they can be used on a large scale in various chemoprevention trials.

Thus, chemoprevention of cancer will become an ideal method or tool in preventing development of malignant disease, instead of treating cancer by chemosuppression in the late stage, and will dominate the cancer investigations for the next decade. Several epidemiologic studies revealed great differences in cancer incidence and distribution for individuals living in different geographical areas, mainly due to environmental or metabolic factors, such as dietary, hormone, or vitamin intakes; thus, a new epidemiology, called "metabolic epidemiology" will emerge in the coming years, and hormones and vitamins can be considered the forerunners of chemopreventive agents against cancer. The development of more sensitive tumor markers in order to detect the early stages and to select and monitor the high-risk candidates for chemoprevention trials will be a very important task for oncologists. Unfortunately, most of these chemoprevention trials are conducted in patients with frank cancer, when it is too late for prevention; it is also an expensive and time-consuming process, from a practical point of view. More research is needed for a better understanding of the action of hormones and vitamins at cellular and molecular levels, in order to develop a rational basis for cancer prevention.

Antiestrogens, triphenylethylene compounds, such as tamoxifen and toremifene, have recently been shown to exert a strong chemosensitizing activity, particularly toremifene and its metabolites. Both toremifene and tamoxifen possess activity to sensitize the breast cancer cells to cytostatic drugs, especially doxorubicin, *in vitro*. Thus, they can reverse the phenomenon of multidrug resistance (MDR), which is associated with overexpression of a membrane protein (P-glycoprotein). This new tricyclic compound, toremifene, is an important antiestrogen in reversing MDR, a phenomenon which, in several cases, hampers the effectiveness of chemotherapeutic drugs. The mechanism of reversing MDR does not appear to be related to its antiestrogenic effect. Since this new hormone antagonist has a long half-life (5 to 6 d), so that high concentrations can be maintained after a single daily oral dose, this new agent may be uniquely suited for use as a clinical modulator of tumor drug resistance in combination with other cytotoxic compounds in humans.[95] In addition to hormones and their antagonists or agonists, vitamins and their synthetic derivatives in combination with cytotoxic drugs may enhance their antitumor activity and reduce their toxic effects, thus playing an important role in combination chemoprevention.

Danazol, a synthetic gonadotropin inhibitor, has been shown to exert significant chemopreventive and chemosuppressive effects on DMBA-induced mammary carcinomas in rats. Danazol therapy has resulted in 66% tumor regression and in 36% tumor disappearance, when administered after the tumor reached 0.5 cm in diameter. Also, danazol exerted a striking inhibition and prevention of mammary carcinogenesis; only 14% from 50 rats developed palpable mammary carcinomas when danazol was concomitantly administered with DMBA. Danazol, by inhibiting endogenous FSH and LH, suppresses ovarian function and induces anovulation and amenorrhea in women and several mammalian species. Hence, danazol may offer a safe and reversible "medical oophorectomy", which is more advantageous and acceptable for patients with metastatic estrogen-sensitive breast cancer.[96]

To date, many LHRH agonists and, lately, antagonists with marked and prolonged antitumor activity have been synthesized and tested; all have induced a "partial hypophysectomy" and clinical castration and consequently will play an important role in chemosuppression and chemoprevention of prostate cancer. Treatment with supraphysiologic doses of LHRH agonists causes pituitary exhaustion and desensitization, inhibition of prolactin secretion, and down-regulation of gonadal gonadotropin receptors with decreased steroidogenesis.[22] The presence of androgen and estrogen receptors in cancer prostatic cells, both in cytosol and nuclear fractions, has been established. Also more recently, specific LHRH receptors in interstitial cells and experimental prostatic tumors have been found, which suggest a direct antitumor effect on prostatic neoplastic cells. Thus, LHRH agonists and antagonists play an important role in treatment and prevention of prostatic cancer.[97] Thus, *in vitro* (cultured cancer cell lines) and various animal tumor studies have revealed that hormones and vitamins exert significant antitumor activity and can prevent the occurrence and development of animal tumors or regress their evolution (skin, prostate, breast, oral, bladder, esophageal, lung, pancreas, endometrial, ovarian, leukemia, thyroid, and central nervous system cancers).[4,11,19,49] Also, recent epidemiologic trials have revealed an overall inverse relation between vitamin (A, β-carotene, retinoids, C, and E) and various types of human cancers (skin, lung, pancreatic, esophageal and gastric, oral, and colorectal cancers, as well as cervical dysplasia and bladder neoplasms), indicating that vitamins influence human carcinogenesis and are potential chemopreventive cancer agents.[50,52,53,89,90]

Interestingly, it seems likely that some vitamins are more protective against a particular type of cancer, such as Vitamin A (retinol) and β-carotene with lung cancer, Vitamin C with gastric, esophageal, and pancreatic cancers, Vitamin E with colon and female reproductive cancers.[50,64,98] A stronger protective effect was found with regard to histologic types of cancer; thus, dietary β-carotene prevents more specifically squamous and small cell carcinoma, whereas retinol is more protective against adenocarcinoma of the lung.[64,89] Endogenous hormonal profiles are also related to an increased risk of hormone-dependent cancers. For instance, an increased breast cancer risk can be associated with adrenal androgen deficiency, ovarian dysfunction, increased 16α-hydroxylation of estradiol, and decreased risk with pregnancy-induced lowering of prolactin levels. Adrenal androgen deficiency seems to be pertinent only in premenopausal cancer patients, whereas ovarian dysfunction seems to be pertinent to both premenopausal and postmenopausal patients and may have a genetic component. Also, increased estradiol hydroxylation seems to have a genetic component. The prolactin effect, however, is clearly environmental rather than genetic and may represent a permissive effect rather than a true risk-promoting effect, Hence, hormonal abnormalities may increase or decrease the cancer risk in some types of cancer.[99]

The exact mechanism(s) by which hormones and vitamins exert their preventive or prophylactic action against cancer is not clearly defined. However, there are several possible mechanisms by which hormones and vitamins can prevent or retard the cancer development, and subsequently decrease the cancer risk. They may inhibit or prevent the transformation of premalignant cells into cancer cells, and subsequently prevent the transformation of premalignant or precancer lesions into malignant lesions or neoplasms. Both hormones and vitamins play an important role in controlling the precancer cell populations and consequently control the homeostatic mechanism of cancer cells. They also may: inhibit the transformation of procarcinogens or dietary carcinogens into ultimate or active carcinogens; inhibit DNA synthesis in premalignant and malignant cells; exert antioxidation effects and also act as free-radical scavengers; maintain the integrity of cell membranes; exert direct cytostatic and/ or cytotoxic effects on cancer cells; control cell differentiation and division; influence host-immune mechanism(s) and act as immunosuppressors or immunoaugmentators; stimulate collagen synthesis, and subsequently increase tumor encapsulation; inhibit metastases; and act as cocarcinogens.

The combination of vitamins and hormones will reduce the toxic effects of conventional radiation and chemotherapy, and consequently enhance their preventive and therapeutic efficacy. This combination chemoprevention will be an important tool in cancer prophylaxis. Also, combination of Vitamin E with selenium will increase their radioprotective and chemopreventive effects. Selenium acts as a true protector by enhancing the capacity of the cell to cope with oxidant stress, while Vitamin E acts as a chain-breaking antioxidant inhibiting the lipid peroxidation and the formation of malonaldehyde, a compound with oncogenic potential. The metabolic functions of Vitamin E and selenium are inter-related, and selenium plays a role in the storage of Vitamin E. Vitamin E action is also related to that of Vitamin C, which appears to increase its antioxidant effect. Vitamin C acts in synergisitic fashion with Vitamin E to inhibit radiogenic transformation.[100]

In addition to synergistic effects of hormones and vitamins in cancer chemoprevention, there is also a relationship between hormones and growth factors, and they may play an important role in the carcinogenic process (chapter 4). Thus, hormones and growth factors, particularly TGF-β, exert important effects in colon cancer by affecting cell proliferation. The therapeutic manipulation of the transforming growth factors, hormones, and vitamins will be useful in the treatment and prevention of cancer.[101] The interplay of hormones, vitamins, and growth factors may enhance or inhibit the cancer development and are critical factors in the induction and prevention of multistage carcinogenesis. Ultimately, they may act by influencing the genome, particularly the oncogene expression, mutations, gene amplification, and DNA transformation, and subsequently cancer chemoprevention may take place at the molecular level. Thus, hormones, vitamins, and growth factors may influence oncogene expression. Hence, the potential for chemoprevention will increase dramatically when specific markers of precancer lesions become detectable by the techniques of molecular biology. Thus, it will be possible to identify high-risk groups and by molecular approaches to modify carcinogenic risk. It has been shown that retinoids and carotenoids have the ability to reverse the progress of preinvasive or even invasive lesions, such as carcinoma *in situ* (CIS) of the cervix, oral leukoplakia, bronchial metaplasia in smokers, and actinic keratoses, and to prevent skin cancer in xeroderma pigmentosum. The effects of retinoids and carotenoids in preneoplastic myeloproliferative lesions and healthy individuals were demonstrated in the administration of a daily 25,000 IU dose of retinol for 9 months in 13 healthy subjects, in which no changes occurred in circulating retinol levels, liver function, cholesterol, bilirubin, or other blood and urine elements. The 25,000 IU or retinol was, therefore, well tolerated, at a chemopreventive level to normal subjects.[102] Also, studies regarding the safety of β-carotene in healthy individuals who take β-carotene for years and for treatment of inherited photosensitivity diseases for more than 15 years at dosages of 180 mg/d or more, showed no adverse effects other than hypercarotinemia. An inverse association of the incidence of prostate cancer with β-carotene intake was observed. Toxicity studies in animals have shown that β-carotene is not carcinogenic, mutagenic, embryotoxic, or teratogenic and does not cause hypervitaminosis A. At present, there are almost 2500 retinoids and over 500 known carotenoids, but only 50 carotenoids have provitamin A activity; β-carotene is the carotenoid with the greatest provitamin A biologic activity.[103] However, other carotenoids, such as α-carotene and γ-carotene found in higher plants in lower amounts, showed even a stronger anticancer activity than β-carotene (in some cancer cell lines); they also should be studied as possible chemopreventive agents.

Randomized clinical trials suggest that tamoxifen reduces the incidence of initial breast cancer in selected high-risk populations and also reduces the incidence of second breast cancer (the new primary cancer).[104] The development of new and more accurate tumor markers for early stages and for measurement of metastatic potential by using monoclonal antibodies (MoAb) against the new proteins as expressed oncogenes will be very helpful in early chemoprevention of cancer. Proto-oncogenes, oncogenes, and tumor suppressor genes, will be important tools for epidemiologic studies and may offer an integrated understanding of cancer treatment and prevention.[105] Although cancer chemoprevention is still an experimental procedure, the use of hormones and vitamins as prophylactic agents will allow us to carry out chemopreventive trials on a a large scale. It has been recently suggested that antiestrogens (tamoxifen) will be a promising chemopreventive drug of breast cancer, since the estrogenic hormones are mainly the promoters of initiated breast cells.[106] This promotional stage is reversible, and the antiestrogens can limit or reverse the promoting estrogenic effect on initiated breast cell populations. The development of new synthetic hormones and vitamin analogs, more effective and less toxic, will be the ideal chemopreventive agents against epithelial cancer, which represent almost 90% of all neoplasms; this will open an exciting field of research and a new strategy for a scientific chemoprevention of cancer. This scientific cancer prevention requires multidisciplinary, broadly based research ranging from molecular biology, cell biology, immunology and genetics to epidemiology. This prevention will be more accurate and will develop more scientific methods to target the high risk groups.

REFERENCES

1. **Wattenberg, L. W.,** Chemoprevention of cancer, *Cancer Res.,* 45, 1, 1985.
2. **Bailar, J. C. and Smith, E. M.,** Progress against cancer?, *N. Engl. J. Med.,* 314, 1226, 1986.
3. **Becker, N., Smith, E. M., and Wahrendorf, J.,** Time trends in cancer mortality in the Federal Republic of Germany: progress against cancer?, *Int. J. Cancer,* 43, 245, 1989.
4. **Lathrop, A. and Loeb, L.,** Further investigations on the origin of tumors in mice. III. On the part played by internal secretion in the spontaneous development of tumors, *J. Cancer Res.,* 1, 1, 1916.

5. **Tomatis, L.,** Environmental cancer risk factors, *Acta Oncol.,* 27, 465, 1988.

6. **Berg, J.,** Can nutrition explain the pattern of international epidemiology of hormone dependent cancers?, *Cancer Res.,* 35, 3345, 1975.

7. **Bertram, J. S., Kolonel, L. N., and Meyskens, F. L.,** Rationale and strategies for chemoprevention of cancer in humans, *Cancer Res.,* 47, 3012, 1987.

8. **Jordan, V. C.,** Chemosuppression of breast cancer with tamoxifen: laboratory evidence and future clinical investigations, *Cancer Invest.,* 6, 589, 1988.

9. **Miller, A. B. and Bulbrook, R. D.,** The epidemiology and etiology of breast cancer, *N. Engl. J. Med.,* 303, 1246, 1980.

10. **Cuzick, J., Wang, D. Y., and Bulbrook, R. D.,** The prevention of breast cancer, *Lancet,* 1, 83, 1986.

11. **Fentiman, I. S.,** The endocrine prevention of breast cancer, *Br. J. Cancer,* 60, 12, 1989.

12. **Tormey, D. C.,** Tamoxifen: transition from the laboratory to clinical preventive chemosuppression, *Cancer Invest.,* 6, 597, 1988.

13. **Powles, T. J., Hardy, J. R., Ashley, S. E., Farrington, G. M., Cosgrove, D., Davey, J. B., Dowsett, M., McKinna, J. A., Nash, A. G., Sinnett, H. D., Tillyer, C. R., and Treleaven, J. G.,** A pilot trial to evaluate the acute toxicity and feasibility of tamoxifen for prevention of breast cancer, *Br. J. Cancer,* 60, 126, 1989.

14. **Pike, M. C., Ross, R. K., Lobo, R.A., Key, T. J., Potts, M., and Henderson, B. E.,** LHRH agonists and the prevention of breast and ovarian cancer, *Br. J. Cancer,* 60, 142, 1989.

15. **Key, T. J. and Pike, M. C.,** The role of oestrogens and progestagens in the epidemiology and prevention of breast cancer, *Eur. J. Cancer Clin. Oncol.,* 24, 29, 1988.

16. **Persson, I., Adami, H. O., Bergkvist, L., Lindgren, A., Pettersson, B., Hoover, R., and Schairer, C.,** Risk of endometrial cancer after treatment with oestrogens alone or in conjunction with progestogens: results of a prospective study, *Br. Med. J.,* 298, 147, 1989.

17. **Mills, P. K., Beeson, W. L., Phillips, R. L., and Fraser, G. E.,** Prospective study of exogenous hormone use and breast cancer in Seventh-Day Adventists, *Cancer,* 64, 591, 1989.

18. **Huggins, C., Moon, R., and Morii, S.,** Extinction of experimental mammary cancer. I. Estradiol-17β and progesterone, *Proc. Natl. Acad. Sci. U.S.A.,* 48, 379, 1962.

19. **Lupulescu, A.,** Chemoprotective effect of progesterone on carcinomas formation in mice and rats, *J. Natl. Cancer Inst.,* 74, 499, 1985.

20. **Asch, R. H., Fernandez, E. O., Smith, C. G., Siler-Khodr, T. M., and Pauerstein, C. J.,** Effects of danazol on gonadotropin levels in castrated rhesus monkeys, *Obstet. Gynecol.,* 53, 415, 1979.

21. **Donaldson, V.,** Danazol, *Am. J. Med.,* 87, 49N, 1989.

22. **Harvey, H. A.,** Luteinizing hormone-releasing hormone agonists in the treatment of breast cancer, in *Endocrine Therapies in Breast and Prostate Cancer,* Osborne, C. K., Ed., Kluwer, Boston, 1988, 39.

23. **Butenandt, A. and Tscherning, K.,** Über Androsteron, ein krystallisiertes männliches sexual Hormon. I. Isolierung und Reindarstellung aus Männerharn, *Hoppe-Seyler's Z. Physiol. Chem.,* 229, 167, 1934.

24. **Baulieu, E.-E., Corpéchot, C., Dray, F., Emiliozzi, R., Lebeau, M.-C., Mauvais-Jarvis, P., and Robel, P.,** An adrenal-secreted "androgen:" dehydroisoandrosterone sulfate. Its metabolism and a tentative generalization on the metabolism of other steroid conjugates in man, *Rec. Prog. Horm. Res.,* 21, 411, 1965.

25. **Schwartz, A. G., Whitcomb, J. M., Nyce, J. W., Lewbart, M. L., and Pashko, L. L.,** Dehydroepiandrosterone and structural analogs: a new class of cancer chemopreventive agents, *Adv. Cancer Res.,* 51, 391, 1988.

26. **Albanes, D.,** Caloric intake, body weight, and cancer: a review, *Nutr. Cancer,* 9, 199, 1987.

27. **Moore, M. A., Thamavit, W., Tsuda, H., Sato, K., Ichihara, A., and Ito, N.,** Modifying influence of dehydroepiandrosterone on the development of dihydroxy-di-n-propylnitrosamine initiated lesions in the thyroid, lung and liver of F344 rats, *Carcinogenesis,* 7, 311, 1986.

28. **Kay, C. R. and Hannaford, P. C.,** Breast cancer and the pill — a further report from the Royal College of General Practitioners' oral contraception study, *Br. J. Cancer,* 58, 675, 1988.

29. **Olsson, H. and Ranstam, J.,** Breast cancer and the pill, *Br. J. Cancer,* 59, 834, 1989.

30. **Olsson, H., Möller, T. R., and Ranstam, J.,** Early oral contraceptive use and breast cancer among premenopausal women: final report from a study in Southern Sweden, *J. Natl. Cancer Inst.,* 81, 1000, 1989.

31. **Bergkvist, L., Adami, H.-O., Persson, I., Hoover, R., and Schairer, C.,** The risk of breast cancer after estrogen and estrogen-progestin replacement, *N. Engl. J. Med.,* 321, 293, 1989.

32. **Vessey, M. P., McPherson, K., Villard-MacKintosh, L., and Yeates, D.,** Oral contraceptives and breast cancer: latest findings in a large cohort study, *Br. J. Cancer,* 59, 613, 1989.

33. **Rohan, T. E. and McMichael, A. J.,** Oral contraceptive agents and breast cancer: a population-based case-control study, *Med. J. Aust.,* 149, 520, 1988.

34. **Murray, P. P., Stadel, B. V., and Schlesselman, J. J.,** Oral contraceptive use in women with a family history of breast cancer, *Obstet. Gynecol.,* 73, 977, 1989.

35. **Dupont, W. D., Page, D. L., Rogers, L. W., and Parl, F. F.**, Influence of exogenous estrogens, proliferative breast disease, and other variables on breast cancer risk, *Cancer*, 63, 948, 1989.
36. **Matthews, K. A., Meilahn, E., Kuller, L. H., Kelsey, S. F., Caggiula, A. W., and Wing, R. R.**, Menopause and risk factors for coronary heart disease, *N. Engl. J. Med.*, 321, 641, 1989.
37. **Ewertz, M.**, Influence of non-contraceptive exogenous and endogenous sex hormones on breast cancer risk in Denmark, *Int. J. Cancer*, 42, 832, 1988.
38. **Bergkvist, L., Adami, H.-O., Persson, I., Bergström, R., and Krusemo, U. B.**, Prognosis after breast cancer diagnosis in women exposed to estrogen and estrogen-progestogen replacement therapy, *Am. J. Epidemiol.*, 130, 221, 1989.
39. **Casagrande, J. T., Hanisch, R., Pike, M. C., Ross, R. K., Brown, J. B., and Henderson, B. E.**, A case-control study of male breast cancer, *Cancer Res.*, 48, 1326, 1988.
40. **Ebeling, K., Nischan, P., and Schindler, C.**, Use of oral contraceptives and risk of invasive cervical cancer in previously screened women, *Int. J. Cancer*, 39, 427, 1987.
41. **Paganini-Hill, A., Ross, R. K., and Henderson, B. E.**, Endometrial cancer and patterns of use of oestrogen replacement therapy: a cohort study, *Br. J. Cancer*, 59, 445, 1989.
42. **MacMahon, B., Trichopoulos, D., Cole, P., and Brown, J.**, Cigarette smoking and urinary estrogens, *N. Engl. J. Med.*, 307, 1062, 1982.
43. The WHO collaboratorive study of neoplasia and steroid contraceptives: endometrial cancer and combined oral contraceptives, *Int. J. Epidemiol.*, 17, 263, 1988.
44. The WHO collaborative study of neoplasia and steroid contraceptives: combined oral contraceptives and liver cancer, *Int. J. Cancer*, 43, 254, 1989.
45. **Press, M. F. and Scully, R. E.**, Endometrial "sarcomas" complicating ovarian thecoma, polycystic ovarian disease and estrogen therapy, *Gynecol. Oncol.*, 21, 135, 1985.
46. **Silverberg, E., Boring, C., and Squires, T.**, Cancer statistics, 1990, *CA*, 40, 9, 1990.
47. **DeCosse, J. J.**, Potential for chemoprevention, *Cancer*, 50 (Suppl. 11), 2250, 1982.
48. **Lupulescu, A.**, Control of epithelial precancer cell transformation into cancer cells by vitamins, *J. Cell Biol.*, 103, 29, 1986.
49. **Moon, R. C., McCormick, D. L., and Mehta, R. G.**, Chemoprevention of animal tumors by retinoids, in *Modulation and Mediation of Cancer by Vitamins*, Meyskens, F. L. and Prasad, K. N., Eds., S. Karger, Basel, 1983, 47.
50. **Stähelin, H. B., Rösel, F., Buess, E., and Brubacher, G.**, Cancer, vitamins, and plasma lipids: prospective Basel study, *J. Natl. Cancer Inst.*, 73, 1463, 1984.
51. **Lippman, S. M. and Meyskens, F. L.**, Vitamin A derivatives in the prevention and treatment of human cancer, *J. Am. Coll. Nutr.*, 7, 269, 1988.
52. **Muñoz, N., Wahrendorf, J., Bang, L. J., Crespi, M., and Grassi, A.**, Vitamin intervention on pre-cancerous lesions of the esophagus in a high risk population in China, *Ann. N.Y. Acad. Sci.*, 534, 618, 1988.
53. **Band, P. R.**, Vitamin A prevention trials in Canada, *Cancer Invest.*, 6, 637, 1988.
54. **Burton, G. W. and Ingold, K. U.**, β-carotene: an unusual type of lipid antioxidant, *Science*, 224, 569, 1984.
55. **Blaner, W. S.**, Retinol-binding protein: the serum transport protein for Vitamin A, *Endocrine Rev.*, 10, 308, 1989.
56. **Willett, W. C., Stampfer, M. J., Underwood, B. A., Sampson, L. A., Hennekens, C. H., Wallingford, J. C., Cooper, L., Hsieh, C., and Speizer, F. E.**, Vitamin A supplementation and plasma retinol levels: a randomized trial among women, *J. Natl. Cancer Inst.*, 73, 1445, 1984.
57. **Fujimaki, Y.**, Formation of gastric carcinoma in albino rats fed on deficient diets, *J. Cancer Res.*, 10, 469, 1926.
58. **Wolf, G.**, Multiple functions of Vitamin A, *Physiol. Rev.*, 64, 873, 1984.
59. **Chopra, D. P. and Wilkoff, L. J.**, Effect of retinoids and estrogens on testosterone-induced hyperplasia of mouse prostate explants in organ culture, *Proc. Soc. Exp. Biol. Med.*, 162, 229, 1979.
60. **Mathews-Roth, M. M.**, Carotenoid pigment administration and delay in development of UV-B-induced tumors, *Photochem. Photobiol.*, 37, 509, 1983.
61. **Stich, H. F., Stich, W., Rosin, M. P., and Vallejera, M. O.**, Use of the micronucleus test to monitor the effect of Vitamin A, beta-carotene and canthaxanthin on the buccal mucosa of betel nut/tobacco chewers, *Int. J. Cancer*, 34, 745, 1984.
62. **Paganini-Hill, A., Chao, A., Ross, R. K., and Henderson, B. E.**, Vitamin A, β-carotene and the risk of cancer: a prospective study, *J. Natl. Cancer Inst.*, 79, 443, 1987.
63. **Connett, J. E., Kuller, L. H., Kjelsberg, M. O., Polk, B. F., Collins, G., Rider, A., and Hulley, S. B.**, Relationship between carotenoids and cancer: the multiple risk factor intervention trial (MRFIT) study, *Cancer*, 64, 126, 1989.
64. **DeVet, H. C.**, The puzzling role of Vitamin A in cancer prevention (review), *Anticancer Res.*, 9, 145, 1989.

65. **Misset, J. L., Santelli, G., Homasson, J. P., Gaget, H., Mathé, G., Gouveia, J., and Sudre, M. C.**, Regression of bronchial epidermoid metaplasia in heavy smokers with etretinate treatment, *Cancer Detect. Prev.*, 9, 167, 1986.

66. **Pastorino, U., Soresi, E., Clerici, M., Chiesa, G., Belloni, P. A., Ongari, M., Valente, M., and Ravasi, G.**, Lung cancer chemoprevention with retinol palmitate, *Acta Oncol.*, 27, 773, 1988.

67. **Wald, N., Thompson, S. G., Densem, J. W., Boreham, J., and Bailey, A.**, Serum beta-carotene and subsequent risk of cancer; results from the BUPA study, *Br. J. Cancer*, 57, 428, 1988.

68. **Suda, D., Schwartz, J., and Shklar, G.**, Inhibition of experimental oral carcinogenesis by topical beta-carotene, *Carcinogenesis*, 7, 711, 1986.

69. **Nomura, A. M., Stemmermann, G. N., Heilbrun, L. K., Salkeld, R. M., and Vuilleumier, J. P.**, Serum vitamin levels and the risk of cancer of specific sites in men of Japanese ancestry in Hawaii, *Cancer Res.*, 45, 2369, 1985.

70. National Cancer Institute, Diet, Nutrition and Cancer Program: Status Report, NIH publication no. 85-2710, National Institutes of Health, National Cancer Institute, Bethesda, MD, 1984.

71. **Slaughter, D. P., Southwick, H. W., and Smejkal, W.**, Field cancerization in oral stratified squamous epithelium: Clinical implications of multicentric origin, *Cancer*, 6, 963, 1953.

72. **Lotan, R. L., Kim, J. S., Maaroui, M., Schantz, S. P., and Hong, W. K.**, Vitamin A, retinoids, and the prevention and treatment of head and neck cancer, *Cancer Bull*, 39, 93, 1987.

73. **Hong, W. K., Endicott, J., Itri, L. M., Doos, W., Batsakis, J. G., Bell, R., Fofonoff, S., Byers, R., Atkinson, E. N., Vaughan, C., Toth, B. B., Kramer, A., Dimery, I. W., Skipper, P., and Strong, S.**, 13-*cis*-retinoic acid in the treatment of oral leukoplakia, *N. Engl. J. Med.*, 315, 1501, 1986.

74. **Alberts, D. S., Coulthard, S. W., and Meyskens, F. L.**, Regression of aggressive laryngeal papillomatosis with 13-*cis*-retinoic acid (Accutane), *J. Biol. Response Mod.*, 5, 124, 1986.

75. **Bosland, M. C.**, The etiopathogenesis of prostatic cancer, *Adv. Cancer Res.*, 51, 1, 1988.

76. **Kolonel, L. N., Hankin, J. H., and Yoshizawa, C. N.**, Vitamin A and prostate cancer in elderly men: enhancement of risk, *Cancer Res.*, 47, 2982, 1987.

77. **Sporn, M. B., Squire, R. A., Brown, C. C., Smith, J. M., Wenk, M. I., and Springer, S.**, 13-*cis*-retinoic acid: inhibition of bladder carcinogenesis in the rat, *Science*, 195, 487, 1977.

78. **McCormick, D. L., Mehta, R. G., Thompson, C. A., Dinger, N., Caldwell, J. A., and Moon, R. C.**, Enhanced inhibition of mammary carcinogenesis by combined treatment with *N*-(4-hydroxyphenyl) retinamide and ovariectomy, *Cancer Res.*, 42, 508, 1982.

79. **McCormick, D. L., Burns, F. J., and Albert, R. E.**, Inhibition of benzo(a)pyrene-induced mammary carcinogenesis by retinyl acetate, *J. Natl. Cancer Inst.*, 66, 559, 1981.

80. **Basu, T. K. and Sasmal, P.**, Plasma Vitamin A, retinol-binding protein, and prealbumin in postoperative breast cancer patients, *Int. J. Vit. Nutr. Res.*, 58, 281, 1988.

81. **Russell, M. J., Thomas, B. S., and Bulbrook, R. D.**, A prospective study of the relationship between serum vitamins A and E and risk of breast cancer, *Br. J. Cancer*, 57, 213, 1988.

82. **Palan, P. R., Romney, S. L., Mikhail, M. Basu, J., and Vermund, S. H.**, Decreased plasma β-carotene levels in women with uterine cervical dysplasias and cancer, *J. Natl. Cancer Inst.*, 80, 454, 1988.

83. **Romney, S. L., Dwyer, A., Slagle, S., Duttagupta, C., Palan, P. R., Basu, Y., Calderin, S., and Kadish, A.**, Chemoprevention of cervix cancer: Phase I-II: a feasibility study involving the topical vaginal administration of retinyl acetate gel, *Gynecol. Oncol.*, 20, 109, 1985.

84. **Calhoun, K. H., Stanley, D., Stiernberg, C. M., and Ahmed, A. E.**, Vitamins A and E do protect against oral carcinoma, *Arch. Otolaryngol. Head Neck Surg.*, 115, 484, 1989.

85. **Ziegler, R. G., Morris, L. E., Blot, W. J., Pottern, L. M., Hoover, R., and Fraumeni, J. F.**, Esophageal cancer among black men in Washington, D.C. II. Role of nutrition, *J. Natl. Cancer Inst.*, 67, 1199, 1981.

86. **Burr, M. L., Samloff, I. M., Bates, C. J., and Holliday, R. M.**, Atrophic gastritis and Vitamin C status in two towns with different stomach cancer death-rates, *Br. J. Cancer*, 56, 163, 1987.

87. **Heilbrun, L. K., Nomura, A., Hankin, J. H., and Stemmermann, G. N.**, Diet and colorectal cancer with special reference to fiber intake, *Int. J. Cancer*, 44, 1, 1989.

88. **McKeown-Eyssen, G., Holloway, C., Jazmaji, V., Bright-See, E., Dion, P., and Bruce, W. R.**, A randomized trial of vitamins C and E in the prevention of recurrence of colorectal polyps, *Cancer Res.*, 48, 4701, 1988.

89. **Fontham, E. T., Pickle, L. W., Haenszel, W., Correa, P., Lin, Y., and Falk, R.**, Dietary vitamins A and C and lung cancer risk in Louisiana, *Cancer*, 62, 2267, 1988.

90. **Knekt, P.**, Serum vitamin E level and risk of female cancers, *Int. J. Epidemiol.*, 17, 281, 1988.

91. **Lipsett, M. B.**, Hormones, nutrition, and cancer, *Cancer Res.*, 35, 3359, 1975.

92. **Wald, N. J., Thompson, S. G., Densem, J. W., Boreham, J., and Bailey, A.**, Serum vitamin E and subsequent risk of cancer, *Br. J. Cancer*, 56, 69, 1987.

93. Serum vitamin E and risk of cancer in Finland, *Nutr. Rev.*, 46, 342, 1988.

94. **Harriman, G. R., Smith, P. D., McDonald, K. H., Fox, C. H., Koenig, S., Lack, E. E., Lane, H. C., and Fauci, A. S.**, Vitamin B$_{12}$ malabsorption in patients with acquired immunodeficiency syndrome, *Arch. Intern. Med.*, 149, 2039, 1989.

95. **DeGregorio, M. W., Ford, J. M., Benz, C. C., and Wiebe, V. J.,** Toremifene: pharmacologic and pharmacokinetic basis of reversing multidrug resistance, *J. Clin. Oncol.,* 7, 1359, 1989.

96. **Peters, T. G., Lewis, D. J., Wilkinson, E. J., and Fuhrman, T. M.,** Danazol therapy in hormone-sensitive mammary carcinoma, *Cancer,* 40, 2797, 1977.

97. **Bollack, C., and Rougeron, G.,** Hormonal therapy trials in prostatic cancer, *Am. J. Clin. Oncol.,* 11 (Suppl. 2), S156, 1988.

98. **Falk, R. T., Pickle, L. W., Fontham, E., Correa, P., and Fraumeni, J.,** Lifestyle risk factors for pancreatic cancer in Louisiana: a case-control study, *Am. J. Epidemiol.,* 128, 324, 1988.

99. **Zumoff, B.,** Hormonal profiles in women with breast cancer, *Anticancer Res.,* 8, 627, 1988.

100. **Borek, C.,** Oncogenes, hormones, and free-radical processes in malignant transformation *in vitro, Ann. N.Y. Acad. Sci.,* 551, 95, 1988.

101. **Conteas, C. N., Desai, T. K., and Arlow, F. A.,** Relationship of hormones and growth factors to colon cancer, *Gastroenterol. Clin. North Am.,* 17, 761, 1988.

102. **Alberts, D. S., McDonald, L., Edwards, L., Peng, Y. M., Xu, M. J., Slymen, D. J., Earnest, D. L., and Ritenbaugh, C.,** Pharmacokinetics and metabolism of retinol administered at a chemopreventive level to normal subjects, *Cancer Det. Prevent.,* 13, 55, 1988.

103. **Bendich, A.,** The safety of β-carotene, *Nutr. Cancer,* 11, 207, 1988.

104. **Fornander, T., Cedermark, B., Mattsson, A., Skoog, L., Aspergren, J., Rutqvist, L., Somell, A., and Hjalmar, M. E.,** Adjuvant tamoxifen in early breast cancer: occurrence of new primary cancers, *Lancet,* 1, 117, 1989.

105. **Yarbro, J. W.,** The new biology of cancer: future clinical applications, *Semin. Oncol.,* 16, 254, 1989.

106. **Love, R. R.,** Prospects for antiestrogen chemoprevention of breast cancer, *J. Natl. Cancer Inst.,* 82, 18, 1990.

Chapter 8

DIET, HORMONES, VITAMINS, AND CANCER

I. SURVEY OF RECENT DATA REGARDING DIET AND CARCINOGENESIS

In recent years, a growing body of evidence, from epidemiologic studies as well as from laboratory animals, suggests a strong relationship between dietary constituents (vitamins, hormones, minerals, and fiber) and the incidence of cancer. By increasing or decreasing these dietary components, or so-called diet manipulation, it is possible to significantly influence cancer risk and development.[1-3] Hence, diet by its components, hormones, vitamins, and minerals, plays an important role in human carcinogenesis, and has received much attention in recent years. Epidemiologic studies estimate that approximately 90% of cancers in the U.S. are of environmental origin, and about 35% (10 to 70%) of all cancers are caused by components of the diet; consequently, the great majority of cancers are avoidable or can be prevented.[4] If correct, this estimate would make diet second only to cigarette smoking as a determinant factor of cancer. However, while natural or additive substances in diet may be carcinogenic, nutritional deficiencies or excesses may promote carcinogenesis. The human diet contains a great variety of natural carcinogens and mutagens, as well as many natural anticarcinogens and antimutagens.[5] Many substances that are potent carcinogens in experimental animals are known to exist in nature and occur as part of the human diet. In addition, many of the substances that are known to inhibit experimental carcinogenesis also exist in the human diet. Thus, in addition to industrially produced carcinogens, there are diets that contain both carcinogens and anticarcinogens.

Although investigators have known for many years that tumor incidence in animals can be affected by nutritional manipulation, the possibility that diet has important causative and protective roles in human carcinogenesis has received major attention only recently. To date, the most important dietary factors associated with cancer causation include fat, alcohol, and nitrates, whereas favorable dietary factors include certain vitamins (A, C, and E, retinoids, carotenoids), certain minerals (selenium and zinc), and fiber. Although natural or added substances in food may be carcinogenic, the quantity and quality of a diet may also render an individual more susceptible to the carcinogen.[6] For instance, unbalanced metabolism resulting from dietary deficiency (few meals daily, alcoholism) or excess (high total dietary fat, obesity, carbohydrates) may promote carcinogenesis. Since diet is a mixture of factors, such as vitamins, fiber, micronutrients, and some hormone-like substances, it is difficult to know which is the causative or preventive factor. The challenge for researchers and epidemiologists addressing the relation between diet and cancer is to identify the specific dietary determinants of cancer and to quantify their effects.

Many nutrients may modify the activity of enzymes, hormones, and vitamins by influencing their biosynthesis and metabolism and by detoxifying or inactivating procarcinogens or cocarcinogens, thus leading to a decrease in carcinogenesis; or they may directly inhibit carcinogen-binding to critical cellular macromolecules. Also, dietary factors may play a role, either by inhibiting the DNA-repair system (carcinogen-induced DNA damage), or possibly by dietary xenobiotics (foreign compounds of no nutritional value found in plants), which may be important in inhibiting carcinogen-induced neoplasms in humans. Some inhibitors of experimentally and human-induced tumors in the human diet include: Vitamin A, retinoids, β-carotenoids, Vitamin C, Vitamin E, indoles, coumarins, flavones, phenols, plant sterols, aromatic isothiocyanates, selenium, and zinc.[7,8] Examples of xenobiotics in edible plants include eugenol, gamma-bisabolene, umbelliferone, limonene, and benzyl isothiocyanate. Their presence induces the body's detoxification mechanisms to excrete any ingested carcinogens. In addition, the reactive forms of carcinogens can potentially be detoxified by binding or "trapping" by cellular nucleophilic molecules, such as methionine, cystine, and glutathione. Some compounds can also inhibit the actions of carcinogens when administered after the carcinogen, such as retinoids, β-carotenoids, and benzyl isothiocyanate.

A variety of animal experiments has demonstrated that selenium supplementation in the diet or water can inhibit experimental carcinogen-induced tumors. The mechanism is unclear, but it is possible that selenium is required for the function of glutathione peroxidase, an enzyme which detoxifies free radicals. Human selenium intake comes mainly from cereal, fish, and meat. Since many dietary mutagens and carcinogens may act through the generation of oxygen radicals, these may also play a major role in DNA damage and mutation, which may be related to cancer. Thus, dietary intake of natural antioxidants (Vitamins C, E) could be an important aspect of the body's defense mechanism against these agents, and many antioxidants are being identified as anticarcinogens (Vitamins E, C and β-carotene). Major epidemiologic evidence links the diet and nutritional status with specific cancers (esophageal, stomach, pancreas, colorectal, rectal, breast, skin, oral, endometrial, ovarian, prostate, cervix, and lung).[9-12]

Dietary factors and food consitituents can be classified from a carcinogenic point of view as initiators (nitrates, alcohol, or pyrolysates), promoters (fat, cholesterol, or obesity), and substances that decrease carcinogenesis (fiber, Vitamins A, E, C, carotenoids, selenium) or protectors. Hence, specific foods and dietary factors are associated with the risk of specific cancers.

A. DIETARY FAT

The most important positive associations have been an intake of total fat, alcohol, and nitrates, which is believed to have either an initiatory or promotive effect. An intake of fresh fruits and vegetables, fiber, and Vitamins A, C, and E is generally protective for all cancers. Normally, foods (dietary patterns) showed a stronger relationship than nutrients, although general nutritional status as reflected by obesity or emaciation showed the strongest relationship for certain cancers.[13] However, besides smoking, alcohol, and nutrition, factors such as hormones and social status have a role in increasing the risk for specific cancers.[14] Furthermore, recent data regarding international epidemiology of hormone-dependent cancers (HDC) suggest that the distribution of the endocrine-dependent cancers (breast, prostate, colorecetal, thyroid) is related to dietary factors. For instance, a predominantly high-protein, high-fat diet imposed in early life can make individuals susceptible to the development of these cancers.[15] Clinical evidence shows associations among breast and colon cancer and endemic goiter. Experimental evidence provides some support for this hypothesis. Thus, caloric restriction has a general inhibitory influence on tumorigenesis, while dietary fat tends to promote carcinogenesis, but only of mammary tumors. The incidence of DMBA-induced mammary tumors in rats increased from about 70 to 95% when the level of dietary fat was raised from 0.5 to 20% by weight.[16]

It is possible that dietary factors act on target cells by modifying the level of hormones. It is known that dietary changes can significantly influence growth hormone, thyroid hormone, and steroid hormone metabolism and biosynthesis. Therefore, a correlation among hormones, vitamins, nutrition, and carcinogenesis should also be made (see Figure 1).

A high fat diet is also associated with a high risk of cancer of the colon, breast, endometrium, and prostate and less strongly with cancer of the ovary and pancreas; in contrast, it is inversely related to cancer of the stomach and less strongly with cancer of the esophagus. Thus, dietary fat is an important etiologic agent in the causation of cancers of the colon, breast, endometrium, and prostate and in protection of the stomach.[17] Recent

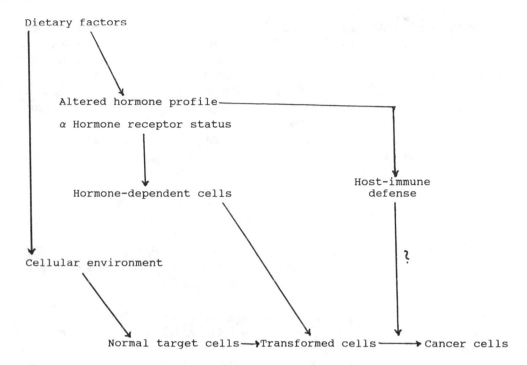

FIGURE 1. Postulated mechanisms by which dietary factors modulate cellular evolution and neoplastic transformation.

epidemiologic studies have also implicated a high-fat and/or low-fiber diet in etiology of colorectal, pancreatic, breast, endometrial/ovarian, and prostatic cancers.[18]

An Australian study of 573 women evaluated associations between obesity and both benign and malignant breast disease, and in particular, investigated the role of estrogens and progesterone. Obesity was strongly associated with the proportions of nonprotein-bound and albumin-bound estradiol, and inversely associated with sex hormone-binding globulin (SHBG) levels and the proportion of SHBG-bound estradiol. Women who gained more than 10 kg from early womanhood had a twofold increase in risk of developing breast cancer, whereas lean women had a greater risk of being treated for benign breast disease. Also, women with breast cancer who are obese, are more likely to develop metastases and have a shorter survival than nonobese women. Thus, there is a strong relationship between obesity, hormones, and risk of breast cancer. Obese women have higher levels of bioavailable estradiol and a lower progesterone level. It is likely that obesity raises estrogen levels by increasing the conversion of estrone and estradiol from their precursors by aromatase enzymes in the lipocytes, and local hormone environment is important in breast cancer development. Avoiding obesity and high-fat diet is a potential preventive method to reduce the morbidity and mortality of cancer.[19]

There is substantial evidence indicating that differences between nations in the incidence of cancer are due, at least in part, to environment factors, such as diet. Descriptive epidemiology and, to a lesser extent, case-control and cohort studies suggest that incidence and mortality rates for cancer, especially some cancers, are positively correlated with total dietary fat. Hence, the existent relationship between dietary fat and hormone metabolism, particularly sex steroids, may explain the increased cancer risk related to sex as well as to group populations who predominantly eat a high fat, so-called "Western diet", and low-fiber foods. Diets high in animal fat, protein and carbohydrates and low in fibers may enhance the cancer risk, whereas diets low in animal fat and protein and abundant in vegetables containing Vitamins A, C, and E may protect against cancer.[20]

Large prospective studies have also shown an association between low serum cholesterol level and cancer mortality, which can be due, at least in part, to an effect of preclinical cancer on serum cholesterol level. These data from a large trial of 361,662 men screened for the multiple risk factor revealed an association between low serum cholesterol level and increased cancer risk that alternates over time, and a low cholesterol serum level is shown to precede death from cancer by at least 2 years.[21] High cholesterol has been implicated in colon and the hormone-sensitive cancers.

Comparative studies of blacks and whites using dietary and nutritional status in the U.S. indicate that blacks eat more nitrate and animal foods and not enough fiber in relation to protein, fat, and carbohydrate. Blacks also have poorer nutritional status with respect to getting enough thiamin (B$_1$), riboflavin (B$_2$), Vitamins A and C, and iron, to being obese (females), and to being underweight (males). This is an agreement with hypotheses regarding the interactions between diet and cancer (associations found in whites) and dose-response relationships reported for some cancers for which blacks have a higher incidence and mortality than whites. There were higher incidence and mortality ratios for black (vs. white) Americans for cancers of the esophagus, larynx, stomach, pancreas, colon, prostate, breast (in women under 40), cervix, lung (for males), and for all sites, and there were lower 5-year relative survival ratios. Dose-response relationships have been reported for esophageal, gastric, colon, pancreatic, and breast cancer. Two Japanese cohort studies conducted over 10 and 16 years, respectively, reported that the recommended Seventh-Day Adventist lifestyle, that of no smoking or drinking, a low meat intake, and a high fruit and vegetable intake, is associated with decreased cancer risk.[22] Similarly, those blacks with Seventh-Day Adventist lifestyle are expected to have a lower cancer incidence and mortality than those blacks not having that lifestyle. One American cohort study, a 4-year followup, reported that eating green and yellow fruits and vegetables was associated with decreased risk in elderly populations. Therefore, both epidemiologic studies and experiments in animals provide convincing evidence that dietary fat appears to have a promoting effect on tumorigenesis. For example, some studies suggest that the development of colon cancer is enhanced by the increased secretion of certain bile steroids that accompanies high level of fat intake and cholesterol. Increasing the intake of total fat increases the incidence of cancer at certain sites, particularly the breast and colon, and conversely, the risk is lower with lower intakes of fat. Experimental studies suggest that when total fat intake is low, polyunsaturated fats are more effective than saturated fats in enhancing tumorigenesis, whereas the data on humans do not permit a clear distinction to be made between the effects of different components of fat.[2,3,6]

B. DIETARY PROTEINS

Dietary proteins have often been associated with cancers of the breast, endometrium, prostate, colorectum, pancreas, and kidney. However, since the major dietary sources of protein (such as meat) contain a variety of other nutrients and nonnutritive components, the association of proteins with cancer at these sites may not be direct, but, rather, could reflect the action of other constituents present in protein-rich foods. Thus, evidence from epidemiologic and laboratory studies suggests that protein diet may be associated with an increased risk of cancers of certain sites. Because of the strong correlation between intakes of fat and protein in the Western diet, it is difficult to reach a firm conclusion about an independent effect of protein.[2,6]

C. CARBOHYDRATES

Carbohydrates and carcinogenesis have been studied less as compared to lipids and proteins and the occurrence of cancer. The principal carbohydrates in foods are sugars, starches, and cellulose. There is little evidence to support a role for carbohydrates per se in

TABLE 1
Components of Dietary
Fiber

Dietary Fiber Found in Plant Cell Wall

Cellulose
Hemicellulose
Lignin
Lipids (waxes)
Pectin
Protein

Dietary Fiber Found Naturally or Used as Food Additives

Mucilages
Gums
Modified cellulose
Algal polysaccharides
Pentosans

the etiology of cancer. Thus, the evidence from epidemiologic studies and laboratory animals is too sparse to suggest a direct role for carbohydrates (except fiber) in carcinogenesis. However, excessive carbohydrate consumption contributes to caloric excess, which in turn has been implicated as a modifier of carcinogenesis.[2,10]

D. DIETARY FIBER

The role of dietary fiber in health and cancer prevention recently has drawn attention. Dietary fiber is not a single substance, but an extremely complex mixture of substances. Usually, dietary fiber is defined as remnants of plant cells resistant to hydrolysis by the alimentary enzymes of man, the group of substances that remain in the ileum but are partly hydrolyzed by bacteria in the colon. Thus, dietary fiber is the sum of lignin and the plant polysaccharides that are not digested by the endogenous secretions of the human digestive tract. The term "dietary fiber" was used in relation to a protective effect against toxemia of pregnancy, and also as a protective factor in ischemic heart disease.[23] Hence, dietary fiber is composed of a variety of polysaccharides including hemicellulose, cellulose, pectic substances, proteins, algal polysaccharides (e.g., agar and carrageen), and lignin. Most foods of plant origin contain both soluble and insoluble dietary fiber. The major components of dietary fiber are found in the plant cell wall (cellulose, hemicellulose, lignin, proteins, lipids), but some are not found as structural components of the plant cell wall and are used as food additives (gums, pectins, and mucilages). Thus, cellulose and hemicellulose are the structural building materials in the plant cell wall, whereas pectins, lignin, and proteins are involved in the plant cell structure and metabolism, and they account for 80 to 90% of the plant cell wall (see Table 1).

The major categories of foods that provide dietary fiber are vegetables (broccoli, carrots, cabbage, onions, and peas), fruits (apples, plums, pears, bananas, oranges, peaches, strawberries, and tomatoes), and whole grain cereals (oatmeal, bran, rice, white flour, brown flour, and rye).[21,23,24] Thus, the hypothesis that a high-fiber diet could prevent certain diseases common in affluent Western societies, such as heart diseases and cancer (colon and rectum) has been under investigation for many years.[25] Since cancer of the colon, like cancer of the breast and uterus, is more common in obese persons, some investigators believe that diet is an important contributing factor to colon cancer.[26] Evidence from population studies suggests that a high-fiber diet is protective while a high-fat diet may increase cancer risk. Evidence to date suggests that dietary fiber is necessary to maintain normal functioning of the gastrointestinal tract and acts as a laxative which is useful in the prevention and treatment of constipation. Thus, the "fiber hypothesis" and its preventive role in certain cancers stimulated a great deal of research in recent years.

Several mechanisms have been proposed for the protective effect of fiber against colon cancer.[27] Fiber may act to reduce transit time in the bowel and thereby decrease the time for exposure to potential carcinogens. Fiber can dilute the concentration of carcinogens in the colon, can affect the production of bile acids and other potential carcinogens in the stool, and can increase short-chain fatty acid production. Studies in animals have also shown that some types of high-fiber ingredients (e.g., cellulose and bran) depress the tumorigenicity of certain chemical carcinogens such as dimethylhydrazine (DMH) or azoxymethane (AOM). DMH produced fewer tumors per rat fed with a high-fiber diet and a higher percentage fed with a low fiber diet. Another study, with DMH in the same strain of rat and incorporating cellulose as the dietary fiber with various kinds of saturated or unsaturated fats, showed a lower tumor incidence and fewer tumors per rat in those groups with cellulose in their diet. A group given fat in the diet without cellulose had a high rate of colon tumor incidence, but a test group receiving cellulose combined with the fat had a lower tumor incidence; the number of tumors per rat was similar to that in rats with cellulose only.[28] Not all kinds of fiber, however, had protective effects. Epidemiologic studies among immigrants, including Poles, Japanese, and Norwegians, showed that from a low incidence in their homeland they shifted to a higher incidence of colon cancer in their adopted land, which implies that mainly dietary factors are responsible for the differences in cancer incidence. Also, studies of Seventh-Day Adventists, who are mainly vegetarians, vs. nonvegetarians showed that vegetarians had less colon and breast cancer, less dietary fat, and higher dietary fiber intake than nonvegetarians or the general population.[29] Allowance for dietary fiber has not been established; however, a dietary fiber intake of up to 30 g/d will be safe and without adverse effects. Although during the last two decades, considerable research has been conducted on the role of dietary fiber in health and disease (colon cancer, heart diseases, and diabetes), the National Research Council Committee on Diet, Nutrition, and Cancer found no conclusive evidence to indicate that dietary fiber (such as that present in fruits, vegetables, grains, and cereals) exerts a protective effect against colorectal cancer in humans. Both epidemiologic and laboratory reports suggest that if there is such an effect, specific components of fiber, rather than total dietary fiber, are more likely to be responsible.[2]

E. DIET AND MICRONUTRIENTS (MINERALS)

Very few epidemiologic studies have been conducted to determine the relationship between minerals and the incidence of cancer in humans. This is due partly to the difficulty of identifying populations with significantly different intakes of the various micronutrients. In contrast, there have been numerous studies in laboratory animals. In these investigations, the carcinogenic effects of many metals, administered at high doses to the animals parenterally, have been well established. However, the results of these studies have shed little light on the potential carcinogenic risk posed by trace elements in the amounts occurring naturally in the diet of humans. The carcinogenic action of these elements is difficult to test in animals because some of them are toxic at levels that exceed dietary requirements, and also it is difficult to control synergistic interactions of the elements with other elements that may contaminate diet, air, and drinking water. This section contains an evaluation of some of those micronutrients that are nutritionally significant and suspected of playing a role in carcinogenesis, such as selenium, zinc, cadmium, iron, copper, iodine, molybdenum, arsenic, and lead.

1. Selenium

Selenium and its role in carcinogenesis, particularly its possible protective effect against cancer, has been recognized for a long time. However, whether selenium can reduce cancer risk is a question that remains unanswered at present. The significance of selenium as a vital element in metal protein synthesis was suggested by the fact that oral administration of selenium can decrease the occurrence of an endemic cardiomyopathy (Keshan's disease).

Epidemiologic studies have revealed an inverse relationship between selenium levels and cancer mortality in the U.S., in both males and females, especially for cancers of the gastrointestinal and genitourinary tract. Also, there is a significant inverse relationship between selenium intake and leukemia as well as with cancer of the colon, rectum, pancreas, breast, ovary, prostate, bladder, lung (males), and skin in serum samples from donors in 19 U.S. states and 22 other countries.[30] In most cases of gastrointestinal cancers and Hodgkin's disease, selenium levels were significantly lower than those in the normal subjects, but there were no differences between normal subjects and patients with cancers at other sites. Although in most studies a reduction by 20 to 30% of cancer risk was found, more comprehensive epidemiologic studies including a great number of participants (50,000 to 100,000) are needed in order to establish a firm conclusion regarding selenium and cancer risk.[31] Experimental studies have revealed in most instances that supplementation of the diet or drinking water with selenium protects against tumors induced by a variety of chemical and viral carcinogens (NMU, DMBA, BP, and UV) found in (skin, mammary, liver, colon, and lung) tumors. In most of these animal tumor models a decrease by 50% in tumor incidence and growth has been reported. However, no effect on transplanted tumors was observed in rodents.

In the majority of studies, the protective effects of selenium were noted only at dietary concentrations of 2 ppm or above, while toxic symptoms, usually weight loss, were generally manifested with dietary levels about 5 ppm, which indicates a fine line between the protective and toxic concentration of selenium. Enhancement of tumor yield caused by selenium deficiency was pronounced only in animals fed a high polyunsaturated fat diet. Thus, there is an interplay of selenium, fat, Vitamin E, proteins (casein), and alcohol, which can complicate the epidemiologic studies. Selenium supplementation must be maintained over the entire life span. Mid-life cessation of selenium supplementation resulted in a subsequent rapid increase of the number of tumors.

The protective and anticarcinogenic mechanism of selenium is complex and still poorly understood. Some studies have suggested that selenium inhibits the initiation phase of carcinogenesis, by enzyme glutathione peroxidase, which exerts protective effects against macromolecules generated by "oxidative stress" as free acid radicals and lipid peroxidation and which are the cause for mutagenic activity of several chemical carcinogens.[31,32] This enzyme, which is selenium dependent, protects cell membranes and tissues against the destructive effects of OH radicals released as by-products of lipid peroxidation. However, others have demonstrated protective effects when given in the late phase, as postcarcinogen. It seems that selenium exerts a direct effect in the proliferation phase of the cell cycle by decreasing the proliferation rate of target cells and will satisfy effects on both initiation and promotion phases of carcinogenesis.[32] Also, selenium exerts stimulatory effects on the immune system (immunopotentiation), by influencing lymphocyte and natural killer (NK) cell activities, as well as interferon, prostaglandin, and interleukin-1 synthesis, and subsequently the antibody synthesis.[33]

In conclusion, both epidemiologic and laboratory studies suggest that selenium exerts some protection against the risk of cancer. However, increasing the selenium intake over 200 μg/d (the upper limit of the range of safe and adequate daily dietary intakes) by the use of supplements is not useful and does not confer more protection than those derived from the consumption of a balanced diet. A correct evaluation of present data revealed a

20 to 30% reduction in cancer risk in most patients. However, it is not certain if all malignant tumors are affected similarly.[31]

2. Zinc

Zinc, a constituent of more than 100 enzymes, is essential for life. Through its function in nucleic acid polymerases zinc plays a predominant role in nucleic acid metabolism, cell replication, tissue repair, and growth. Severe zinc deficiency in animals and humans results in depressed immune functions.[34] However, there are few epidemiologic data concerning dietary zinc and cancer. Some studies have suggested that higher levels of dietary zinc are associated with an increase in the incidence of cancer at different sites, including the breast and stomach. Other studies have reported lower levels of zinc in the serum and tissue of patients with esophageal, bronchogenic, and other cancers, compared to corresponding levels in controls. Experiments in animals have shown that zinc can either enhance or retard tumor growth. Zinc deficiency appears to retard the growth of transplanted tumors, whereas it enhances the incidence of some chemically induced cancers. Thus, the epidemiologic data concerning zinc are too sparse, and the findings of laboratory experiments are too contradictory to permit any conclusion to be drawn regarding the role of zinc in cancer risk and prevention.

3. Iron

Iron deficiency was associated with cancers of the upper alimentary tract including the esophagus and the stomach. In epidemiologic studies conducted in Sweden, iron deficiency was associated with Plummer-Vinson syndrome, which in turn was associated with increased risk for cancer of the upper alimentary tract. Improved nutrition, especially with iron and vitamins in the diet, has been associated with the virtual elimination of new cases of Plummer-Vinson syndrome in areas of Sweden where it had formerly been highly endemic.[35] Some evidence suggests that iron deficiency may be related to gastric cancer through an indirect mechanism. Although some epidemiologic and clinical reports suggest that heavy exposure to iron by inhalation increases the risk of cancer, there is no evidence to indicate that high levels of dietary iron increase the risk of cancer in humans. Hence, the data are not sufficient to draw a firm conclusion about the role of iron in carcinogenesis.

4. Copper

Copper is an essential nutrient that is widely distributed in foods and probably in public water supplies. The intake of copper varies in different countries; however, more recent studies indicate that the average copper intake for U.S. adults is ≈ 1 mg/d. In addition to epidemiologic studies that showed an increased risk for bronchogenic carcinoma for copper miners in cases where exposure to radiation was discussed as a likely cause, there is little evidence pertaining to the role of dietary copper in the etiology of human cancers.[36] Experiments in animals have indicated that pharmacologic doses of copper salts added to the diet of animals provided some protection against chemically induced liver tumors, but there are no studies to indicate whether the nutritional copper status of animals influences their susceptibility to cancer. Thus, the evidence does not permit any conclusion to be drawn about the role of dietary copper in carcinogenesis.

5. Iodine

Iodine is an essential micronutrient in the diet and is an integral component of thyroid hormones. The mean daily intake of iodine in the U.S. is estimated to range between 60 and 680 μg/d. The recommended dietary allowance is 150 μg/d, but many diets furnish iodine in excess of this amount. Epidemiologic evidence showed that thyroid cancer occurred more frequently in areas of endemic goiter, especially papillary carcinoma. Comparative studies show a relationship between the iodine intake and histologic types of thyroid cancers; thus, in iodine-deficient populations, the risk of follicular thyroid carcinoma is increased, whereas in the populations with high dietary iodine intake, a higher incidence of papillary carcinoma is found.

However, experimental studies in rats and mice have revealed a strong relationship between the iodine-deficient diet and induction of hyperplastic-parenchymatous goiter as well as the occurrence of thyroid neoplasms, both follicular and papillary carcinomas, with local metastases in some instances.[37] It seems that iodine deficiency induced goiter and thyroid neoplasms by an increased secretion of TSH (thyrotropic-stimulating hormone). Hypophysectomy and some steroid hormones, such as cortisone, progesterone, and dexamethasone decreased their formation, whereas estrogens enhanced it. Ultrastructural and autoradiographic studies revealed that most experimental and human thyroid cancers occurred from a pre-existent goiter which can be transformed cytologically into thyroid malignancy. There are intermediate histologic types between experimental or endemic goiter and thyroid neoplasms.[37] A second type of cancer associated with iodine deficiency is breast cancer in females. Although experimentally induced iodine deficiency seems to predispose rats to the development of preneoplastic and neoplastic lesions in mammary tissue and to reduce the induction time of chemically induced mammary tumors by DMBA or thyroid tumors by 2-acetylaminofluorene (2-AAF) or thyroid irradiation, there is no clear evidence that the risk of cancers of the breast, ovary, and endometrium is related to dietary iodine deficiency in humans.[2,38] Thus, iodine deficiency is associated with an increased risk for thyroid cancer in humans.

6. Molybdenum

Molybdenum, especially molybdenum deficiency, has indirectly been implicated in the etiology of cancer, especially cancer of the esophagus, in some areas of China. Also, data from one report of laboratory experiments suggests that molybdenum supplementation of the diet may reduce the incidence of nitrosamine-induced tumors of the esophagus and forestomach.[39] However, the epidemiologic and laboratory evidence is too meager to assess the validity of the association of molybdenum with cancer. It is postulated that molybdenum acts by its precursor called molybdopterin which is very labile. Estimation of molybdopterin in various foods will be valuable for epidemiologic studies.

7. Cadmium

Cadmium, which was regarded only as a toxic substance for many years, is now recognized as an element with a possible physiologic function. Per capita intake of cadmium in the U.S. ranges from 26 to 61 μg/d. A correlative study of per capita cadmium intakes with cancer mortality rates in 27 countries found significant direct association with leukemia, cancers of the intestine, female breast, uterus, prostate, and skin, and an inverse association with liver cancer.[40] It has been suggested that cadmium may act as a selenium antagonist to prevent its uptake and lower its physiologic activity as an anticarcinogen. Occupational exposure to cadmium has been associated with an increase in the risk of renal and prostate cancer. Data from laboratory experiments suggest that cadmium given in drinking water is not carcinogenic in mice, whereas i.m. injections of cadmium salts induced sarcomas and Leydig cell tumors in Wistar rats. However, the evidence from epidemiologic and laboratory studies does not permit any firm conclusions regarding the carcinogenic effects of dietary exposure to cadmium.

8. Arsenic

Arsenic is considered to be an essential element for growth in animals. Epidemiologic studies regarding the exposure to arsenic and cancer risk has been reviewed by the International Agency for Research on Cancer (IARC) and the National Academy of Sciences and there has been reported to be an association of cancers of the skin, lung, and liver (hemangioendotheliomas) with chronic arsenism in different parts of the world.[2,41] Experimental studies indicate that arsenic does not appear to induce tumors in laboratory animals despite extensive testing in animals of various species. It is possible that humans are more sensitive to the carcinogenic effects of arsenic than other species. Mutagenic activity and chromosome breakage in leukocytes and lymphocytes have also been reported in patients exposed to arsenic.[41] Despite epidemiologic evidence that drinking water heavily contaminated with arsenic increases the risk of skin cancer in humans as well as the risk of lung cancer by inhaling arsenic, there is no sufficient information to determine the effects of the normally low levels of dietary arsenic on cancer risk.

9. Lead

Lead is not known to be essential to human nutrition, although a requirement for trace amounts of lead (29 ng/g diet) has recently been demonstrated in rats for the maintenance of growth, reproduction, and hemopoiesis. The only epidemiologic study that correlates lead levels in drinking water supplies and cancer mortality, suggests a direct correlation of lead with cancers of the stomach, small intestine, large intestine, ovary, and kidney, as well as with myeloma, all lymphomas, and all leukemias.[42] Experimental studies showed that ingestion of high levels of lead compounds (subacetate and acetate) induced renal tumors in Swiss mice and Wistar rats. Thus, experiments in animals indicate that exposure to large amounts of some lead compounds may pose a carcinogenic risk to humans. However, there is little direct epidemiologic evidence to support this conclusion.

At the intracellular level, the Na/K ratio has been found to be associated with cancer risk, though the mechanism by which these monovalent ions affect carcinogenesis is unknown. Although there are numerous studies in laboratory animals which demonstrate the carcinogenic effects of many metals administered in high doses to the animals particularly, very few epidemiologic studies have been conducted to determine the relationship between minerals and the incidence of cancers to humans (such as selenium, iodine, and arsenic).

This section contains an evaluation of some micronutrients that are nutritionally significant and suspected of playing a role in carcinogenesis. The interpretation of these findings is difficult, since most of epidemiologic studies are conflicting due in part to their distribution among diets and individuals of different geographic areas. Further studies are needed to confirm their validity.

F. Diet and Vitamins

In recent years, a growing body of evidence has pointed toward increasing some dietary components (certain vitamins, fiber, and minerals) while decreasing others (fat and total calories) as possibly influencing the incidence of cancer. Of all the dietary components examined, perhaps the most studied in the experimental animals and epidemiologically have been Vitamin A and carotenoids, Vitamin B_1 (thiamin), Vitamin H (biotin), and Vitamin E (α-tocopherol).

1. Vitamin A and Carotenoids

It has long been demonstrated that Vitamin A has effects on cellular differentiation, and neoplastic transformation is a disorder mainly of cellular differentiation; thus, Vitamin A plays an important role in carcinogenesis. Vitamin A deficiency enhances the induction of lung and urinary bladder carcinomas in the rat. It is also well documented that several compounds with Vitamin A activity and synthetic retinoids can prevent breast, skin, and bladder cancer in experimental animals, and they can suppress the malignant transformation of cultured cells by viruses, chemicals, or radiation.[43] Furthermore, antimutagenic activity of β-carotene has been demonstrated *in vitro* and *in vivo*, whereas no effect was seen with retinol when both compounds were examined. Since β-carotene has no known toxicity, this compound is now receiving more thorough study in laboratory models of carcinogenesis. Two carotenoids (canthaxanthin and phytoene) which cannot be converted to Vitamin A in the animal body have also demonstrated an anticancer effect in the laboratory, showing that anticarcinogenic effect may not be related to provitamin A activity.[44] Most epidemiologic studies demonstrate a decreased cancer risk for populations with greater consumption of foods high in retinol or carotenoids, especially green and yellow vegetables. It is also possible that substances present in vegetables other than carotenoids may be responsible for the anticancer effect. However, serum retinol levels are not a good indicator of Vitamin A status except in cases of extreme deficiency or excess. Thus, lack of an inverse association between plasma retinol and cancer incidence does not completely rule out the role of Vitamin A in cancer prevention.

It is also interesting that in all studies where plasma/serum carotene level was strongly associated with lower incidence of lung cancer, Vitamin A blood levels did not show this association. This suggests that the cancer preventive effect of β-carotene is not mediated through an elevation of plasma Vitamin A levels. A recent study of persons aged 66 years or older found decreasing cancer mortality with increasing intake of carotene-containing fruits and vegetables. Hence, it seems prudent that dietary recommendations include daily portions of foods rich in β-carotene, such as carrots, spinach, broccoli, sweet potatoes. Since many dietary and biochemical epidemiologic studies have shown an inverse association between β-carotene and the risk of cancer, the determinant factors of plasma levels of β-carotene and retinol are important predictors for cancer risk. Another recent study conducted on a large number (over 1750) of patients with nonmelanoma skin cancer showed that dietary carotene and female sex were positively related to β-carotene levels, while cigarette smoking was negatively related. Use of vitamins, beta blockers or other antihypertensive drugs was also associated to β-carotene levels, but with much smaller changes in these levels. Retinol levels were positively related to male sex and use of vitamins, diuretics, beta blockers, and menopausal estrogens, and negatively related to current cigarette smoking and use of nitrates.[45] Higher levels of serum retinol (Vitamin A) may be associated with a decreased risk of cancer, although the epidemiologic evidence is less consistent than that for β-carotene.[46] Since hepatic secretion of retinol-binding protein (RBP) maintains fairly constant levels of retinol over a wide range of dietary retinol intake, the only factors which are clearly associated with higher retinol levels in humans are male sex and oral contraceptives. These findings are useful for epidemiologic trials as well as for better understanding the human pharmacology of retinol and β-carotene.

2. Vitamin B₁ (Thiamin)

Many nondietary factors may have a depleting effect on tissue thiamin. Among nondietary factors, some metabolic anomalies may interfere with homeostasis of the internal milieu, transport, and transformation of nutrients to substrates. Glucose-6-phosphate dehydrogenase (G_6PDH) deficiency is the most common enzyme producing deficiency of human beings. A recent study showed a Vitamin B₁ deficiency of 15%, 75%, and 60% among normal, and G_6PDH-deficient males and females among young Egyptians from the oasis. Biochemical thiamin deficiency of various degrees was reported among Austrian school girls and boys, where 50 to 75% of the studied individuals had some degree of deficiency. Differences between sexes with regard to Vitamin B₁ status were observed in several epidemiologic studies in some European countries and in the U.S. Thiamin deficiency normally occurs due to an inadequate intake of the vitamin, which could be due to seasonal variations, antithiamin effects of tea and coffee, or improper vitamin utilization such as cases with Wernicke's encephalopathy or with pentosuria. Thus, Vitamin B₁ deficiency is more widespread and should be detected earlier, especially among vulnerable groups.[47]

3. Vitamin H (Biotin)

Vitamin H (Biotin) deficiency results in a scaly dermatitis, alopecia, and neurologic impairment. The principal dietary sources of biotin, a water-soluble vitamin, are products of animal origin, particularly liver, milk, and egg yolk. Overt deficiency is rare, but has been shown to occur during parenteral nutrition, after prolonged ingestion of uncooked egg white, and in patients with biotinidase deficiency. Animal studies clearly demonstrate impaired immune function and a high rate of teratogenesis even with moderately severe biotin deficiency. Epidemiologic studies between strict vegetarian (vegans), lacto-ovovegetarian, or mixed-diet (nonvegetarian) groups showed a significantly greater biotin excretion in the vegetarian group than in either lacto-ovovegetarians or mixed-diet groups. Also, in children, the biotin excretion rates in both the vegetarian and the lacto-ovovegetarian groups were significantly greater than in the mixed-diet group. However, the biotin nutritional status of vegans is not impaired.

There is considerable interest in whether biotin deficiency may occur more commonly than realized and produce nonspecific but important manifestations, such as abnormalities of amino acid metabolism.[48]

4. Vitamin E (α-Tocopherol)

Vitamin E (α-tocopherol) and its status are important due to its potential role in cancer risk; interest in Vitamin E has increased in recent years. Data on normal blood levels in different populations are a useful adjuvant in studying this relationship between Vitamin E, cancer risk, and different diets. Because serum tocopherol levels are influenced independently of body Vitamin E stores, some investigators recommend that a tocopherol-lipid ratio be used to assess Vitamin E status. It was found that the ratio of tocopherol to cholesterol, plus triglyceride was almost as powerful in identifying inadequate Vitamin E status as tocopherol-total lipid ratio. The tocopherol-cholesterol ratio had the highest sensitivity and specificity of the ratios of tocopherols to individual lipids.[49]

A recent study estimated serum α-tocopherol levels and ratios of α-tocopherol to cholesterol plus triglyceride and to cholesterol (in subjects aged 4 to 74 years) of Mexican Americans (MA), Cubans, and Puerto Ricans (PR). No differences between sexes were found. PR had lower mean α-tocopherol and α-tocopherol-lipid ratios and higher prevalences of α-tocopherol (<11.6 μmol/l) than did MA or Cubans in several age groups. MA and Cuban adolescents had lower α-tocopherol levels than children had. Mean α-tocopherol levels and α-tocopherol-lipid ratios increased and prevalences of α-tocopherol (<11.6 μmol/l) decreased during adulthood in all three ethnic groups.[50] Further research is needed to explore why serum α-tocopherol levels decrease during adolescence. It would also be useful to measure serum levels of other tocopherol isomers, such as γ-tocopherol. Serum γ-tocopherol would be of particular interest because the U.S. food supply is estimated to contain two to three times as much γ-tocopherol as α-tocopherol. Although γ-tocopherol normally accounts for 10% of total circulating tocopherol, in some circumstances it can account for a larger proportion.[51] Further research is also needed to explore why PR had lower serum α-tocopherol levels than MA or Cubans. It would be interesting to assess if the trend in cancer risk in these three ethnic groups can be related to the differences in their α-tocopherol levels.

Vitamin E, being an antioxidant, can protect against cellular damage (see chapter 7). Additionally, α-tocopherol has been shown to inhibit endogenous nitrosation reactions leading to the formation of carcinogenic nitrosamines, and then α-tocopherol should be protective. Supportive evidence for the protective role of Vitamin E in human cancer comes from the observation that administration of Vitamin E and Vitamin C to volunteers on Western diets causes dramatic reduction in fecal mutagenicity which can play an important role in colon carcinogenesis. Association of low levels of Vitamins A and E appears to enhance the risk of low levels of selenium, suggesting that they act synergistically in cancer prevention, and assessments of any of these nutrients alone could be misleading.[52]

II. CANCERS RELATED TO DIETARY FACTORS

Animal experimentation as well as epidemiologic studies have repeatedly provided evidence that nutrition plays an important role in carcinogenesis. According to current knowledge, it is assumed that 35% of cancers in the U.S. (with a possible range of 10 to 70%) may be caused by components of the diet. Thus, this estimate would make diet second only to cigarette smoking as a determinant factor of cancer in this country. Several experimental, ecologic, migrant, and international epidemiologic studies strongly suggest that some cancers, such as breast, prostate, colon, ovarian, endometrial, lung, and skin, are related to dietary factors, change in diet behavior, and socioeconomic factors. This can explain the great differences in geographic prevalence of cancer in some areas, great risk for certain types of cancers in some races or groups of people, predominant diets (vegetarians, lacto-vegetarians, and omnivores) as well as sex or socioeconomic status in general. Reduction in dietary fat presents an opportunity for disease prevention. International regression analyses suggest that two- to fivefold risk reductions may be possible after some appropriate period of time, not only for breast cancer but also for cancers of the colon, prostate, ovary, endometrium, and rectum, and for coronary heart disease. International comparisons suggest an association between cancer and dietary fat with about a fourfold risk reduction corresponding to a 60% reduction in total fat.

A. BREAST CANCER

Dietary fat has been suggested as an etiologic factor in human breast cancer because of the high correlation between national per capita fat consumption and incidence of breast cancer. The association between dietary fat and breast tumors was first described in 1942, and since then, a large number of animal studies have confirmed the effect of fat on mammary carcinogenesis.[53] This effect occurs during the promotional phase of carcinogenesis and appears to be independent of total caloric intake. It is not clear how the fat exerts its effect on the cells, although many hypotheses have been suggested.[54] Thus, prolonged survival of rats with mammary tumors after they have been placed on a low-fat diet has been reported.

Several epidemiologic studies, primarily correlation studies and case-control studies, have shown an association between dietary fat and risk for breast cancer in humans, but numerous studies of this relationship are still conflicting. Breast cancer has also been associated with a low-fiber diet and with low plasma levels of Vitamin E. Breast cancer patients in Japan have been reported to have a better prognosis than those in the U.S., and the difference in dietary fat was one of the suggested explanations for this difference in prognosis. Studies in humans suggest that high-fat intake is an important factor in the prognosis of breast cancer, and recommend a reduction of fat intake as a component in the treatment of both breast cancer and benign breast disease.[55] Recent studies regarding dietary habits and prognostic factors for breast cancer compared patients having tumors poor in estrogen receptor with those having ER-rich tumors, and showed that women with ER-rich tumors had a low fat diet and higher carbohydrate intake and also a high retinol intake, as compared to women with low ER, who had a Western diet (high fat intake and low intake of carbohydrates and fiber). Thus, dietary patterns affect certain prognostic factors in breast cancer, such as tumor size and ER content of the tumor.[56]

In addition, a relationship between dietary fat, estrogen level, and the causation of the breast cancer suggests that in women treated surgically for breast cancer, a major component in the treatment to prevent recurrence should be a strict low-fat diet to decrease the body weight.[13] It is of interest that black women have a lower total caloric and fat intake than white women. It is postulated that the obesity in black women is due to their lower physical activity in relation to their caloric (food) intake, and that this has important implications for breast and other hormone-related cancer development.[9] Also, there is some good evidence that women who have breast cancer and who are obese, are more likely to develop metastases and have a shorter survival than nonobese women.[13] Recent case-control studies regarding the role of nutritional factors and dietary patterns in the etiology of benign breast disease (BBD) revealed a trend for increasing saturated fatty acid consumption with increasing ductal atypia, which is a precancerous mastopathy or *in situ* carcinoma. Women with atypical lesions (Grades ≥III) reported a higher intake especially of foods containing ≥10% fat. These findings lend support to the hypothesis that dietary fat is a risk factor for breast cancer.[57]

Other case-control studies also were designed to re-evaluate the association of breast morphology seen on mammograms with breast cancer risk and to assess the relation of diet, especially intake of fat and Vitamin A, to the high risk of breast cancer. These findings showed that risk increased regularly with the extent of nodular and homogenous densities on the mammogram. A higher risk of 5.5 was found in women in whom 60% or more of the volume of the breast showed either nodular or homogenous densities. Increasing carotenoid and fiber intakes were associated with a reduction of the extent of densities on the mammograms, but retinol intake seemed to have little or no effect on mammographic features. These data suggest that elevation in saturated fat intake may be related to an increase in breast cancer risk through effects of dietary factors on breast tissue morphology.[58]

A recent cohort study regarding dietary habits and breast cancer incidence among Seventh-Day Adventist women showed a strong relationship to risk in these studies. Thus, age at menopause, maternal history of breast cancer, and obesity were all significantly related to risk. However, increasing consumption of high-fat animal products was not consistently associated with increased risk of breast cancer. Neither is there any demonstrable relationship between dietary habits (vegetarian vs. nonvegetarian) during the childhood and early teenage years, and subsequent, adult risk of breast cancer.[29] This is interesting, since almost 50% of the Adventists follow a strict vegetarian or lacto-ovovegetarian diet, as compared to 50% who currently follow a nonvegetarian diet. Also, previous studies indicate that Adventist women experience somewhat lower cancer risk than comparable populations.[29]

However, several epidemiologic data suggest an association of a fourfold risk reduction corresponding to a 60% reduction in total fat. Under reasonable dietary measurement assumptions, available case-control studies suggest a positive relationship between total fat intake and breast cancer risk. Also experimental data indicate a positive association between fat intake and rodent mammary tumors. Thus, a reduction in dietary fat presents an opportunity for disease prevention of major public health potential. International regression analyses suggest that two- to fivefold risk reductions may be possible after some appropriate period of time, not only for breast cancer but also for colon, prostate, ovarian, endometrial, and rectal cancer and for coronary heart diesase.[59] Hence, dietary fat reduction has major potential for reducing the risk of diseases, including several prominent cancers and coronary heart disease, that are the most common in our society and pose the most elevated risk in other societies.

Dietary fat reduction is advocated in dietary recommendations of the National Academy of Sciences and the National Cancer Institute.[2,3,10] Interestingly, results of cross-cultural and regional correlation studies have shown that breast cancer mortality correlates positively with the consumption of milk products. Thus, in Italy and France, a positive association between consumption of dairy products (including yogurt) and breast cancer was observed. Feeding of fermented milk products diminished the development of sarcoma 180 and Ehrlich ascites tumors in rodents. A case-control study in the Netherlands showed that consumption of fermented milk products (yogurt, buttermilk, and Gouda cheese) significantly decreased the breast cancer risk, and supports the hypothesis that high consumption of fermented milk and fermented milk products may protect against breast cancer. However, no statistically significant differences for daily intake of milk between breast cancer patients and controls were observed.[60]

It is likely that alteration of intestinal bacterial activity may influence the formation and withdrawal of estrogenic compounds or may alter bile acid metabolism in the enterohepatic cycle. Furthermore, microorganisms provided by cultured dairy products may stimulate the immunologic activity in the host. A relationship between breast cancer and breast-feeding (lactation) in both premenopausal and postmenopausal women has been recently shown in an Australian case-control study. It has been suggested that lactation may play a modest direct or indirect part in reducing the risk of breast cancer.[61]

Hormonal factors have been assumed to influence breast cancer risk by altering the number of cells at risk. Such alterations are most likely to take place in the lobules, since it is lobular tissue that responds most markedly to the known hormonal changes during the menstrual cycle, during pregnancy, and after menopause. International epidemiologic studies found an association between breast cancer risk factors, histologic types of invasive breast carcinoma, and all hormonally related socioeconomic and geographic risk factors. These risk factors exert their effect by selectively increasing the number of lobular cells at risk. An epidemiologic study conducted in 2728 patients from 14 countries, including the U.S., revealed that lobular and tubular carcinomas occurred with increased relative frequency in most high-risk groups. As a general trend, the higher the overall relative risk, the higher the proportion of lobular and tubular carcinomas. The proportion of these types increased with age to a maximum at 45 to 49 years and decreased in the following decade. Therefore, factors related to childbearing and menstruation and some socioeconomic and geographic risk factors, which presumably act through hormonal mechanisms, influence breast cancer risk by altering the number of lobular cells. Since epithelial proliferation in the lobules occurs mainly during the luteal phase of the menstrual cycle when the progesterone stimulation is longer, the effect of combined oral contraceptives is stronger in low-risk populations, where the growth potential is not counteracted by nutritional factors.[62]

Recently, an association between depot medroxyprogesterone (Depo-Provera) and risk of breast cancer showed a moderate increased breast cancer risk, particularly in women aged 25 to 34 who had used the drug for 6 years or longer. Women who had used it for 2 years or longer before age 25 had also an increased risk of breast cancer. Thus, this study from New Zealand where medroxyprogesterone has been used more extensively than in any other developed country suggests that Depo-Provera may increase the risk of breast cancer in young women by a factor of risk of 1.0.[63] Studies conducted by the World Health Organization (WHO) regarding the risk of breast cancer in women using medroxyprogesterone at centers in Thailand, Kenya, and Mexico found a similar relative risk of 1.0. The mechanism of action of medroxyprogesterone is still unknown. Medroxyprogesterone was found to induce mammary tumors only in beagles and the relevance of this finding was debated.

B. PROSTATE CANCER

This is the second most common cancer among men in the U.S. ranking only behind lung cancer. Among men, 20% of all newly diagnosed cancers are prostate cancers, and they comprise 11% of all male cancer deaths. Various factors have been investigated in regard to etiology of this cancer, including dietary factors. Diets rich in animal fat appear to be associated with increased risk for prostate cancer. In ecologic studies there is a strong positive correlation between dietary fat consumption and prostatic cancer incidence worldwide. In the U.S. prostatic cancer mortality rates are highest in counties with the highest fat consumption. Also, prostatic cancer is increasing in Japan, which is experiencing increases in fat consumption, as well as among Japanese and Polish immigrants in the U.S. Studies among Seventh-Day Adventist vegetarians showed lower rates for prostate cancer. A recent cohort study of diet, lifestyle, and prostate cancer in Adventist men demonstrated a strong protective relationship by the increased consumption of various fruits and vegetables, in particular, beans, lentils, peas, tomatoes, and dried fruits (dates, raisins). These significantly decreased prostate cancer risk.[22]

Investigations regarding the relationship between dietary factors, in particular β-carotene, animal fat, and prostate cancer risk showed a decreased risk and protective effects for high levels of β-carotene intake and an increased risk for animal fat intake. Consumption of high-fat milk was associated with increased risk. Men who reported drinking three or more glasses of milk daily had a relative risk (RR) of 2.49, compared with men who never drank whole milk.[12] Experimental studies showed that a high corn oil diet promotes more rapid appearance of hormonally induced prostate adenocarcinomas in rats.[64] Correlative studies of sex hormone plasma levels, diet, and prostate cancer in Seventh-Day Adventists and omnivores demonstrated higher plasma levels of testosterone and estradiol for the omnivores. Also, differences in sex hormone levels and dietary habits were found in 171 pairs of twins, and fat intake correlated with differences in testosterone levels.[65]

Since prostate cancer is a hormonally dependent disease it would be possible to achieve a decreased risk by changing the hormonal milieu through dietary modifications in human populations. Another prospective study of diet and prostate cancer among men of Japanese ancestry in Hawaii found that increased consumption of rice and tofu both were associated with a decreased risk of prostate cancer, while consumption of seaweeds was associated with an increased risk of prostate cancer.[14] Several species of seaweeds have been shown to contain mutagenic compounds which are also carcinogenic in laboratory animals.

Although several potential dietary risk factors for prostate cancer have been tentatively identified, including meat, fish, eggs, milk, cheese, rice, fat, and protein, the exact role of dietary factors in the etiology of prostate cancer remains unknown. However, environmental factors play a major role in the etiology of prostate cancer. The incidence rate of prostate cancer is approximately ten times higher among Japanese in Hawaii than those in Japan. The black-to-white incidence and mortality ratios for prostate cancer are 1.60 and 2.09, respectively. Obesity appears to be involved in addition to high-fat, low-fiber diets. Excess of Vitamin A appears to be important and so does poor zinc status, especially the zinc-retinol binding protein-Vitamin A axis.[9]

C. COLORECTAL CANCER

This is one of the most common malignant lesions in the U.S. as well as in the Western world rather than in the underdeveloped countries. Also, it increases in frequency with increasing age and rarely occurs before the age of 50. Such factors as diet, hormones, and longer life expectancy may contribute to the higher incidence seen in the U.S. Other risk factors for colorectal cancer are hereditary diseases, ulcerative colitis, Crohn's disease, and the presence of polyps. Environmental factors, especially dietary factors, play a major role in the etiology of colorectal cancers. Recent epidemiologic case-control studies revealed that consumption of fresh fruits and raw vegetables and a preference for whole grain breads were protective for the colon cancer but not for the rectum; while fatty foods increased risk at both proximal and distal ends of the colorectum, but not at the intervening subsites; and barbecued/cured meats increased risk only in the right colon. Beef, milk, alcohol, and cigarette smoking appeared to play little or no role in the etiology of these tumors at any subsite. A relatively consistent but small association with obestiy over the subsites of the colorectum was observed.[67]

Although colon and rectal cancers are often combined in epidemiologic studies, many investigations in which they have been examined separately conclude that different etiological factors prevail at the two sites and even at the various subsites within the colon. Thus, the typical Western diet, which contains more fat and less fiber than diet in underdeveloped countries, may result in slower movement of fecal material through the large bowel, which allows prolonged contact of the carcinogen with the colonic mucosa, thus increasing the risk of colorectal cancers. A high-fat diet may increase the production of acid and neutral steroids, and their metabolites which resemble some carcinogens. Also, a high-fat diet causes an increased secretion of bile acids in the gut, which may be linked to the development of colon cancer.[68] A high-fat, high-protein diet may lead to increased fecal steroids, but no active carcinogens from these have been isolated; while a low-fiber diet which decreases fecal bulk leads to increased large bowel concentrations of carcinogens and cocarcinogens, which can induce a malignant tumor.[20]

The most consistent risk factor for colorectal cancer was dietary protein, which was associated with a two- to threefold relative risk for colon cancer and for rectal cancer in women for all levels of consumption above the baseline. For male colon cancer, the corresponding relative risk was similar, but for male rectal cancer, risk was elevated only at old ages. There was an increased risk of colon and rectal cancer in both sexes associated with alcohol consumption. A reduced risk of rectal cancer was associated with Vitamin C but not with Vitamin A. The level of total dietary intake is suggested to influence the rate of colon cell renewal and, therefore, to influence the rate at which cell transformation or at which malignant progression is likely to occur. Female sex hormones influence not only bile acid (BA) production, but also other aspects of gut physiology, so that the female colon is more susceptible to dietary-associated carcinogenesis at a younger age. In addition, the bacterial populations may be directly influenced by female hormones, as may colon mucosal cells.

Rectal carcinoma will be influenced in part by micronutrients, particularly by Vitamin C.[69] A significant inverse association of dietary fiber and colon cancer risk among low-fat intake men was also found. Thus, a high-fiber diet exerts a protective effect against colorectal cancer. A significant negative association between Vitamin C intake and the risk of colon cancer has also been found. Cereals and legumes show a slight decrease in relative risk of colon cancer, and higher consumption of fruit and green and deep yellow vegetables is associated with consistently decreased risk of colon cancer. Rectal cancer is not associated with dietary fiber intake, and this is consistent with the findings of other case-control studies, even though this is not a valid explanation.[70]

In a recent chemoprevention trial on large bowel neoplasia, 58 patients with familial adenomatous polyposis were treated with 4 g of ascorbic acid (Vitamin C)/d plus 400 mg of α-tocopherol (Vitamin E)/d alone or with a grain fiber supplement (22.5 g/d) for rectal polyps. The results from this randomized, double-blind, placebo-controlled study show an inhibition of benign large bowel neoplasia by wheat fiber supplements (22.5 g/d), compared with 12.2 g/d in the low-fiber placebo group. High doses of Vitamin C (4 g/d) or α-tocopherol (400 mg/d) in combination with the low-fiber placebo have no effect. Thus, dietary grain fiber and total dietary fat act as competing variables in the genesis of large bowel neoplasia. Familial adenomatous polyposis, a premalignant autosomal dominant disorder, is characterized by a multitude of adenomatous polyps and progression to cancer in almost 100% of patients if not treated.[71] At present, it is widely believed that dietary fiber or its components inhibit, while dietary fat or its components stimulate colon carcinogenesis.[1,2]

Earlier studies of ascorbic acid (4 g/d) in patients with adenomatous polyposis suggested that this agent can reduce polyp formation. Both Vitamins C and E are antioxidants and have been shown to inhibit experimental colon tumors and to reduce human fecal mutagenic activity. Recent evidence has been accumulated for the role of sex hormones on the risk and development of colorectal cancer. A recent study conducted by the Cross Cancer Institute in Northern Alberta, regarding the relationship of parity, exogenous female hormones, and colorectal cancer, evaluated 528 colon cancer and 192 rectal cancer patients. This study indicated that parity may have a protective effect against the development of colorectal cancer, similar to the effects reported in the case of breast, endometrial, and ovarian tumors.[72] Previous studies suggest a possible role of sex hormones (endogenous and exogenous) in the risk of colorectal cancer. Nuns have experienced higher than expected rates of colon cancer as well as other hormone-dependent cancers, such as those of breast, ovary, and uterine corpus. Lactation, menstrual history, and oral contraceptives (OC) exert a role on colorectal risk cancer. Parity appears to exert its predominant effect on risk of cancer of the right colon.[73] It has been postulated that endogenous estrogens increase colon cancer incidence through increased bile acid production, while progestins, pregnancy, and high-dose oral contraceptives decrease colon cancer incidence through reduced bile acid production.

D. OVARIAN CANCER

Ovarian cancer is responsible for more cancer deaths in women than any other site in the female genital system. Among high-risk factors for ovarian cancer are exposure to diethylstilbestrol (DES), use of contraceptive estrogens, early menopause, obesity, and having a history of breast cancer. Factors identified as decreasing a woman's risk of developing ovarian cancer include childbearing and oral contraceptive use. Recently, the intake of foods high in fat has been associated with an increased risk of ovarian cancer, while other foods which are high in fiber and Vitamin A have been shown to decrease risk of the disease.[74] A recent case-control study, regarding dietary intake from 85 first primary ovarian cancer cases and 492 population-based controls, revealed that calories, fat protein, fiber, and Vitamins A and C do not appreciably alter the risk of developing ovarian cancer. However, high intake of β-carotene appears to confer protection against ovarian cancer.[75]

E. ENDOMETRIAL CANCER

Endometrial cancer is associated with body weight, as it occurs more frequently in obese women. This can be explained by increased aromatization of androgens to estrogens in adipose tissue, which is the major source of estrogens in postmenopausal women. However, the relationship between obesity and endometrial cancer risk is similar in premenopausal women when circulating estrogens are chiefly ovarian in origin.[76] Thus, the link between nutrition and endometrial cancer is more complex, including the sex hormone-binding globulins (SHGB). International epidemiologic studies show a positive and strong correlation between total fat consumption per capita and incidence of endometrial cancer, and this correlation is with both unsaturated and saturated fat. Furthermore, mortality rates from endometrial cancer are lower in selected populations, such as Seventh-Day Adventists with a chiefly vegetarian diet.[29]

A recent study, regarding the risk of endometrial cancer in relation to nutrition and diet, found a strong and positive association of obesity with the risk of endometrial cancer, and other conditions related to body weight, such as early menarche, diabetes mellitus, or hypertension. The risk of endometrial cancer was elevated in subjects with a greater fat intake (butter, margarine, and oil), and lowered in subjects with a frequent intake of green vegetables, fruit, and whole-grain foods; thus, the risk of endometrial cancer appeared inversely related to indices of β-carotene and fiber intake. No significant difference was noted between cases and controls in the frequency of intake of carrots, meat, eggs, ham and cheese. Alcohol consumption was somewhat larger among the cancer cases, but not significant. Thus, there is a strong, positive relationship between obesity, high dietary fat, and risk of endometrial cancer, and an inverse relationship to β-carotene and fiber intake.[77] However, case-control and dose-response studies show a relative risk (RR) of cervix cancer with a low intake of Vitamins A and C.

F. LUNG CANCER

Lung cancer is also significantly influenced by dietary factors. There is strong and extensive epidemiologic evidence to indicate that there is an inverse relationship between the risk of lung cancer and the previous consumption of foods which contain carotenoids (particularly β-carotene) and Vitamin A. Also, there is an inverse relationship between serum β-carotene and Vitamin A levels and lung cancer.[78] Serum zinc is one of the factors involved in the mobilization of Vitamin A from the liver, and low levels of zinc are correlated with low levels of serum Vitamin A; thus, low levels of serum zinc are found in cases of lung cancer. Some studies indicate that people with low levels of β-carotene in their blood are approximately four times more likely to develop squamous cell carcinoma of the lung than are individuals with normal levels. These studies also demonstrate that low levels of Vitamin E increase the risk of all types of lung cancer by about two and one half times.

Although it is not known how Vitamin E and β-carotene prevent cancer, it is possible that these substances protect cell membranes. A recent study performed for serum levels of β-carotene, Vitamin A, and zinc in 64 histologically confirmed male lung cancers compared with 63 randomly selected male hospital controls, showed significantly lower levels of β-carotene and Vitamin A in lung cancer patients. The mean zinc serum levels were not statistically significant between cancer patients and controls. The level of β-carotene, Vitamin A, or zinc were not significantly influenced by either the extent of the cancer or the cancer cell types.[79]

In addition, a case-control study of diet and mesothelioma in Louisiana was performed on 37 patients with malignant mesothelioma of the pleura (n = 32) or peritoneum (n = 5). The results revealed that patients with mesothelioma had less frequent consumption of cruciferous vegetables and all vegetables combined, than did the controls. Estimation of β-carotene showed that carotene intake was also signficantly lower in cancer patients. Dose-dependent reductions in risk were seen with increasing consumption of vegetables, especially of cruciferous vegetables. The results indicate that consumption of vegetables or some vegetable-related constituents may have a protective effect on developing mesothelioma after a lifetime exposure to asbestos.[80] Experimental studies also have revealed that diets enriched in dried cruciferous vegetables (cabbage and collards) significantly decrease the number of pulmonary metastases in mice injected intravenously with mammary tumor cells. Thus, cruciferous vegetables represent a dietary constituent that can influence the metastic process.[81] An inverse relationship exists between the consumption of high amounts of cabbage and the risk of stomach, breast, and colon cancers. A reduction in the mammary cancer incidence induced by DMBA in rats and fed by diets containing cabbage and cauliflower has been reported.[8]

Therefore, cruciferous vegetables represent an important dietary constituent which inhibits cancer development as well as the metastatic process, and thus plays a chemopreventive and possibly chemotherapeutic role in the carcinogenic process. It is possible that by isolation and purification of the active principles from cruciferous vegetables a more scientific and fruitful approach to cancer chemoprevention and treatment will be achieved.

G. SKIN CANCER

Skin cancer is affected by high-fat diets. Thus, papilloma growth in mice induced by topical application of DMBA and fed with a high-fat diet after promotion by 12-O-tetra-decanoyl-phorobol-13-actate (TPA), was more rapid compared with those fed a low-fat diet. Therefore, a high-fat diet acts as a co-promoter of skin tumors in mice.[82]

H. OTHER CANCERS

Other cancers, such as esophageal, gastric and pancreatic are also linked to diet and nutritional status.

1. Esophageal Cancer

Esophageal cancer has an increased risk following diets low in fiber, high in fat, and low in vegetables and fruits. Diets low in Vitamins A, C, and riboflavin (B_2), but high in pickled, moldy foods, and alcohol, as well as few meals, poor weight, and poor nutritional status also increase the risk of esophageal cancer.

2. Gastric Cancer

Gastric cancer risk is higher in individuals eating highly spiced, smoked, salted, or pickled foods. Diets high in nitrates and fried foods and low in fiber and Vitamin C also increase the risk.

3. Pancreatic Cancer

Pancreatic cancer incidence is higher following high-fat diets, high sugar, coffee, white bread, alcohol, and meat (2.5 relative risk); also, a high risk is seen in individuals eating low vegetable and low fruit diets and in females with diabetes.

III. POSSIBLE MECHANISM(S) OF ACTION OF DIET ON CARCINOGENESIS

Extensive basic sciences and epidemiologic literature provide evidence that dietary factors play an important role in cancer development and prevention, and foods may be classified as initiators, promoters, or protectors of specific cancers, There are various types of animal tumors and human cancers which can be strongly affected in their incidence and progression by changes of dietary components or dietary habits; thus, these neoplasms can be called diet-related cancers. Also descriptive epidemiology reveals that their geographic distribution is related to predominance of dietary factors, socioeconomic factors, hormones, migration and cultural background, which vary from country to country, and subsequently to the incidence of cancer. Cancer risk factors are strongly influenced by modifications in dietary components, and thus some cancers can be decreased in their incidence, retarded or prevented. Hence, dietary intake can play a significant role in cancer prevention and possibly may act as cancer chemopreventors or chemotherapeutic agents.

However, the exact mechanism(s) by which dietary factors influence cancer incidence and development remains largely unknown. Additional laboratory and epidemiologic studies are needed in order to clarify the mechanism of dietary factors at cellular and biochemical levels so that more confident dietary recommendations and interventional strategies may be formulated. Research in this area should also be focused on detection of the early stages or premalignant stages, in which it is easier to prevent or reverse the cancer evolution.

Several mechanisms have been proposed by which dietary components may increase or decrease the risk of cancer. Some possible mechanisms have already been proposed, based on data coming from animal tumor models, biochemical, and epidemiologic studies. Certain dietary factors may act as carcinogen promoters or cocarcinogens, while others are anticarcinogens or cancer protective. Some dietary factors are also antimutagens and anticarcinogens, while others are mutagenic. Many dietary components may act through the generation of oxygen radicals, antioxidation, which may also play a role in DNA damages and mutation (and possibly promotion). Certain vitamins, such as Vitamin C, Vitamin E, and β-carotene, are strong antioxidants and thus exert their cancer chemopreventive and chemotherapeutic effects. Cell proliferation, cell renewal, and cell differentiation, which are the cornerstones of neoplastic transformation, are also strongly influenced by dietary factors, especially Vitamins A and E. An increase in the production of bile acids and also the synthesis of acid and neutral steroids and their metabolites, which resemble carcinogens, may be linked to the development of cancer, particularly colorectal cancer. Another possible mechanism is changing the intestinal flora and many colonic bacteria which are involved in hormone steroid synthesis as well as deconjugation and reabsorption of steroid hormones and their metabolites excreted by the biliary system or reabsorbed into circulation through the enterohepatic system.

Hormones and hormone-like substances appear to act as a pathogenic bridge between diet and hormone-sensitive cancers. Dietary fat and endogenous hormones are believed to be the major etiologic factors in development and progression of hormone-dependent cancers.

It is well known that diet can influence hormonal activity. For example, androgens can be converted into estrogens by the fecal microflora. Higher levels of dietary cholesterol increase the concentration of neutral sterols and bile acids which may act as tumor promoters. Increased levels of bile acids and neutral steroids were found in populations with higher rates of colon cancer. Conversion of androgens into estrogens in extragonadal tissues, such as adipose tissue, by the aromatization process, is also affected by dietary factors. Dietary fat increases the excretion and synthesis of bile acids, as well as certain neutral steroids which can be synthesized by intestinal bacterial flora, and free acids. These compounds, although not primary carcinogens, are potent promoters, particularly of colon carcinogenesis in several animal models. However, little is known about how such compounds act to promote tumors, but the bile acids, neutral steroids, and free fatty acids have been shown to damage the colonic mucosa and increase the proliferative activity of colon epithelium.

Higher levels of dietary cholesterol increase the concentration of fecal neutral steroids, which are metabolites of cholesterol and may act as carcinogenic promoters. Evidence suggests that their tumor-promoting effect may be mediated by increasing the turnover of intestinal mucosal cells. Colonic flora, with an increased enzymatic capacity for transforming bile acids and neutral sterols to potential carcinogens, have been found in populations with high rates of colon cancers and in ominvores as compared to vegetarians.

It has been observed that estrogens are synthesized by intestinal flora and this synthesis may be increased by adding fat to the diet. Changes in colonic flora mediated by diet may increase the deconjugation and reabsorption of estrogens excreted by the biliary system. Adipose tissue can convert androstenedione to estrone, and thus increase the circulating levels of estrogens in postmenopausal women. Postmenopausal women, omnivores, who generally consume substantial amounts of dietary fat, had higher urinary excretion of estriol and total estrogens, and higher plasma levels of estrone and estradiol than vegetarian women. Feeding a high-fat, Western diet to black South African women who typically consumed a low-fat, vegetarian diet, caused an apparent decrease in levels of LH, FSH, and prolactin, and only a small increase in estradiol levels. Among premenopausal women, inconsistent association of diet and sex hormones have been observed. Although premenopausal American women who were omnivores were found to have higher levels of plasma estrone and estradiol than vegetarians; studies among vegetarian and nonvegetarian Seventh-Day Adventist teenagers and among teenage girls in four countries with large differences in breast cancer rates, found no significant associations between plasma or urinary estrogen levels and dietary factors. Hence, the relation between dietary factors and hormonal levels among premenopausal women remains incompletely defined.[83]

Thus, obesity may increase the risk of breast cancer only in older women. Recent experimental work suggests that the incidence of mammary tumors in rats is related to total fat intake but that at least a small amount of polyunsaturated fat is necessary for this effect to be manifested. It has also been suggested that fat may affect breast cancer risk by altering prolactin secretion. The existence of such a mechanism is supported by some experimental studies. It has been previously reported that prolactin (PRL) plays an important role in carcinogenesis (see chapter 2). However, little is known regarding the role of PRL in carcinogenesis and in other organs such as liver and skin.

Our recent studies have revealed that long-term administration of PRL markedly enhanced the induction and development of squamous cell carcinomas by a chemical carcinogen, methylcholanthrene (3-MCA), in Swiss male albino mice. Prolactin also stimulated the DNA synthesis in cancer cells by at least twofold and played an important role in cell differentiation and division of epithelial neoplastic cells. Cytologic studies revealed a transformation of squamous cell carcinomas toward a trabecular-hepatoid type with increased number of mitoses and advanced nuclear abnormalities, phagolysosomes, and glycogen granules; also, cell surface studies by scanning electron microscopy showed the predominance of rounded cells covered by numerous thick microvilli and blebs with an intense stromal reaction. Hence, prolactin exerts significant stimulatory effects on carcinoma formation as well as in the cytodifferentiation of neoplastic cells toward more anaplastic, undifferentiated cells. These findings demonstrate that PRL is an important hormone in cancer cell growth and differentiation.[84]

Other hormones, such as glucagon and insulin, also exert an important role in controlling tumor cell biology and neoplastic transformation. Long-term administration of glucagon markedly enhances carcinoma formation in mice induced by a chemical carcinogen, 3-MCA. The number and size of squamous cell carcinomas (SCC) were almost threefold greater compared to those in mice treated with 3-MCA alone. DNA synthesis was estimated by the incorporation and the percentage of [^{3}H]-thymidine-labeled cells, which were also two- to threefold higher in glucagon and 3-MCA-treated mice than in those treated with MCA only. Ultrastructural and scanning electron microscopic studies revealed the predominance of acinar-cystoid and secretory types of tumors, with large and dense secretory granules (zymogen-like granules), markedly dilated endoplasmic reticulum cisternae, and lysosomes; scanning electron microscopic observations also revealed that tumor cells of MCA and glucagon-treated tumors exhibited characteristic secretory features on their cell surfaces, with marked increase in blebs and microvilli. These findings demonstrate that glucagon in pharmacologic doses significantly enhances cancer formation, and changes the cytodifferentiation of cancer cells and, thus, plays an important role in controlling tumor cell biology and carcinogenesis.[85]

Long-term insulin administration also enhances the incidence and development of tumors chemically induced by 3-MCA in mice. Autoradiographic studies with [^{3}H]-thymidine show a significant increase in DNA synthesis, and high resolution autoradiography especially shows that [^{3}H]-thymidine is distributed particularly over dense or heterochromatin, also called genetic chromatin of cancer cells. Ultrastructural and scanning electron microscopic studies revealed the predominance of less differentiated tumors, with numerous vacuoles, laminated concentric myelin figures, and rounded cells covered with several elongated microvilli and blebs, as compared to polygonal cells covered with sparse and thin microvilli and horny pearls. An intense stromal reaction around tumor cells can also be seen following insulin and MCA treatment.

These findings demonstrate that insulin in pharmacologic doses stimulates cancer development and cancer cell differentiation.[86] These findings also indicate that hormones, such as prolactin, progesterone, insulin, and glucagon, which are important factors for growth and differentiaiton of epithelial mammary tissue from normal subjects as well as patients with breast cancer, also play an important role in tumor formation outside of their target cells, acting possibly as direct tumor promoters. Thus, estrogens promote hepatocarcinogenesis previously initiated by diethylnitrosamine in rats; progesterone promotes mammary carcinogenesis induced by 7,12-dimethyl-benzanthracene (DMBA) in rats and hepatocarcinogenesis in rats, and testosterone promotes radiation-induced prostate carcinomas in rats.[87] In our investigations, prolactin, glucagon, and insulin markedly promoted the epithelial carcinoma formation, whereas progesterone inhibited it.

Micronutrients, such as calcium (Ca), selenium (Se), and zinc (Zn), are related also to diet and play an important role in carcinogenesis. Thus, colonic epithelial cell proliferation was significantly reduced after oral administration of calcium for 2 to 3 months to ten asymptomatic members of kindreds with hereditary colon cancer without polyposis. It is assumed that ionized fatty acids and bile acids were converted to insoluble calcium compounds, and subsequently the toxic and cancer-promoting effects of these compounds were mitigated.

Increased dietary calcium could also result in a decrease of $1\alpha,25$-hydroxy Vitamin D_3, which has a trophic effect on the small intestine. It is not known whether calcium binds to fiber components in the diet, which may independently affect proliferative activity.[88] Selenium (Se) is an essential trace element that has a key role in the activity of glutathione peroxidase, an enzyme that protects against oxidative tissue damage on the cellular level. Selenium decreases the proliferation rate of target cells. Both internationally and within the U.S. geographic areas with low selenium levels in the soil or in the serum have higher cancer rates, than areas with higher selenium levels. Blood selenium levels are usually depressed in patients with cancer; they are significantly lower among women with breast cancer than in controls. Selenium exerts its anticarcinogenic effect by its antioxidant activity, which is mediated through the activity of glutathione peroxidase, and probably enhances immune defenses.[1,3,31] Zinc (Zn), especially dietary zinc, is associated with an increase in the incidence of cancer at certain sites. Usually serum zinc levels in cancer patients were found lower by other investigators. Results in experimental animals are inconclusive. Zinc is an essential constituent in more than 100 enzymes and is essential for life.[2,79] Its role in carcinogenesis should be explored.

Vitamins, particularly Vitamins A, β-carotene, and Vitamins C and E, play a role in carcinogenesis. Vitamin A has a major physiologic role to control cell differentiation. Since loss of cell differentiation is a basic feature of cancer, there is ample reason to suspect that intake of Vitamin A may be related to cancer incidence. However, the interpretation of most epidemiologic studies regarding Vitamin A and cancer is difficult. Most preformed Vitamin A comes mainly from animal sources, whereas plants (yellow and green vegetables) contain carotenoids, namely, β-carotene, a dimer which is partially cleaved after absorption to form two molecules of Vitamin A. Their mechanism(s) of action is different. Vitamin A (retinol) exerts its anticarcinogenic effect mainly by regulating cell differentiation and also influencing host immunologic defense, while β-carotene is an antioxidant and may protect against oxidative reactions by quenching singlet oxygen and trapping free radicals, thus limiting damage to DNA.

Vitamin C exerts its anticarcinogenic effect by many possible mechanisms, such as influencing the maintenance of the integrity of the intercellular matrix, enhancement of immune mechanisms, promotion of tumor encapsulation, and producing an antioxidative effect. Vitamin C blocks the conversion of nitrates and nitrogen-containing compounds to carcinogens under conditions found in the stomach and in food stored under normal conditions.[1,2,7]

Vitamin E, (α-tocopherol), has received popular attention as an inhibitor of cancer. It exerts its antitumor effect by being an important intracellular antioxidant that reduces mutations in some bacterial testing systems. Vitamin E and selenium may reduce the peroxidation of polyunsaturated fatty acids which may result in damage to macromolecules, suggesting that an interaction between the type of dietary fat and antioxidant consumption may be related to the risk of cancer.[1,2,50,51]

Increasing immune host-defense mechanism can be achieved by Vitamins A, β-carotene, Vitamin C, Vitamin E, and selenium. Diet components can affect both cellular-mediated and humoral-mediated immunity. Thus, overfeeding in cancer can act by stimulation of mitotic activity, alteration of hormonal levels, or reduction of immune competence.

IV. COMMENTS AND CONCLUSIONS

By some estimates, as much as 90% of all cancers in humans have been attributed to various environmental factors, including diet. It has been suggested that diet constitutes the greatest lifestyle contribution to cancer mortality, accounting for approximately 35% of cancer deaths. It also has been estimated by many epidemiologists that diet is responsible for 30 to 40% of cancers in men and 60% of cancers in women. It has also been suggested that a significant proportion (40 to 50%) of the deaths from cancer could be prevented by dietary means and that dietary modifications would have the greatest effect on the incidence of cancers of the stomach, colon, rectum, and esophagus and, to a lesser extent, on cancers of the breast, endometrium, prostate, lung, pancreas, and kidney. The evidence reviewed by the Committee on Diet, Nutrition, and Cancer suggests that cancers of most major sites are influenced by dietary patterns.[1-3,6,10] Hence, data from basic sciences and descriptive epidemiology strongly indicate that dietary factors play an important role in cancer incidence and distribution as well as in cancer prevention.

A new prophylaxis, called nutritional cancer prophylaxis, would have as a main goal to identify the anticancer agents among foods, food additives, and drugs and to establish guidelines for the protection of individuals or population groups against cancer by nutritional means.[27] These findings have led the National Cancer Institute (NCI) to recommend a reduction of fat intake to 25% of total calories and an increase of fiber consumption to 20 to 30 g/d. Thus, a high-fiber, low-fat diet rich in fruits and vegetables would be more protective against cancer as compared to a high-fat, low-fiber diet, mainly used in developed countries or so-called Western diet.[1,2,24] To date, the most important dietary factors associated with cancer causation include fat, alcohol, and nitrates. Thus, alcohol may itself be carcinogenic or may promote its effects through malnutrition and other side-effects and mechanisms, such as alterations of steroid hormone metabolism or synthesis of sex hormone-binding globulin in the liver.[77]

Epidemiologic studies provide good evidence that alcoholic beverages are carcinogenic to the human liver, esophagus, nasopharynx, and larynx. There is some evidence that alcohol, when ingested in the form of beer, may be a carcinogenic for the colon and rectum. There is also tenuous evidence suggesting a link between cancer of the lung, urinary bladder, stomach, and pancreas and alcohol consumption. The mechanism of carcinogenic effect of alcohol is not understood. However, it has been shown that alcohol can profoundly alter the metabolism of nitrosamines, which are potent carcinogens, and may also act as a tumor promoter following initiation by nitrosamines.[89]

Other specific dietary deficiencies (hormones, vitamins, and minerals) may create a sensitized ''environment'' for the combined activities of initiatory and promotional factors. Initiatory factors, such as nitrosamines, and promotional factors including physical (irritant vegetable components) or chemical (alcohol, tobacco) also play an important role in esophageal and colon carcinogenesis.[90] The etiology of both esophageal and colon cancers is probably multifactorial. Thus, a high-fat, high-protein diet may lead to increased fecal steroids, and a low-fiber diet with decreased fecal bulk may lead to increased large bowel concentrations of carcinogens and cocarcinogens and ultimately to the development of a malignant tumor.[24]

An important role of dietary minerals and micronutrients in carcinogenesis is also foreseeable in years to come. These minerals include selenium, zinc, calcium, sodium, potassium, iron, and fluoride. The mechanism by which each of these minerals alters cancer risk has not been established; however, micronutrients may prove to be the primary determinants of risk contained in human cancer.[91,92] In addition to the fact that some dietary factors exert carcinogenic activity per se, compounds, such as hydrazynes, metabolites of mold (mycotoxins), metabolites of bacteria (carcinogenic nitrosamines), pose a potential risk for cancer. There is also a great risk in cooking and manufacturing procedures of foods. Thus, mutagens have been found in charred meat and fish, and smoking of food enhances the mutagenic and carcinogenic activity in foods. A great number of food additives (nearly 3000 in the U.S.), only a few of which have been tested for carcinogenicity, as well as a vast number of extensively used pesticides and insecticides find their way into foods, such as vegetables, meat, fat, and fruits, which are basic components of our daily diet and can pose a great carcinogenic risk.

Despite the fact that epidemiologic studies provide some important data from populations with homogenous dietary habits, and since we cannot distinguish various degrees of susceptibility, it is more likely that populations whose diets have changed or are changing are of great importance to carcinogenesis. Some of the epidemiologic trials are conflicting. This may be due to the fact that epidemiology at present is mainly a descriptive, nonexperimental science which studies the cases and relations between diet, vitamins, and micronutrients in a noncontrolled environment. A new epidemiology based on data from cell and molecular biology, biochemistry, immunology,and tumor biology, called metabolic epidemiology, combines the laboratory methodology with epidemiologic approaches, and will become particularly useful for elucidating dietary and nutritional mechanisms in cancer.

It has been demonstrated that nutritional modification by dietary factors, vitamins, and hormones can prevent the development of several animal and human cancers, slow their progression, or cause them to regress. Since diet is a complex mixture of fat, proteins, fibers, sterols, vitamins, carbohydrates, and micronutrients, it is difficult to establish whether the reduction of carcinogenic risk or protective effects against cancer belong to the total diet or to some of its components only. Thus, the role of diet in cancer prevention remains unclear.

By isolation and purification of the active principals from various dietary components (fat, vegetables) a more scientific and fruitful approach for cancer prevention will be achieved. Hence, specific foods which provide the most protective effects and tumor sites which are most influenced should be identified. There is strong supportive evidence that dietary factors exert their protective effects by altering hormone synthesis and metabolism, hormone receptor production, host immune defenses, cell proliferation and turnover, and certain vitamins and micronutrients (Figure 1). Data from international epidemiology reveals a relation between distribution of hormone-dependent cancers and dietary factors. It is suggested that most hormone-dependent cancers are also dietary-related cancers. Thus, breast, prostate, colorectal, thyroid, and endometrial/ovarian cancers are related to dietary pattern and diet behavior. It is known that dietary modification can significantly influence the synthesis of growth hormone (GH), follicle-stimulating hormone (FSH), luteinizing hormone (LH), prolactin, thyroid hormones, steroid hormones (estrogen, progesterone, testosterone), and probably hypothalamic-releasing factors. Generally, caloric restriction exerts an inhibitory effect, whereas obesity and excess of calories exert a strong promoting tumor effect. It is interesting that dietary factors can influence or prevent not only primary cancer, but also its metastatic process. Isolation and purification of more potent anticarcinogenic and antimutagenic agents from plants, particularly cruciferous vegetables, will be of particular interest for cancer chemoprevention and chemotherapy.

Diet and its specific aspects will be the major factor of current interest in the next decade, and may turn out to exceed even cigarette smoking as the leading avoidable cause of cancer deaths.[93] Recent data revealed an association between serum nutrients, such as selenium, α-tocopherol, lycopene, β-carotene, retinol and bladder cancer. Thus, in serum collected from 25,802 persons, 35 bladder cancers developed among participants, and a signficant decrease of selenium followed by lycopene was found. Alpha-tocopherol, β-carotene and retinol were similar among cancer patients and controls.[94] Lycopene is the carotenoid responsible for the red pigment in fruits and vegetables, such as tomatoes. It can play a protective role in other cancers, such as in cancers of the pancreas and rectum, but not in prostate cancer. Also, recently in a case-control study in Toronto, it was demonstrated that an increased consumption of vegetables is associated with a decreased relative risk of lung cancer.[95] Thus, a correlation of diet, hormones, vitamins, and carcinogenesis should always be made. Due to the increased numbers of chemicals in our environment which can get into our foods, as well as the extensive use of hormones as oral contraceptives and drugs, concern is being expressed by laymen. TV media as well as some scientific journals are disseminating information regarding the role of dietary factors as carcinogens. Many patients are asking their physicians what kinds of foods, hormones, and vitamins they have to eat or use in order to avoid cancer risk or to prevent cancer development. Therefore, oncologists and epidemiologists should use dietary modifications or dietary manipulation more often for decreasing cancer risk and cancer prevention. Currently, a high-fiber, low-fat diet rich in vegetables and fruits (with high vitamin content) is the chief recommendation for decreasing cancer risk and preventing cancer formation.

REFERENCES

1. **Willett, W. C. and McMahon, B.,** Diet and cancer — an overview, *N. Engl. J. Med.,* 310, 633, and 697, (Part I, Part II) 1984.
2. Am. Inst. Cancer Res., Natl. Acad. Sci., Diet, Nutrition, and Cancer, *Natl. Acad. Press,* Washington, D.C., 1982, 3.
3. **Schatzkin, A., Baranovsky, A., and Kessler, L. G.,** Diet and Cancer, *Cancer,* 62, 1451, 1988.
4. **Doll, R. and Peto, R.,** The causes of cancer; quantitative estimates of avoidable risks of cancer in the United States today, *J. Natl. Cancer Inst.,* 66, 1191, 1981.
5. **Ames, B. N.,** Dietary carcinogens and anticarcinogens, *Science,* 221, 1256, 1983.
6. **Byers, T. and Graham, S.,** The epidemiology of diet and cancer, *Adv. Cancer Res.,* 41, 1, 1984.
7. **Carr, B. I.,** Chemical carcinogens and inhibitors of carcinogenesis in the human diet, *Cancer,* 55, 218, 1985.
8. **Wattenberg, L. W.,** Inhibition of neoplasia by minor dietary constituents, *Cancer Res.,* 43 (Suppl. 5), 2449s, 1983.
9. **Hargreaves, M. K., Baquet, C., and Gamshadzahi, A.,** Diet, nutritional status, and cancer risk in American Blacks, *Nutr. Cancer,* 12, 1, 1989.
10. **Weinhouse, S.,** The role of diet and nutrition in cancer, *Cancer,* 58, 1791, 1986.
11. **Kune, G. A. and Kune, S.,** The nutritional causes of colorectal cancer: an introduction to the Melbourne Study, *Nutr. Cancer,* 9, 1, 1987.
12. **Mettlin, C., Selenskas, S., Natarajan, N., and Huben, R.,** Beta-carotene and animal fats and their relationship to prostate cancer risk, *Cancer,* 64, 605, 1989.
13. **Hill, M. J.,** Dietary fat and human cancer, *Anticancer Res.,* 7, 281, 1987.
14. **Severson, R. K., Nomura, A. M., Grove, J. S., and Stemmermann, G. N.,** A prospective study of demographics, diet, and prostate cancer among men of Japanese ancestry in Hawaii, *Cancer Res.,* 49, 1857, 1989.
15. **Berg, J.,** Can nutrition explain the pattern of international epidemiology of hormone dependent cancers?, *Cancer Res.,* 35, 3345, 1975.
16. **Carroll, K. K.,** Experimental evidence of dietary factors and hormone dependent cancers, *Cancer Res.,* 35, 3374, 1975.
17. **Nauss, K. M., Jacobs, L. R., and Newberne, D. V.,** Dietary fat and fiber: relationship to caloric intake, body growth, and colon carcinogenesis, *Am. J. Clin. Nutr.,* 45, 243, 1987.
18. **Kaul, L., Heshmat, M. Y., Kovi, J., Jackson, M. A., Jackson, A. G., Jones, G., Edson, M., Enterline, J., and Perry, S. L.,** The role of diet in prostate cancer, *Nutr. Cancer,* 9, 123, 1987.
19. **Ingram, D., Nottage, E., Ng, S., Sparrow, L., Roberts, A., and Willcox, D.,** Obesity and breast disease: the role of the female sex hormones, *Cancer,* 64, 1049, 1989.
20. **Sian, M. S.,** Diet and nutritional factors in the aetiology of colon cancer, *Anticancer Res.,* 7, 293, 1987.
21. **Sherwin, R. W., Wentworth, D. N., Cutler, J. A., Hulley, S. B., Kuller, L. H., and Stamler, J.,** Serum cholesterol levels and cancer mortality in 361,662 men screened for the multiple risk factor intervention trial, *JAMA,* 257, 943, 1987.
22. **Mills, P. K., Beeson, W. L., Phillips, R. L., and Fraser, G. E.,** Cohort study of diet, lifestyle, and prostate cancer in Adventist men, *Cancer,* 64, 598, 1989.
23. Council Report, Dietary fiber and health, *JAMA,* 262, 542, 1989.
24. **Greenwald, P. and Lanza, E.,** Role of dietary fiber in the prevention of cancer, in *Important Advances in Oncology,* DeVita, V. T., Hellman, S., and Rosenberg, S. A., Eds., Lippincott, Philadelphia, 1986, 37.

25. **Cleave, T. L.,** The neglect of natural principles in current medical practice, *J. R. Nav. Med. Serv.,* 42, 55, 1956.

26. **Burkitt, D. P.,** Colon cancer: emergence of a concept, in *Medical Aspects of Dietary Fiber,* Spiller, G. A. and Kay, R. M., Eds., Plenum Press, New York, 1980, 75.

27. The Surgeon General's Report on Nutrition and Health, Public Health Service, U.S. Department of Health and Human Services Publication, 88-50210, Washington, D.C., 1988.

28. **Trudel, J. L., Senterman, M. K., and Brown, R. A.,** The fat/fiber antagonism in experimental colon carcinogenesis, *Surgery,* 94, 691, 1983.

29. **Mills, P. K., Beeson, W. L., Phillips, R. L., and Fraser, G. E.,** Dietary habits and breast cancer incidence among Seventh-Day Adventists, *Cancer,* 64, 582, 1989.

30. **Clark, L. C.,** The epidemiology of selenium and cancer, *Fed. Proc.,* 44, 2584, 1985.

31. **Voigtmann, R.,** Mindert Selen das Krebsrisiko beim Menschen?, *Dtsch. Med. Wochenschr.,* 114, 573, 1989.

32. **LeBoeuf, R. A. and Hoekstra, W. G.,** Changes in cellular glutathione levels: possible relation to selenium-mediated anticarcinogenesis, *Fed. Proc.,* 44, 2563, 1985.

33. **Kiremidjian-Schumacher, L. and Stotzky, G.,** Selenium and immune responses, *Environ. Res.,* 42, 277, 1987.

34. **Poswillo, D. E. and Cohen, B.,** Inhibition of carcinogenesis by dietary zinc, *Nature (London),* 231, 447, 1971.

35. **Larsson, L. G., Sandström, A., and Westling, P.,** Relationship of Plummer-Vinson disease to cancer of the upper alimentary tract in Sweden, *Cancer Res.,* 35, 3308, 1975.

36. **Newman, J. A., Archer, V. E., Saccomanno, G., Kuschner, M., Auerbach, O., Grondahl, R. D., and Wilson, J. C.,** Histologic types of bronchogenic carcinoma among members of copper-mining and smelting communities, *Ann. N.Y. Acad. Sci.,* 271, 260, 1976.

37. **Lupulescu, A. and Petrovici, A.,** *Ultrastructure of the Thyroid Gland,* Williams & Wilkins, Baltimore, 1968, 35.

38. **Edington, G. M.,** Dietary iodine and risk of breast, endometrial, and ovarian cancer, *Lancet,* 1, 1413, 1976.

39. **Luo, X. M., Wei, H. J., Hu, G. G., Shang, A. L., Liu, Y. Y., Lu, S. M., and Yang, S. P.,** Molybdenum and esophageal cancer in China, *Fed. Proc. Fed. Am. Soc. Exp. Biol.,* 40, 928, 1981.

40. International Agency for Research on Cancer (IARC), Case reports and epidemiological studies, in IARC Monographs on the Evaluation of the Carcinogenic Risk of Chemicals to Humans, Vol. 23, Some Metals and Metallic Compounds, International Agency for Research on Cancer, Lyon, France, 1980, 101.

41. **Nordenson, I., Beckman, G., Beckman, L., and Nordström, S.,** Occupational and environmental risks in and around a smelter in Northern Sweden. II. Chromosomal aberrations in workers exposed to arsenic, *Hereditas,* 88, 47, 1978.

42. **Berg, J. W. and Burbank, F.,** Correlations between carcinogenic trace metals in water supplies and cancer mortality, *Ann. N. Y. Acad. Sci.,* 199, 249, 1972.

43. **Hennekens, C. H., Stampfer, M. J., and Willett, W. C.,** Micronutrients and cancer chemoprevention, *Cancer Detect. Prev.,* 7, 147, 1984.

44. **Mathews-Roth, M. M.,** Carotenoid pigments and protection against photosensitization: how studies in bacteria suggested a treatment for a human disease, *Perspect. Biol. Med.,* 28, 127, 1984.

45. **Nierenberg, D. W., Stukel, T. A., Baron, J. A., Dain, B. J., Greenberg, E. R., and the Skin Cancer Prevention Study Group,** Determinants of plasma levels of beta-carotene and retinol, *Am. J. Epidemiol.,* 130, 511, 1989.

46. **Nierenberg, D. W., Peng, Y. M., and Alberts, D. S.,** Methods for the determination of retinoids, alpha-tocopherol, and carotenoids in human serum, plasma, and other tissues, in *Nutrition and Cancer Prevention: the Role of Micronutrients,* Micozzi, M. and Moon, T., Eds., Marcel Dekker, New York, 1989, 181.

47. **Hussein, L., Arafah, A., and Yamamah, G.,** The Vitamin B_1 status among young Egyptians from the oasis in relation to glucose-6-phosphate dehydrogenase deficiency, *Int. J. Vitam. Nutr. Res.,* 59, 52, 1989.

48. **Lombard, K. A., and Mock, D. M.,** Biotin nutritional status of vegans, lactoovovegetarians, and non-vegetarians, *Am. J. Clin. Nutr.,* 50, 486, 1989.

49. **Thurnham, D. I., Davies, J. A., Crump, B. J., Situnayake, R. D., and Davis, M.,** The use of different lipids to express serum tocopherol: lipid ratios for the measurement of Vitamin E status, *Ann. Clin. Biochem.,* 23, 514, 1986.

50. **Looker, A. C., Underwood, B. A., Wiley, J. A., Fulwood, R., and Sempos, C. T.,** Serum α tocopherol levels of Mexican Americans, Cubans, and Puerto Ricans aged 4-74y, *Am. J. Clin. Nutr.,* 50, 491, 1989.

51. **Behrens, W. A. and Madère, R.,** Alpha- and gamma-tocopherol concentrations in human serum, *J. Am. Coll. Nutr.,* 5, 91, 1986.

52. **Salonen, J. T., Salonen, R., Lappetelainen, R., Mäenpää, P. H., Alfthan, G. and Puska, P.,** Risk of cancer in relation to serum concentrations of selenium and Vitamins A and E: matched case-control analysis of propsective data, *Br. Med. J.,* 290, 417, 1985.

53. **Tannenbaum, A.,** The genesis and growth of tumors. III. Effect of a high-fat diet, *Cancer. Res.,* 2, 468, 1942.

54. **Welsch, C. W.,** Enhancement of mammary tumorigenesis by dietary fat: review of potential mechanisms, *Am. J. Clin. Nutr.,* 45, 192, 1987.

55. **Boyar, A. P., Rose, D. P., Loughridge, J. R., Engle, A., Palgi, A., Laakso, K., Kinne, D., and Wynder, E. L.,** Response to a diet low in total fat in women with postmenopausal breast cancer: a pilot study, *Nutr. Cancer,* 11, 93, 1988.

56. **Holm, L.-E., Callmer, E., Hjalmar, M.-L., Lidbrink, E., Nilsson, B.,and Skoog, L.,** Dietary habits and prognostic factors in breast cancer, *J. Natl. Cancer Inst.,* 81, 1218, 1989.

57. **Lubin, F., Wax, Y., Ron, E., Black, M., Chetrit, A., Rosen, N., Alfandary, E., and Modan, B.,** Nutritional factors associated with benign breast disease etiology: a case-control study, *Am. J. Clin. Nutr.,* 50, 551, 1989.

58. **Brisson, J., Verreault, R., Morrison, A. S., Tennina, S., and Meyer, F.,** Diet, mammographic features of breast tissue, and breast cancer risk, *Am. J. Epidemiol.,* 130, 14, 1989.

59. **Prentice, R. L., Pepe, M., and Self, S. G.,** Dietary fat and breast cancer: a quantitative assessment of the epidemiological literature and a discussion of methodological issues, *Cancer Res.,* 49, 3147, 1989.

60. **Van't Veer, P., Dekker, J. M., Lamers, J. W., Kok, F. J., Schouten, E. G., Brants, H. A., Sturmans, F., and Hermus, R. J.,** Consumption of fermented milk products and breast cancer: a case-control study in the Netherlands, *Cancer Res.,* 49, 4020, 1989.

61. **Siskind, V., Schofield, F., Rice, D., and Bain, C.,** Breast cancer and breast-feeding: results from an Australian case-control study, *Am. J. Epidemiol.,* 130, 229, 1989.

62. **Stalsberg, H., Thomas, D. B., Noonan, E. A., and the WHO Collaborative Study of Neoplasia and Steroid Contraceptives,** Histologic types of breast carcinoma in relation to international variation and breast cancer risk factors, *Int. J. Cancer,* 44, 399, 1989.

63. **Paul, C., Skegg, D. C., and Spears, G. F.,** Depot medroxyprogesterone (Depo-Provera) and risk of breast cancer, *Br. Med. J.,* 299, 759, 1989.

64. **Carroll, K. K. and Noble, R. L.,** Dietary fat in relation to hormonal induction of mammary and prostatic carcinomas in Nb rats, *Carcinogenesis,* 8, 851, 1987.

65. **Bishop, D. T., Meike, A. W., Slattery, M. L., Stringham, J. D., Ford, M. H., and West, D. W.,** The effect of nutritional factors on sex hormone levels in male twins, *Genet. Epidemiol.,* 5, 43, 1988.

66. **Kolonel, L. N., Yoshizawa, C. N., and Hankin, J. H.,** Diet and prostatic cancer: a case-control study in Hawaii, *Am. J. Epidemiol.,* 127, 999, 1988.

67. **Peters, R. K., Garabrant, D. H., Yu, M. C., and Mack, T. M.,** A case-control study of occupational and dietary factors in colorectal cancer in young men by subsite, *Cancer Res.,* 49, 5459, 1989.

68. **Bruckstein, A. H.,** Update on colorectal cancer: risk factors, diagnosis and treatment, *Postgrad. Med.,* 86, 83, 1989.

69. **Potter, J. D. and McMichael, A. J.,** Diet and cancer of the colon and rectum: a case-control study, *J. Natl. Cancer Inst.,* 76, 557, 1986.

70. **Heilbrun, L. K., Nomura, A., Hankin, J. H., and Stemmermann, G. N.,** Diet and colorectal cancer with special reference to fiber intake, *Int. J. Cancer,* 44, 1, 1989.

71. **DeCosse, J. J., Miller, H. H., and Lesser, M. L.,** Effect of wheat fiber and Vitamins C and E on rectal polyps in patients with familial adenomatous polyposis, *J. Natl. Cancer Inst.,* 81, 1290, 1989.

72. **Davis, F. G., Furner, S. E., Persky, V., and Koch, M.,** The influence of parity and exogenous female hormones on the risk of colorectal cancer, *Int. J. Cancer,* 43, 587, 1989.

73. **Potter, J. D. and McMichael, A. J.,** Large bowel cancer in women in relation to reproductive and hormonal factors: a case-control study, *J. Natl. Cancer Inst.,* 71, 703, 1983.

74. **Snowdon, D.,** Diet and ovarian cancer, *JAMA,* 254, 356, 1985.

75. **Slattery, M. L., Schuman, K. I., West, D. W., French, T. K., and Robison, L. M.,** Nutrition intake and ovarian cancer, *Am. J. Epidemiol.,* 130, 497, 1989.

76. **Henderson, B. E., Casagrande, J. T., Pike, M. C., Mack, T., Rosario, I., and Duke, A.,** The epidemiology of endometrial cancer in young women, *Br. J. Cancer,* 47, 749, 1983.

77. **LaVecchia, C., DeCarli, A., Fasoli, M., and Gentile, A.,** Nutrition and diet in the etiology of endometrial cancer, *Cancer,* 57, 1248, 1986.

78. **Palmer, S.,** Diet, nutrition and cancer, *Prog. Food Nutr. Sci.,* 9, 283, 1985.

79. **Kune, G. A., Kune, S., Watson, L. F., Pierce, R., Field, B., Vitetta, L., Merenstein, D., Hayes, A., and Irving, L.,** Serum levels of β-carotene, Vitamin A, and zinc in male lung cancer cases and controls, *Nutr. Cancer,* 12, 169, 1989.

80. **Schiffman, M. H.., Pickle, L. W., Fontham, E., Zahm, S. H., Falk, R., Mele, J., Correa, P., and Fraumeni, J. E.,** Case-control study of diet and mesothelioma in Louisiana, *Cancer Res.,* 48, 2911, 1988.

81. **Scholar, E. M., Wolterman, K., Birt, D. F., and Bresnick, E.,** The effect of diets enriched in cabbage and collards on murine pulmonary metastasis, *Nutr. Cancer,* 12, 121, 1989.

82. **Birt, D. F., Pelling, J. C., Tibbels, M. G., and Schweickert, L.,** Acceleration of papilloma growth in mice fed high-fat diets during promotion of two-stage skin carcinogenesis, *Nutr. Cancer,* 12, 161, 1989.

83. **Goldin, B. R., Aldercreutz, H., Dwyer, J. T., Swenson, L., Warram, J. H., and Gorbach, S. L.,** Effect of diet on excretion of estrogens in pre- and postmenopausal women, *Cancer Res.,* 41, 3771, 1981.

84. **Lupulescu, A.,** Enhancement of epidermal carcinoma formation by prolactin in mice, *J. Natl. Cancer Inst.,* 74, 1335, 1985.

85. **Lupulescu, A.,** Glucagon control of carcinogenesis, *Endocrinology,* 113, 527, 1983.

86. **Lupulescu, A.,** Effect of prolonged insulin treatment on carcinoma formation in mice, *Cancer Res.,* 45, 3288, 1985.

87. **Takizawa, S. and Hirose, F.,** Role of testosterone in the development of radiation-induced prostate carcinoma in rats, *Gann,* 69, 723, 1978.

88. **Lipkin, M. and Newmark, H.,** Effect of added dietary calcium on colonic epithelial-cell proliferation in subjects at high risk for familial colonic cancer, *N. Engl. J. Med.,* 313, 1381, 1985.

89. **Driver, H. E. and Swann, P. F.,** Alcohol and human cancer, *Anticancer Res.,* 7, 309, 1987.

90. **Pera, M., Cardesa, A., Pera, C., and Mohr, U.,** Nutritional aspects in oesophageal carcinogenesis, *Anticancer Res.,* 7, 301, 1987.

91. **Nelson, R. L.,** Dietary minerals and colon carcinogenesis, *Anticancer Res.,* 7, 259, 1987.

92. **Nomura, A., Heilbrun, L. K., Morris, J. S., and Stemmermann, G. N.,** Serum selenium and the risk of cancer by specific sites: case-control analysis of prospective data, *J. Natl. Cancer Inst.,* 79, 103, 1987.

93. **Lerman, C., Rimer, B., and Engstrom, P. F.,** Reducing avoidable cancer mortality through prevention and early detection regimens, *Cancer Res.,* 49, 4955, 1989.

94. **Helzlsouer, K. J., Comstock, G. W., and Morris, J. S.,** Selenium, lycopene, α-tocopherol, β-carotene, retinol, and subsequent bladder cancer, *Cancer Res.,* 49, 6144, 1989.

95. **Jain, M., Burch, J. D., Howe, J. R., Risch, H. A., and Miller, A. B.,** Dietary factors and risk of lung cancer results from a case-control study, Toronto, 1981—1985, *Int. J. Cancer,* 45, 287, 1990.

INDEX

A

T

W

X

Y

Z